Drug Discovery and Development in Pharmaceuticals

Drug Discovery and Development in Pharmaceuticals

Edited by Erica Helmer

hayle
medical

New York

Hayle Medical,
750 Third Avenue, 9ᵗʰ Floor,
New York, NY 10017, USA

Visit us on the World Wide Web at:
www.haylemedical.com

ISBN: 978-1-63241-470-0

Cataloging-in-Publication Data

Drug discovery and development in pharmaceuticals / edited by Erica Helmer.
    p. cm.
Includes bibliographical references and index.
ISBN 978-1-63241-470-0
1. Drug development. 2. Drugs. 3. Pharmacology. 4. Pharmacy. 5. Pharmaceutical industry.
I. Helmer, Erica.
RM301.25 .D78 2017
615.19--dc23

Table of Contents

Preface

Drug discovery and development is the process whereby medication is designed, developed and manufactured through new chemical entities. This book on drug discovery and pharmaceutical development discusses topics related to scientific experimentation related to pharmaceutical agent development and quality control. This book includes contributions of experts and scientists which will provide innovative insights into this field. It brings forth some of the most innovative concepts and elucidates the unexplored aspects of this field. This book is a vital tool for all researching and studying drug discovery and development. It is a complete source of knowledge on the present status of this important field.

The researches compiled throughout the book are authentic and of high quality, combining several disciplines and from very diverse regions from around the world. Drawing on the contributions of many researchers from diverse countries, the book's objective is to provide the readers with the latest achievements in the area of research. This book will surely be a source of knowledge to all interested and researching the field.

In the end, I would like to express my deep sense of gratitude to all the authors for meeting the set deadlines in completing and submitting their research chapters. I would also like to thank the publisher for the support offered to us throughout the course of the book. Finally, I extend my sincere thanks to my family for being a constant source of inspiration and encouragement.

Editor

Coumarin compounds of *Biebersteinia multifida* roots show potential anxiolytic effects in mice

Hamid Reza Monsef-Esfahani[1], Mohsen Amini[2], Navid Goodarzi[3,4], Fatemeh Saiedmohammadi[1,5], Reza Hajiaghaee[6], Mohammad Ali Faramarzi[7], Zahra Tofighi[1] and Mohammad Hossein Ghahremani[4,5]*

Abstract

Background: Traditional preparations of the root of *Biebersteinia multifida* DC (Geraniaceae), a native medicinal plant of Irano-Turanian floristic region, have been used for the treatment of phobias as anxiolytic herbal preparation.

Methods: We utilized the phobic behavior of mice in an elevated plus-maze as a model to evaluate the anxiolytic effect of the plant extract and bio-guided fractionation was applied to isolate the active compounds. Total root extract, alkaline and ether fraction were administered to mice at different doses 30 and 90 min prior to the maze test. Saline and diazepam were administered as negative and positive controls, respectively. The time spent in open and closed arms, an index of anxiety behavior and entry time, was measured as an index of animal activity.

Results: The total root extract exhibited anxiolytic effect which was comparable to diazepam but with longer duration. This sustained effect of the crude extract was sustained for 90 min and was even more after injection of 45 mg/kg while the effect of diazepam had been reduced by 90 min. The anxiolytic effect factor was only present in the alkaline fraction and displayed its effect at lower doses than diazepam while pure vasicinone as the previously known alkaloid did not shown anxiolytic effect. The effect of the alkaline fraction was in a dose dependent manner starting at 0.2 mg/kg with a maximum at 1.0 mg/kg. Bio-guided fractionation using a variety of chromatographic methods led to isolation and purification of three coumarin derivatives from the bioactive fraction, including umbelliferone, scopoletin, and ferulic acid.

Conclusion: For the first time, bio-guided fractionation of the root extract of *B. multifida* indicates significant sustained anxiolytic effects which led to isolation of three coumarin derivatives with well-known potent MAO inhibitory and anti-anxiety effects. These data contribute to evidence-based traditional use of *B. multifida* root for anxiety disorders.

Keywords: Biebersteinia multifida, Coumarin, Anxiolytic, Scopoletin, Umbelliferone

Background

Biebersteinia multifida DC (Geraniaceae), a native plant of Irano-Turanian floristic regions [1], is known traditionally as Chelleh-Dagh or Adamak in Iran. All four species of Biebersteinia distributed geographically from central Asia to Greek in temperate mountain zones. Among these pharmacologically active species, only *B. multifida* and *B. orphanidis* have tuberous roots. In folk medicine, the tuberous roots of *B. multifida* have been used topically for the relief of inflammation and pain of musculoskeletal disorders [2,3] and orally in the treatment of nocturia in children and of phobia and anxiety in humans and domestic animals [4] with no systematic approach to characterize the observed ethnopharmacological effects. Thus far, isolation of an alkaloid, vasicinone, and number of polysaccharides and peptide substances has been reported [5]. Flavonoids including 7-glucosides of apigenin, luteolin, and tricetin, as well as the 7-rutinoside of apigenin and luteolin have been isolated from its leaves which in part are responsible for antioxidant and antihemolytic activities [6-8]. Recently, essential oil composition of *B. multifida*

* Correspondence: mhghahremani@tums.ac.ir
[4]Nanotechnology Research Centre, Faculty of Pharmacy, Tehran University of Medical Sciences, Tehran, Iran
[5]Department of Pharmacology and Toxicology, Faculty of Pharmacy, Tehran University of Medical Sciences, Tehran, Iran
Full list of author information is available at the end of the article

was studied which exhibited that the main components were (E)-nerolidol, phytol, 6,10,14-trimethyl-2- pentadecanone and hexadecanoic acid [9].

Ethnopharmacological studies have revealed that the root extract of this plant has anti-inflammatory and analgesic activities that confirm the traditional use of *B. multifida* for the treatment of joint disturbances as well as in restoring bone fractures [10]. However, no report has yet been made on the anti-anxiety effects of the plant.

The elevated plus-maze has been developed as an ethological model of provoked anxiety and its use for the study of animal anxiety-like behavior has been pharmacologically validated and widely used for rats and mice [11-13]. In the present study, we have utilized the phobia behavior of mice in the elevated plus-maze as a model to evaluate the anxiolytic effect of the plant. For this purpose, the anxiolytic effects of the total root extract of *B. multifida* and its fractions were evaluated in mice and the chemical composition of the active fraction was identified.

Materials and methods
Chemicals
All chemicals were obtained from Merck (Darmstadt, Germany). Solvents used in chromatography methods were HPLC-grade. Diazepam (purity: not less than 98.0%) was obtained from Chemidarou Pharmaceutical Company (Tehran, Iran). Vasicinone (purity ≥97%) was a generous gift from Dr. Vahid Ziaee in Department of Medicinal Chemistry, Tehran University of Medical Sciences.

Plant materials
The plant materials were collected from the region of Ruine, located in North Khorasan Province of Iran following the national rule on biodiversity by local agent of Iran Department of Environment. A voucher specimen has been deposited at the Herbarium of the Faculty of Pharmacy, Tehran University of Medical Sciences (Voucher No. 6691 TEH) by Prof. GR Amin. The root of the plant was used in this study.

Chromatographic apparatus
A high performance liquid chromatography (HPLC) instrument equipped with K-1001 pump (Knauer, Germany), a D-14163 manual injector valve (Rheodyne), and a K-2600 UV detector for peak detection was used in the analytical studies. Another HPLC instrument (Knauer, Germany) including preparative K-1800 pumps (Double), two switching valves and a K-2501 UV detector were used for preparative purification. Solvents were filtered through a Millipore system and separation was performed on Knauer Eurosphere 100 C18 columns (150 mm × 4.0 mm, I.D. 5 μm) and (120 mm × 16 mm, I.D. 5 μm) for analytical and preparative HPLC, respectively.

Spectroscopy instruments
The ^{1}H-NMR and ^{13}C-NMR spectra of the isolated compounds were measured in DMSO-d_6 or CDCl$_3$ at 500 and 125 MHz, respectively, using a Bruker AC 500 spectrophotometer (Germany). Mass spectra were prepared on Finnigan-Mat TSQ-70 spectrometer (CA, USA). Fourier-transform infrared (FTIR) spectra were obtained with a Nicolet Magna-FTIR 550 spectrometer (WI, USA).

Extraction procedures
The roots were collected from the field, cleaned, dried for two weeks in the shade, then powdered and stored in airtight containers. The total extract was prepared from the powdered root refluxed with methanol for 72 hours using a Soxhlet apparatus, followed by filtration. The filtrate was concentrated using low-pressure distillation at 45°C and evaporated to dryness. We obtained 690±1 g of total extract solids from 4900 g powdered root (14.08%). To prepare the fractions, an aliquot of 300 g of the extract solids were re-suspended in 1400 mL of water/acetic acid (95:5) solution and further extracted with light petroleum ether (4 × 1000 mL) to separate the lipophilic compounds (ether fraction, 4.3% of total extract). The remaining aqueous part was treated with ammonia 25% and sequentially partitioned in chloroform and ethyl acetate (4 × 1000 mL for each of them). The solvent was removed under reduced pressure and the total alkaline residue (1.6%) was used for the experiments (alkaline fraction). All extracts were analyzed by thin layer chromatography (TLC). Plant total extract was prepared in 1% carboxymethylcellulose (CMC) in saline prior to animal testing. The alkaline and ether fractions were dissolved in saline containing 2% DMSO.

Pharmacological studies
Male Swiss white mice, 20–25 g, were obtained from the Animal Care Facility (Faculty of Pharmacy, Tehran, Iran). The animals were housed six per cage in a temperature-controlled (22 ± 1°C) colony room. They were maintained in a 12h light/dark schedule with *ad libitum* food and water except during experimental procedures. All trials were carried out in the light phase. Subjects were experimentally naïve and each mouse was used only once. Animals were allowed 7 days to acclimatize to the laboratory environment including handling before testing began. All procedures were carried out in accordance with institutional guidelines for animal care and use. The protocol (No. 357) had been approved by the Committee of Ethics of the Faculty of Sciences of Tehran University.

Plant extracts and fractions were injected intraperitoneally (*i.p.*) in a single dose. Control groups received vehicle in saline (saline group) or diazepam 1 mg/kg, as a known anti-anxiety drug. The elevated plus maze consisted two open arms (6 × 30 × 2 cm) and two closed arms (6 × 30 × 10 cm), having an open roof, elevated 40 cm with a central platform of 8 × 8 cm. The test was performed 30 and 90 min after injection. Each mouse was placed in the central platform facing toward a closed arm and the cumulative time spent in open or closed arms was recorded for 5 min. The percent time spent was used as the measure of plus-maze performance. The ratio of percent time spent in open to closed arm (Ratio = % time spent in open arms/% time spent in closed arms) was indexed as the anxiolytic effect of various groups. Based on this calculation, when the animal had equal preference for open and closed arms at ratio = 1, this was an indicator of loss of anxiety. A ratio < 1 indicated that the animal avoided the open arm, indicating anxiety behavior. The entry time into each arm and the total entry time for each mouse were used as an index of activity for each animal. There were 4 mice in each group and the experiment was repeated 3 times, independently (n = 12).

Isolation, purification, and structure elucidation
The alkaline fraction (2 g) was subjected to column chromatography (100 g silica gel) for clean-up and initial fractionation. Elution with 1200 mL of $CHCl_3$/EtOAC (80:20) gave a fraction that contained major compounds of the chloroform extraction. This fraction was further purified by HPLC to yield compounds 1 and 2 as described below. Compound 3 eluted from the column with an Rf value greater than 1 and 2. This compound was further purified by preparative TLC by $CHCl_3$/EtOAC (65:35) as the mobile phase.

For further purification, the $CHCl_3$/EtOAC (80:20) fraction from column chromatography was subjected to preparative HPLC. Initially, a small amount of the fraction was injected into the analytical HPLC and the composition of the mobile phase was optimized by varying the percent of acetonitrile in phosphate buffer for separation of compounds 1 and 2. The best purification was obtained using the following conditions: acetonitrile/0.1 M phosphate buffer/glacial acetic acid (6:94:1 v/v/v), pH 4.15; flow rate: 1.2 mL/min; detector wavelength 300 nm. After optimizations using analytical HPLC, scale-up was performed for preparative separation. A flow rate of 14 mL/min was applied for preparative separation; other conditions were identical with the analytical method. The $CHCl_3$/EtOAC (80:20) fraction was subjected to preparative HPLC and pure compounds 1 (32 mg) and 2 (12 mg) were separated collected in the mobile phase. The purity of these two compounds was re-checked by analytical HPLC and structure elucidation of the purified compounds was carried out by spectroscopic methods (MS, FTIR, ^{1}H and ^{13}C-NMR).

Statistical analysis
The data obtained from independent pharmacological experiments were pooled and reported as mean ± SEM. The data were analyzed by one-way ANOVA followed by Tukey post hoc multiple comparison. $P < 0.05$ was considered significant.

Results
The anxiolytic effect of total extract in mice
In animals receiving the total extract of the roots and tested 30 min after injection, the time spent in open arm was prolonged compared to the animals that received saline (Figure 1). The effect was first seen at a dose of 25 mg extract/kg body weight and increased in a dose dependent

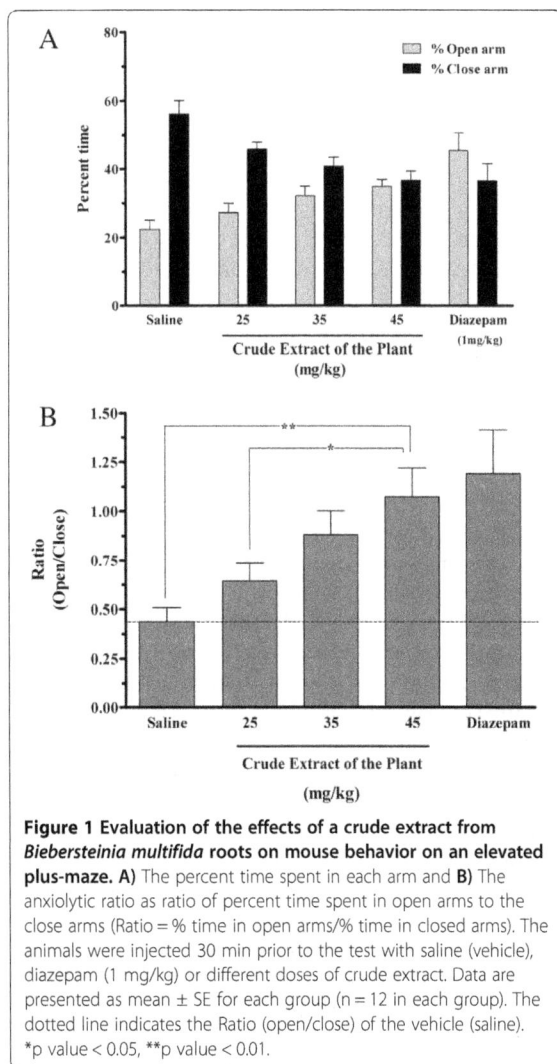

Figure 1 Evaluation of the effects of a crude extract from *Biebersteinia multifida* roots on mouse behavior on an elevated plus-maze. A) The percent time spent in each arm and **B)** The anxiolytic ratio as ratio of percent time spent in open arms to the close arms (Ratio = % time in open arms/% time in closed arms). The animals were injected 30 min prior to the test with saline (vehicle), diazepam (1 mg/kg) or different doses of crude extract. Data are presented as mean ± SE for each group (n = 12 in each group). The dotted line indicates the Ratio (open/close) of the vehicle (saline). *p value < 0.05, **p value < 0.01.

Table 1 The effect of total extract of *Biebersteinia multifida* on the behavior of mice on an elevated plus-maze

Treatment	Total entry		Percent entry into open arms	
	30 min	90 min	30 min	90 min
Saline	14.5 ± 1.5^a	14.5 ± 0.9	41.2 ± 3.8	39.2 ± 4.3
Diazepam (1 mg/kg)	24.2 ± 2.7	18.3 ± 2.2	57.2 ± 3.55	44.2 ± 2.4
Extract (25 mg/kg)	15.7 ± 1.3	16.1 ± 1.3	41.2 ± 2.4	46.4 ± 2.2
Extract (35 mg/kg)	12.4 ± 1.3	14.3 ± 0.8	43.1 ± 1.7	44.2 ± 3.5
Extract (45 mg/kg)	16.4 ± 1.0	12.8 ± 1.4	50.5 ± 2.2	52.1 ± 2.8
Extract (50 mg/kg)	15.5 ± 3.6	10.0 ± 2.2	48.8 ± 1.9	44.0 ± 12.3
Extract (75 mg/kg)	8.2 ± 1.2	ND^b	53.0 ± 6.2	ND

^{a}The data are presented as mean $\pm$ SE (n = 12).
^{b}ND not determined.
The table indicates the total entry and percent entry into open arms as an indicator of the activity of the animal. The entry to each arm was measured at 30 and 90 min after administration of the total extract.

manner to its maximum level at 45 mg/kg, where the animals spent equal time in the open and closed arms. The effect of 45 mg/kg of the total extract was comparable to that of diazepam at 1 mg/kg, where the mice showed a slightly more, but not significant, preference for the open arm (Figure 1A). At lower dose (10 mg/kg), the animals behaved similar to those given the saline treatment. At higher doses (50 and 75 mg/kg), the animals continued to show equal preference for the open and closed arms. The extract had very little effect on the activity of the animals at the doses used. As indicated in Table 1, the total entries into the closed and open arms are equal in all groups. In animals receiving 50 and 75 mg/kg of the extract, the entries were lower and they were mostly in sleep (Table 1). To compare the anxiolytic effect in various groups, we calculated the ratio of percent time spent in open arm to closed arm (see *Materials and Methods*) for each group (Figure 1B). The ratio = 1 indicates an equal preference for the open and the closed arms, representing loss of anxiety; and the ratio lower than 1 implies less preference for the open arm and an increase in anxiety behavior. This ratio in animals receiving 25 mg/kg of the total extract was higher (0.64±0.09) than in the saline group (0.44±0.07), indicating a trend toward preference for the open area although the difference was not statistically significant (Figure 1B). The anxiolytic ratio increased with increases in the dose of total extract and reached 1.07±0.15 in the mice that received 45 mg/kg of the total extract (p < 0.01 compared to saline), suggesting a lack of anxiety. This ratio was comparable to that obtained with diazepam (1.19±0.22, p < 0.01 compared to saline, Figure 1B). In order to evaluate the duration of anxiolytic effect, we also tested the effect of total extract 90 min after injection. As seen in Figure 2, the anxiolytic effect of the plant extract was sustained for 90 min. This anxiolytic ratio was even higher at 90 min after injection of 45 mg/kg of the total extract (p < 0.05 compared to 30 min, Figure 2). On the other hand, the effect of diazepam had been reduced considerably by

90 min. This observation suggests a longer duration of action for the extract compared to that of diazepam (Figure 2).

The anxiolytic effect of alkaline and ether fractions
To further isolate the active compounds in *B. multifida*, the total root extract was fractionated as mentioned in *Materials and Methods*. Alkaloids of this plant may be responsible for its pharmacological activities [10]; thus we examined the anxiolytic activity of the alkaline and ether (lipophilic compounds) fractions of the root extract. Figure 3 shows the effects of various doses of the alkaline fraction on animal performance on elevated plus-maze 30 min after injection. An increase in tendency toward presence in the open arm was seen as the dose of the alkaline fraction was increased (Figure 3). The anxiolytic ratio calculated for these experiments

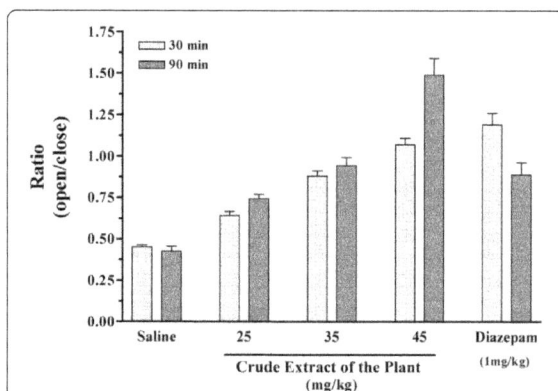

Figure 2 The time dependency of the anxiolytic effect of total extract. Effects were analyzed by performing the test at 30 min and 90 min after injection. The animals were injected 30 min prior to the plus maze test with saline (vehicle), diazepam (1 mg/kg) and different doses of crude extract of the plant. The ratio of percent time spent in open arms to close arms was calculated and plotted as mean $\pm$ SE for each group (n = 12 in each group).

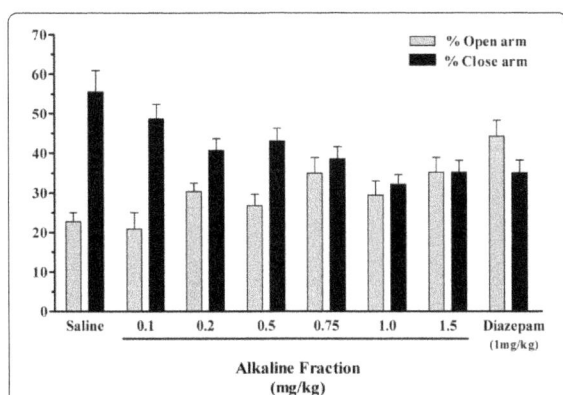

Figure 3 The effect of an alkaline fraction of a *Biebersteinia multifida* root extract on the behavior of mice on an elevated plus-maze by the percent time spent in each arm. The animals were injected 30 min prior to the test with saline (vehicle), diazepam (1 mg/kg) or different doses of alkaline fraction. Data are presented as mean ± SE for each group (n = 12 in each group).

indicated that this effect was dose dependent; it began at a dose of 0.2 mg/kg and the maximum effect was obtained at 1.0 mg/kg of the alkaline fraction. The activity of the animals indicated as total entries into the arms show no significant differences among the various groups (Table 2). We also studied the effect of the alkaline fraction 90 min after injection. As Figure 4 shows, unlike the diazepam treated group, the anxiolytic effect of alkaline fraction continued to be seen 90 min after injection, suggesting a sustained effect for this fraction.

We also tested the ether fraction of plant extract, which contained lipophilic compounds. At doses of 3 and 6 mg/kg of the ether fraction, the animals showed no significant anxiolytic effects compared to saline treated group (Figure 5A). The 3 and 6 mg of ether fraction were equivalent to 69.7 and 139.5 mg of total extract, respectively. The effect of the ether fraction was

similar to saline and did not show any anxiolytic effect at either 30 or 90 min after injection (Figure 5B).

Collectively, the alkaline fraction produced an anxiolytic effect in a dose dependent manner starting at 0.2 mg/kg and reaching a maximum effect at 1.0 mg/kg. This effect was comparable to that seen for diazepam (1.0 mg/kg). Doses of 0.2 and 1.0 mg/kg of alkaloid fraction were equivalent to 12.5 and 62.5 mg/kg of the total root extract.

Isolation, purification, and structure elucidation of chemicals present in the alkaline fraction

The alkaline fraction that showed the anxiolytic effect was subjected to different chromatography methods, as mentioned in *Materials and Methods*, which led to isolation and purification of three compounds.

Structure elucidation of compounds 1, 2, and 3 was carried out by spectroscopic methods (MS, FTIR, ^{1}H and ^{13}C-NMR) and by comparison of acquired data with those reported in the literature [14-17]. Compounds 1, 2, and 3 were identified as umbelliferone, scopoletin, and ferulic acid, respectively (Figure 6, Additional file 1: Table S1 and Additional file 2: Figure S1, Additional file 3: Figure S2, Additional file 4: Figure S3, Additional file 5: Figure S4, Additional file 6: Figure S5, Additional file 7: Figure S6) as the major components of alkaloid fraction.

Discussion

The anti-inflammatory and analgesic activities of *B. multifida* have been reported before [10]. We have employed a bio-guided fractionation to study the anxiolytic effect of the extracts. This approach has been successfully applied as a valuable strategy for the finding of new lead compounds in phytochemical studies [18].

The use of the elevated plus-maze to study animal anxiety-like behavior has been comprehensively studied and pharmacologically validated for rats [11] and mice

Table 2 The effect of alkaline fraction of *Biebersteinia multifida* on the behavior of mice on an elevated plus-maze

Treatment	Total entry		Percent entry to open arms	
	30 min	90 min	30 min	90 min
Saline	14.2 ± 1.7[a]	8.8 ± 1.5	41.5 ± 3.3	39.9 ± 3.6
Diazepam (1 mg/kg)	32.2 ± 4.1	25.8 ± 6.2	60.5 ± 2.4	54.0 ± 6.4
Alkaline fraction (0.1 mg/kg)	19.2 ± 1.2	15.4 ± 1.7	42.3 ± 4.1	41.7 ± 6.9
Alkaline fraction (0.2 mg/kg)	14.8 ± 0.7	13.8 ± 1.4	48.8 ± 2.3	36.2 ± 2.5
Alkaline fraction (0.5 mg/kg)	13.8 ± 1.64	9.5 ± 1.3	41.0 ± 4.4	37.7 ± 4.9
Alkaline fraction (0.75 mg/kg)	16.5 ± 1.5	12.1 ± 1.1	51.2 ± 3.9	51.6 ± 3.6
Alkaline fraction (1.0 mg/kg)	23.0 ± 1.7	13.0 ± 4.3	48.4 ± 2.0	59.9 ± 3.1
Alkaline fraction (1.5 mg/kg)	18.2 ± 2.7	ND[b]	51.5 ± 2.7	ND

[a]The data are presented as Mean ± SE (n = 12).
[b]ND not determined.
The table indicates the total entry and percent entry into open arms as an indicator of the activity of the animal. The entry to each arm was measured at 30 and 90 min after administration of the alkaline fraction.

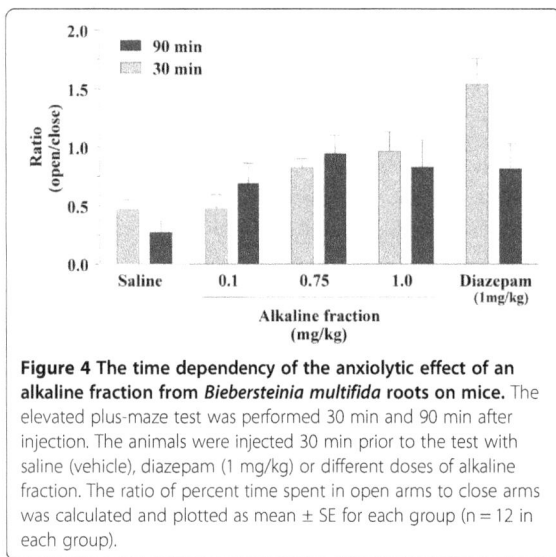

Figure 4 The time dependency of the anxiolytic effect of an alkaline fraction from *Biebersteinia multifida* roots on mice. The elevated plus-maze test was performed 30 min and 90 min after injection. The animals were injected 30 min prior to the test with saline (vehicle), diazepam (1 mg/kg) or different doses of alkaline fraction. The ratio of percent time spent in open arms to close arms was calculated and plotted as mean ± SE for each group (n = 12 in each group).

[13]. In various studies, the open arm entry to total entry or open time ratio were used as an indicator of anxiety behavior in mice and rats [11,13]. Since locomotion is an important factor in the elevated plus-maze, the total entry time has been used as an indicator of activity [11,13]. In this study, the time spent in each arm, the open and closed time ratio, was used to evaluate the anxiety behavior, while the total entry time considered as an index of animal activity.

A bio-guided phytochemical analysis of *B. multifida* has not previously been reported. Although other reports have thus far identified a number of flavonoids, a few polysaccharides and one alkaloid (vasicinone) from root extract, in which vasicinone considered as the responsible molecule for observed pharmacological activities [5-7,9], there were no direct relation between the isolated compounds to traditional use of *B. multifida*. Thus, to identify the active anxiolytic components, the total extract is fractioned into alkaline and ether fractions and subjected to anxiety alleviation studies. The anxiolytic compounds act readily in alkaline fraction form while the ether fraction showed little anxiolytic effect. This bio-guided fractionation indicates that the active compounds are present in the alkaline fraction. Furthermore, the results suggest that the alkaloid extract has a sustained anxiolytic effect compared to that observed with diazepam. Diazepam is a known anxiolytic used as control in various pharmacological studies. In this study, our results indicate a strong anti anxiety effect in animals receiving diazepam (Figures 1 and 2). Interestingly, the anxiolytic effect of diazepam has been reduced considerably by 90 min (Figure 2). Thus compared to diazepam, the plant extract has a longer duration of action.

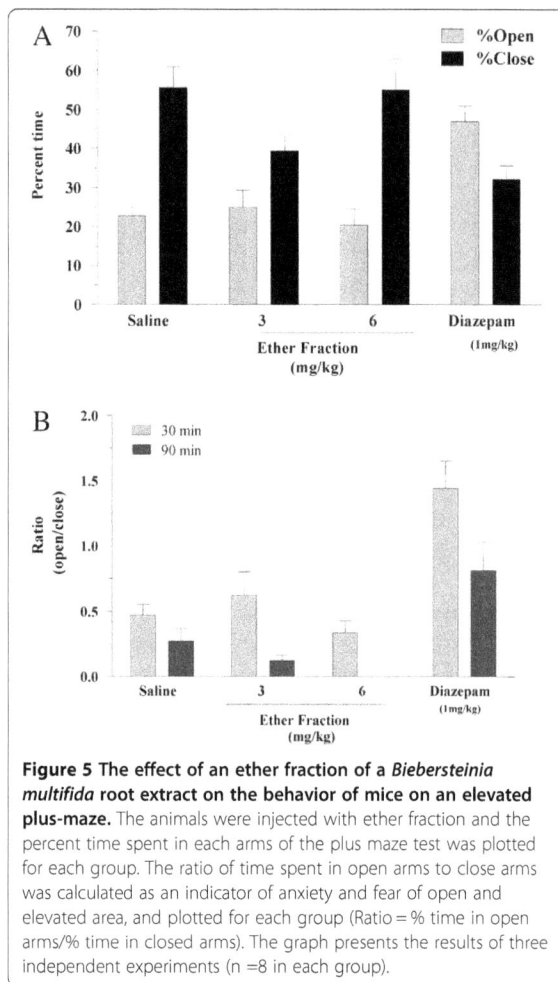

Figure 5 The effect of an ether fraction of a *Biebersteinia multifida* root extract on the behavior of mice on an elevated plus-maze. The animals were injected with ether fraction and the percent time spent in each arms of the plus maze test was plotted for each group. The ratio of time spent in open arms to close arms was calculated as an indicator of anxiety and fear of open and elevated area, and plotted for each group (Ratio = % time in open arms/% time in closed arms). The graph presents the results of three independent experiments (n =8 in each group).

Before any further chromatographic studies, the effects of pure vasicinone -as the suspected active compound in the alkaloid fraction- on mouse performance is tested by the same experimental procedure as described above. The analysis of vasicinone, at doses as high as 10 mg/kg, had no significant effect on open time ratio (data not shown). Thus, the alkaline fraction is further characterized for the major components present which lead to isolation and structure elucidation of three compounds of coumarin derivatives including umbelliferone, scopoletin, and ferulic acid. However the presence of ferulic acid after alkaline

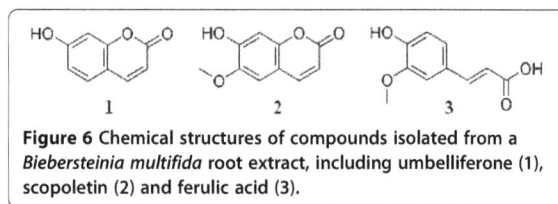

Figure 6 Chemical structures of compounds isolated from a *Biebersteinia multifida* root extract, including umbelliferone (1), scopoletin (2) and ferulic acid (3).

extraction could be a consequence of ring opening of scopoletin after extraction.

According to previous reports, coumarin derivatives, including scopoletin and umbelliferone, are potent inhibitors of monoamine oxidases (MAOs) [19,20]. Scopoletin shows MAO inhibition activity in a dose-dependent fashion, with IC_{50} values of 19.4 μg/mL [19]. In addition, daphnoretin a bicoumarin of scopoletin and umbelliferone exhibits significant anxiolytic activity in EPM model [21-23]. It has been also suggested that coumarin derivatives interact with the benzodiazepine binding site of the GABA-A receptor [24]. This may explain the effects observed in the present study and may confirm at least a partial role of these coumarins anxiolytic effects of *B. multifida*.

In addition to the anxiolytic effect, scopoletin is also a known potent anti-inflammatory agent [25,26], which can explain, in part, the anti-inflammatory and anti-nociceptive effects of *B. multifida* extracts. The ability of low molecular weight substances to cross the blood–brain barrier could explain the reported central anti-nociceptive effect [10]. However, this needs further specific pure substance studies in validated pharmacological models.

In conclusion, for the first time, bio-guided fractionation of the root extract of *B. multifida* indicates significant sustained anxiolytic effects which led to isolation of three coumarin derivatives of those scopoletin and umbelliferone with known MAO inhibitory and anti-anxiety effects. These data contribute to evidence-based traditional medicines using root of *B. multifida* for anxiety disorders.

Additional files

Additional file 1: Table S1. NMR chemical shift assignments of umbelliferone (1), scopoletin (2) and ferulic acid (3).

Additional file 2: Figure S1. Mass spectrum of Umbelliferone.

Additional file 3: Figure S2. FTIR spectrum of Umbelliferone.

Additional file 4: Figure S3. Mass spectrum of Scopoletin.

Additional file 5: Figure S4. FTIR spectrum of Scopoletin.

Additional file 6: Figure S5. Mass spectrum of Ferulic acid.

Additional file 7: Figure S6. FTIR spectrum of Ferulic acid.

Competing interests

The authors declare that they have no conflicts of interest.

Authors' contributions

HRM participated in the design of the study and carried out the phytochemical studies. MA carried out the structure elucidation. NG carried out the extraction, isolation and HPLC analysis and wrote the manuscript. FS carried out the animal studies and drafted the manuscript. RH participated in extraction and chromatography studies. MAF participated in the phytochemical analysis. ZT participated in experimental coordination and helped to draft the manuscript. MHG designed the study, performed the statistical analysis and finalized the manuscript. All authors read and approved the final manuscript.

Acknowledgments

This study was financially supported by a grant from Research Council of Tehran University of Medical Sciences and a grant from Center of Excellence for Toxicology, Ministry of Health and Medical Education of Iran. We gratefully acknowledge Professor Gholam Reza Amin, head of the Herbarium of Faculty of Pharmacy, Tehran University of Medical Sciences, and Dr. Vahid Ziaee for providing synthetic Vasicinone generously.

Author details

[1]Department of Pharmacognosy, Faculty of Pharmacy, Tehran University of Medical Sciences, Tehran, Iran. [2]Department of Medicinal Chemistry, Faculty of Pharmacy, Tehran University of Medical Sciences, Tehran, Iran. [3]Department of Pharmaceutics, Faculty of Pharmacy, Tehran University of Medical Sciences, Tehran, Iran. [4]Nanotechnology Research Centre, Faculty of Pharmacy, Tehran University of Medical Sciences, Tehran, Iran. [5]Department of Pharmacology and Toxicology, Faculty of Pharmacy, Tehran University of Medical Sciences, Tehran, Iran. [6]Pharmacognosy & Pharmaceutics Department of Medicinal Plants Research Center, Institute of Medicinal Plants, ACECR, Karaj, Iran. [7]Department of Pharmaceutical Biotechnology, Faculty of Pharmacy & Biotechnology Research Center, Tehran University of Medical Sciences, Tehran, Iran.

References

1. Muellner AN, Vassiliades DD, Renner SS: **Placing Biebersteiniaceae, a herbaceous clade of Sapindales, in a temporal and geographic context.** *Plant Syst Evol* 2007, **266**:233–252.
2. Amin G: *Popular Medicinal Plants of Iran*. 1st edition. Tehran: Research Deputy, Ministry of Health, Treatment and Medical Education; 1991.
3. Amirghofran Z: **Medicinal plants as immunosuppressive agents in traditional Iranian medicine.** *Iran J Immunol* 2010, **7**:65–73.
4. Aboutorabi H: *Ethnobotanic and phytochemical study of plants in Rouin region. PharmD Thesis.* Tehran: Tehran University of Medical Sciences; 2001.
5. Arifkhodzhaev AO, Rakhimov DA: **Polysaccharides of saponin-bearing plants. V. Structural investigation of glucans A, B, and C and their oligosaccharides from Biebersteinia multifida plants.** *Chem Nat Compd* 1994, **30**:655–660.
6. Greenham J, Vassiliades DD, Harborne JB, Williams CA, Eagles J, Grayer RJ, Veitch NC: **A distinctive flavonoid chemistry for the anomalous genus Biebersteinia.** *Phytochemistry* 2001, **56**:87–91.
7. Omurkamzinova VB, Maurel ND, Bikbulatova TN: **Flavonoids of Biebersteinia multifida.** *Chem Nat Compd* 1991, **27**:636–637.
8. Nabavi SF, Ebrahimzadeh MA, Nabavi SM, Eslami B, Dehpour A: **Antihemolytic and antioxidant activities of Biebersteinia multifida.** *Eur Rev Med Pharmacol Sci* 2010, **14**:823–830.
9. Javidnia K, Miri R, Soltani M, Khosravi AR: **Essential oil composition of biebersteinia multifida DC. (Biebersteiniaceae) from Iran.** *J Essent Oil Res* 2010, **22**:611–612.
10. Farsam H, Amanlou M, Dehpour AR, Jahaniani F: **Anti-inflammatory and analgesic activity of Biebersteinia multifida DC. root extract.** *J Ethnopharmacol* 2000, **71**:443–447.
11. Pellow S, Chopin P, File SE, Briley M: **Validation of open: closed arm entries in an elevated plus-maze as a measure of anxiety in the rat.** *J Neurosci Methods* 1985, **14**:149–167.
12. Rabbani M, Sajjadi SE, Jalali A: **Hydroalcohol extract and fractions of Stachys lavandulifolia vahl: effects on spontaneous motor activity and elevated plus-maze behaviour.** *Phytother Res* 2005, **19**:854–858.
13. Lister RG: **The use of a plus-maze to measure anxiety in the mouse.** *Psychopharmacology* 1987, **92**:180–185.
14. Yan J, Tong S, Sheng L, Lou J: **Preparative isolation and purification of two coumarins from Edgeworthia chrysantha Lindl by high speed countercurrent chromatography.** *J Liq Chromatogr Related Technol* 2006, **29**:1307–1315.
15. Aplin RT, Page CB: **The constituents of native umbelliferae. Part I. Coumarins from dill (Anetheum graveolens L.).** *J Chem Soc C* 1967, 2593:2596.
16. Torres R, Urbina F, Morales C, Modak B, Delle Monache F: **Antioxidant properties of lignans and ferulic acid from the resinous exudate of Larrea nitida.** *J Chil Chem Soc* 2003, **48**:61–63.

17. Dobhal MP, Hasan AM, Sharma MC, Joshi BC: **Ferulic acid esters from Plumeria bicolor.** *Phytochemistry* 1999, **51**:319–321.

18. Pieters L, Vlietinck AJ: **Bioguided isolation of pharmacologically active plant components, still a valuable strategy for the finding of new lead compounds?** *J Ethnopharmacol* 2005, **100**:57–60.

19. Yun BS, Lee IK, Ryoo IJ, Yoo ID: **Coumarins with monoamine oxidase inhibitory activity and antioxidative coumarino-lignans from Hibiscus syriacus.** *J Nat Prod* 2001, **64**:1238–1240.

20. Seon HJ, Xiang HH, Seong SH, Ji SH, Ji HH, Lee D, Myung KL, Jai SR, Bang YH: **Monoamine oxidase inhibitory coumarins from the aerial parts of Dictamnus albus.** *Arch Pharm Res* 2006, **29**:1119–1124.

21. Herrera-Ruiz M, Gonzalez-Carranza A, Zamilpa A, Jimenez-Ferrer E, Huerta-Reyes M, Navarro-Garcia VM: **The standardized extract of Loeselia mexicana possesses anxiolytic activity through the gamma-amino butyric acid mechanism.** *J Ethnopharmacol* 2011, **138**:261–267.

22. Navarro-García VM, Herrera-Ruiz M, Rojas G, Zepeda LG: **Coumarin derivatives from Loeselia mexicana. Determination of the anxiolytic effect of daphnoretin on elevated plus-maze.** *J Mex Chem Soc* 2007, **51**:193–197.

23. Kumar D, Bhat ZA, Kumar V, Shah MY: **Coumarins from Angelica archangelica Linn. and their effects on anxiety-like behavior.** *Prog Neuropsychopharmacol Biol Psychiatry* 2013, **40**:180–186.

24. Singhuber J, Baburin I, Ecker GF, Kopp B, Hering S: **Insights into structure–activity relationship of GABAA receptor modulating coumarins and furanocoumarins.** *Eur J Pharmacol* 2011, **668**:57–64.

25. Moon PD, Lee BH, Jeong HJ, An HJ, Park SJ, Kim HR, Ko SG, Um JY, Hong SH, Kim HM: **Use of scopoletin to inhibit the production of inflammatory cytokines through inhibition of the IκB/NF-κB signal cascade in the human mast cell line HMC-1.** *Eur J Pharmacol* 2007, **555**:218–225.

26. Meotti FC, Ardenghi JV, Pretto JB, Souza MM, D'Ávila Moura J, Cunha A Jr, Soldi C, Pizzolatti MG, Santos ARS: **Antinociceptive properties of coumarins, steroid and dihydrostyryl-2- pyrones from Polygala sabulosa (Polygalaceae) in mice.** *J Pharm Pharmacol* 2006, **58**:107–112.

2

Alteration in brain-derived neurotrophic factor (BDNF) after treatment of mice with herbal mixture containing Euphoria longana, Houttuynia cordata and Dioscorea japonica

Songhee Jeon[1], Chia-Hung Lee[2], Quan Feng Liu[2], Geun Woo Kim[3], Byung-Soo Koo[4*] and Sok Cheon Pak[5]

Abstract

Background: Literature data indicate that brain-derived neurotrophic factor (BDNF), cyclic-AMP response element-binding protein (CREB) and phospho-CREB (pCREB) may have a place in depression. BDNF belongs to the neurotrophin family that plays an important role in proliferation, survival and differentiation of different cell populations in the mammalian nervous system. The herbal mixture used in the present study consists of *Euphoria longana*, *Houttuynia cordata* and *Dioscorea japonica*. The purpose of the present study was to determine the neuroprotective effect of herbal mixture. We also tested the hypothesis that administration of herbs reverses memory deficits and promotes the protein expression of BDNF in the mouse brain.

Methods: Mice were randomized into four different treatment groups (n = 10/group). Normal and stress groups received regular lab chow without stress and under stress conditions, respectively, for 3 weeks. The animals in the stress group were immobilized for 4 hours a day for 2 weeks. Different doses of herbal mixture (206 and 618 mg/kg) were administered for 3 weeks to those mice under stress conditions. Mice were analyzed by behavioral tests and immunoblotting examination in the hippocampus and cortex. An additional in vitro investigation was performed to examine whether herbs induce neurotoxicity in a human neuroblastoma cell line, SH-SY5Y cells.

Results: No significant toxicity of herbs on human neuroblastoma cells was observed. These herbs demonstrated an inductive effect on the expression of BDNF, pCREB and pAkt. For spatial working memory test, herbal mixture fed mice exhibited an increased level of spontaneous alternation (p < 0.01) compared to those in stress conditions. Moreover, herbal mixture produced highly significant (p < 0.01) reduction in the immobility time in the tail suspension test. Mice in the herbal mixture groups demonstrated lower serum corticosterone concentration than mice in the stress group (p < 0.05). Effects of the oral administration of herbal mixture on protein levels of BDNF in the hippocampi and cortices were significant.

Conclusions: Our study showed that herbal mixture administration has antidepressant effects in mice. It is proposed that adverse events such as stress and depression can modulate the expression of molecular players of cellular plasticity in the brain.

Keywords: Stress, Depression, BDNF, Memory, *Euphoria longana*, *Houttuynia cordata*, *Dioscorea japonica*

* Correspondence: koobs@dongguk.ac.kr
[4]Department of Korean Neuropsychiatry, Dongguk University Ilsan Oriental Hospital, Goyang, Republic of Korea
Full list of author information is available at the end of the article

Background

Specific data from the Global Burden of Disease 2010 study confirmed that mental and substance use disorders account for 7.4% of disease burden worldwide which is greater than HIV/AIDS and tuberculosis (5.3%), diabetes (2%) or transport injuries (3.3%) [1]. Depression in particular is projected to become the leading cause of disability and the second leading contributor to the global burden of disease in approximately 10 years [2]. As a heterogeneous disorder with unclear etiology, depression includes disturbance of neurogenesis, genetic predisposition, deficiency of monoamines, hypercortisolemia, reduction of neurotrophins, inflammation and oxidative stress [3].

It has been proposed that brain-derived neurotrophic factor (BDNF), as one of neurotrophins, may be a key player in depression since it is involved in regulation of neuronal differentiation, survival, function and plasticity [4]. This neurotrophic hypothesis of depression claims that decreased levels of BDNF contribute to the hippocampal atrophy seen in depressed patients [5]. Depressive symptoms are also associated with decreased serum level of BDNF [6]. These evidences have already led to clinical trials of antidepressant medications for treating major depression, although there are some gaps in the clinical outcomes depending on the classes of psychotropic drugs and uncertainty about whether drugs that specifically target depressive symptoms are feasible and safe. The transcription of BDNF is dependent on cyclic-AMP response element-binding protein (CREB).

CREB is a transcriptional factor implicated in the control of adaptive neuronal responses. It has been found that calcium ions in neurons bind to a calcium response element within the BDNF gene which triggers phosphorylation of CREB and subsequent activation of BDNF transcription [7]. Depression is accompanied by down-regulated and decreased phosphorylated CREB (pCREB). A growing number of clinical and experimental studies have demonstrated that structural and functional modifications of hippocampus from antidepressant treatments most likely require the transcription and protein expression of CREB, despite some inconsistencies in its mRNA and protein levels depending on the brain regions where such molecule is expressed [7]. CREB is regulated by several pathways including protein kinase B (PKB/Akt).

Antidepressant medications are effective at treating depression, but discontinuation rates are high because adverse effects are common [8]. For example, selective serotonin reuptake inhibitors (SSRIs) frequently cause gastrointestinal problems, insomnia, headache, anxiety and sexual dysfunction although they are the most commonly prescribed antidepressants [9]. Considering the side effects of synthetic antidepressants, natural plants can be alternative sources of new antidepressant drugs due to their more tolerable and less toxic properties.

Therefore, the current study was performed as the progress toward finding reliable alternatives to depression.

Three different ingredients of traditional Korean medicine for depression were selected to observe the effects of them in cell culture and animal experiment. *Euphoria longana* Lam., especially a dried longan seed extract, contain high levels of antioxidant polyphenolic compounds [10]. Longan seed extracts are found to possess anticancer properties by inducing apoptosis [11]. *Houttuynia cordata* Thunb. is a single species of its genus and the whole plant of *H. cordata* is used for the treatment of diabetes [12]. Reported pharmacological activities of plant include anti-cancer [13], anti-inflammatory [13] and antioxidant [14]. The rhizome of *Dioscorea japonica* Thunb. has been used to strengthen stomach function, improve anorexia, eliminate diarrhea, dilute sputum, and moisturize skin in traditional Chinese medicine [15]. An ethanol extract of the rhizome of *D. japonica* showed considerable cytotoxic activity against some human tumor cell lines [16]. These three natural plants have been used as traditional herbal medicines in the treatment of neurological disorders in Korea. However, few studies have evaluated their antidepressant effects. The effects of these three herbs on BDNF, pCREB and pAkt are currently unknown. In this experiment, one human neuroblastoma cell line was used to investigate the neuroprotective effect of herbs. We also tested the hypothesis that administration of herbs reverses memory deficits and promotes the protein expression of BDNF in the mouse brain. To test the hypothesis, three different settings of neuronal cell culture, behaviour study and their brains have been used in the present study.

Methods

Preparation of herbal extracts

All medicinal herbs used were purchased from DY Herb (Seoul, Korea). Each herb was boiled in 30% ethanol mixed filter-purified drinking water for 2 h at 100°C in a reflux condenser. For the cellular experiment, aqueous extract of each herb was freeze-dried and the dried extract was reconstructed with distilled water and filtered through 0.2 μm filter (Millipore, MA, USA). In addition, the resulting dry powder of each herb was mixed with the same ratio and added into the feed in the animal studies.

Cell culture

Human neuroblastoma SH-SY5Y cells were obtained from American Type Culture Collection (Rockville, MD, USA). Cells were maintained in Dulbecco's modified Eagle's minimum essential medium (DMEM, Invitrogen, Carlsbad, CA, USA) supplemented with 10% fetal bovine serum (FBS, Invitrogen, Carlsbad, CA, USA), 100 unit/ml penicillin and 100 μg/ml streptomycin (Gibco-BRL, Rockville, MD, USA) with further addition of trypsin-

EDTA (Gibco-BRL, Rockville, MD, USA) in condition of 95% air and 5% CO_2 at 37°C.

Cell viability assay

Cell viability was determined by 3-(4,5-dimethylthizaol-2-yl)-2,5-diphenyltetrazolium bromide (MTT, Abcam, Cambridge, MA, USA) assay. SH-SY5Y cells were seeded in 12-well plates (Corning Incorporated, USA) at a density of 5×10^3 cells/well, stabilized at 37°C for 16 h in DMEM medium supplemented with FBS and cultured with the indicated concentrations of herbs for 24 h. The medium was removed and the cells were incubated with 2 mg/ml of MTT solution. After incubation for 4 h at 37°C and 5% CO_2, the supernatants were removed and dimethyl sulfoxide (DMSO, Sigma, USA) was added. The reactants were measured in terms of optical density (OD) at 580 nm with a microplate reader (UV max, Molecular Devices, USA). The optical densities were converted into percentages using the following formula: Cell viability (%) = OD sample/OD negative control × 100. Negative control cells were treated with complete DMEM alone.

Quantification of BDNF/pCREB/pAkt expression by Western blot analysis

SH-SY5Y cells were maintained in serum-free medium with herbs at 30 μg/ml for 24 h. Cells were then washed twice with ice-cold PBS and lysed in lysis buffer containing 62.5 mmol/L Tris–HCl, pH 6.8, 2% SDS, 20% glycerol, 10% 2-mercaptoethanol and protease inhibitors. After incubation for 30 min on ice, cell lysates were centrifuged and protein concentrations were determined using bicinchoninic acid method (Pierce). Samples of cell lysate containing 50 μg of total protein were separated by 4-12% SDS-PAGE and transferred onto nitrocellulose membrane (Amersham Pharmacia Biotech, Buckinghamshire, UK) by electroblotting. After blocking with 5% skim milk in Tris-buffered saline (50 mmol/L Tris–HCl, pH 7.6, 150 mmul/L NaCl, 0.1% Tween-20) for more than 30 min, the membranes were incubated for 16 h at 4°C with primary antibodies (anti-BDNF, anti-phosphorylated-CREB, anti-phosphorylated-Akt, β-actin antibody) and further incubated with horseradish peroxidase-conjugated secondary antibodies for 1 h. The membranes were visualized by an enhanced chemiluminescence system (ECL kit; Pierce, Rockford, IL, USA). Densitometric analysis was performed by Quantity One (Bio-Rad, Hercules, CA) to scan the signals. Further assay was carried out to detect BDNF protein expression in the hippocampus and cortex. The treated hippocampal and cortical tissues removed and homogenized in lysis buffer containing 50 mM Tris-base (pH 7.5), 150 mM NaCl, 2 mM EDTA, 1% glycerol, 10 mM NaF, 10 mM Na-pyrophosphate, 1% NP-40 and protease inhibitors (0.1 mM phenylmethylsulfluoride, 5 μg/ml aprotinin, and 5 μg/ml leupeptin). Thirty μg of tissue lysate

were electrophoresed using SDS-polyacrylamide gels and transferred to nitrocellulose membranes, which were then incubated with anti-BDNF (Cell signaling technology, Beverly, MA, USA) for 16 h at 4°C. After washing with TBS-T (0.05%), the blots were incubated with horseradish peroxidase-conjugated anti-rabbit or anti-mouse IgG, and the bands were visualized using the ECL system (Thermo Fisher Scienctific, USA). Band images were obtained by using a Molecular Imager ChemiDoc XRS$^+$ (Bio-Rad, Hercules, CA, USA) and band intensity was analyzed using Image Lab™ software version 2.0.1 (Bio-Rad).

Experimental animals

Protocols for animal use were reviewed and approved by the Institutional Animal Care and Use Committee at the Dongguk University Ilsan Hospital and were in accordance with National Institute of Health guidelines. Healthy male ICR mice (20–26 g, 6 weeks old) were obtained from OrientBio (Seoul, Korea) and were allowed 1 week for quarantine and acclimatization. Animals were housed under the conditions of constant temperature (22 ± 1°C), relative humidity (55 ± 1%) and 12 h light/12 h dark cycle (light on at 7:00 am). They were housed in polycarbonate cages and given tap water and commercial rodent chow (Samyang Feed, Daejeon, Korea) ad libitum. Forty mice were blindly randomized into four different treatment groups (n = 10/group). Normal and stress groups received regular lab chow without stress and under stress conditions, respectively, for 3 weeks. The animals in the stress group were immobilized for 4 h a day for 2 weeks by being gently inserted into a flexible triangle shaped vinyl screen that was closed and secured with nonallergic adhesive tape. Different doses of herbal mixture (206 and 618 mg/kg which are equivalent to the recommended adult human dose of 1000 and 3000 mg/kg, respectively) were administered for 3 weeks to those mice under stress conditions. The herbal mixture of *E. longana*, *H. cordata* and *D. japonica* was in a ratio of 1:1:1 by weight. Lab chow with or without herbal mixture was prepared for a mouse to have 1 g/kg/day which is equivalent to 7 g/60 kg/day for human and was gamma-irradiated. In order to examine the nutritional status, body weight was evaluated in mice that were fed with normal or herb mixture diet. At the end of experiment period, all animals were immediately decapitated, and their hippocampus and cortex of brains were collected and frozen at –80°C for following analysis. Blood was collected from the heart by cardiac puncture prior to the excision of brain, then after centrifugation serum aliquots were stored at –70°C for further corticosterone determination. The concentration of serum corticosterone was measured with the Corticosterone EIA Kit (Enzo Life Sciences, Farmingdale, NY, USA) in accordance with the manufacturer's instructions.

Step-through passive avoidance test

The apparatus (AP model; O'Hara Co., Tokyo, Japan) for the step-through passive avoidance test consisted of two compartments, an illuminated compartment [100 mm · 120 mm · 100 mm; light at the top of compartment (27 W, 3000 lx)] and a dark compartment (100 mm · 170 mm · 100 mm). The compartments were separated by a guillotine door. During the training trial, a mouse was placed in the safe, illuminated compartment. As the compartment was lit, the mouse stepped through the opened guillotine door into the dark compartment. The time spent in the illuminated compartment was defined as the latency time. Three seconds after the mouse entered the dark compartment, a foot shock (0.3 mA, 50 V, 50 Hz ac for 3 seconds) was delivered to the floor grids in the dark compartment. The mouse could escape from the shock only by stepping back to the safe illuminated compartment. Mice remaining in the light chamber for more than 120 seconds during the learning stage were excluded from the following retention trial. The retention trials were carried out at 24 h after the training trial to evaluate the retention of avoidance memory. The latency time was measured for up to 300 seconds without delivering a foot shock. It was judged that the mouse retained the avoidance memory when it stayed in the illuminated safe compartment for 300 seconds.

Y-maze test

This behavioral test was performed at 48 h after the passive avoidance test. The maze was made of black painted wood; each arm was 40 cm long, 12 cm high, 3 cm wide at the bottom and 10 cm wide at the top. The arms converged at an equilateral triangular central area that was 4 cm at its longest axis. Each mouse was placed at the centre of the apparatus and allowed to move freely through the maze for 8 min. The series of arm entries was recorded visually. Alternation was defined as successive entry into the three arms on overlapping triplet sets. Alternation behavior (%) was calculated as the ratio of actual alternations to possible alternations (defined as the number of arm entries minus two) multiplied by 100.

Forced swimming test

Mice were placed in a Plexiglas cylinder 25 cm in height with a 15 cm internal diameter containing water at a temperature of $25 \pm 1°C$ and a depth of 10 cm so they could not escape and could not touch the bottom. Water was changed between each swim session to prevent possible effects of an alarm substance released by mice during the swim session. There were two swim sessions. The first was 15 min pre-test swim for 3 days in a row and a second 5 min swim test. The pre-test facilitates the development of immobility during the test session and increases the sensitivity for detecting antidepressant behavioral effects. The 5 min swim test was used for analysis of behavior such as swimming, climbing and immobility.

Tail suspension test

Mice both acoustically and visually isolated were suspended individually by their tails 40 cm above the tabletop with the use of an adhesive tape placed approximately 1 cm from the tip of the tail. After a few minutes of vigorous activity, the mice hung passively and completely motionless. The total immobility period in number of seconds was scored throughout the 6 min test. Mice were considered immobile with the absence of any limb or body movements, except for those caused by respiration. A

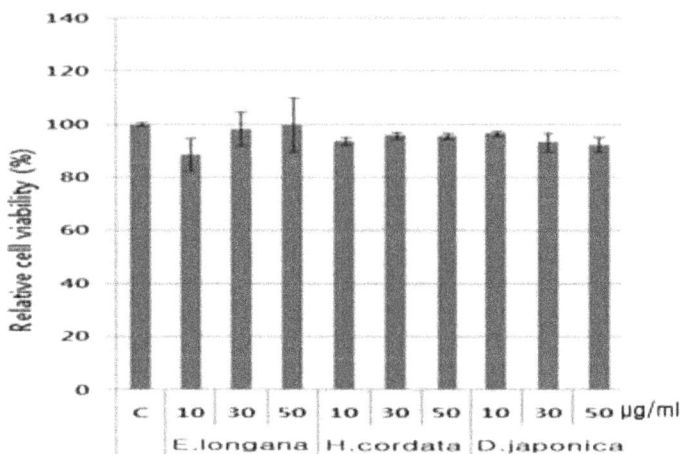

Figure 1 Effect of herbs on the cell viability measured by MTT assay. The human neuroblastoma SH-SY5Y cells were incubated at concentrations of 10, 30 and 50 μg/ml of each herb for 24 h. Values are presented as means ± SEM of six determinations.

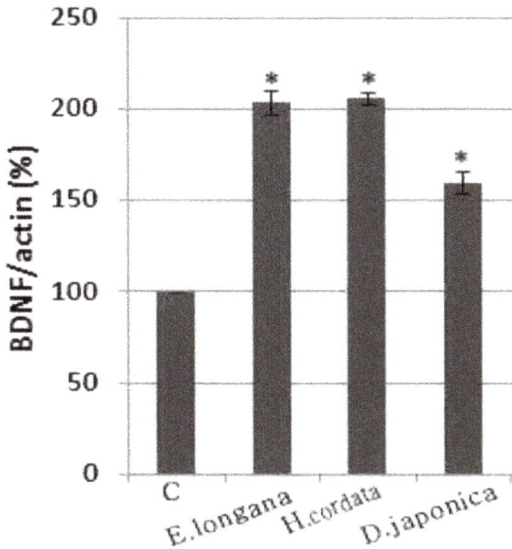

Figure 2 Measurement of BDNF level in neuroblastoma SH-SY5Y cells. To evaluate the protein level of BDNF expression, cells were incubated with 30 μg/ml herb. For the control, nonincubated cells were analyzed. The BDNF level in cell lysates was measured by immunoblotting. Data are presented as means ± SEM of three determinations. *P < 0.05 vs. control.

decrease in the duration of immobility is indicative of an antidepressant-like effect [17].

Data analysis
All statistical analyses were conducted with SPSS (ver. 19, Somers, NY, USA). Values are expressed as means ± SEM. All data were analyzed using Student's t-test. Statistical significance was accepted at a p value less than 0.05.

Results
Effect of herbs on cell viability
In order to measure the cytotoxicity of herbs on SH-SY5Y neuroblastoma cells, a cell viability using MTT assay was utilized. Cells were treated with herbs at concentrations of 10, 30 and 50 μg/ml for 24 h (Figure 1). The percentages of viable cells were as follows: E. longana 10 μg/ml, 88.53 ± 6.3%; 30 μg/ml, 98.25 ± 6.4%; 50 μg/ml, 99.73 ± 10.1%; H. cordata 10 μg/ml, 93.76 ± 1.6%; 30 μg/ml, 95.83 ± 1.2%; 50 μg/ml, 95.61 ± 1.0%; and D. japonica 10 μg/ml, 96.58 ± 0.9%; 30 μg/ml, 93.22 ± 3.4%; 50 μg/ml, 92.38 ± 2.8%. No significant toxicity of herbs on SH-SY5Y was observed at the indicated concentrations.

Effect of herbs on BDNF/pCREB/pAkt expression
We looked at the inductive effects of herbs on the expression of BDNF, pCREB and pAkt in cell extracts. For the control, nonincubated SH-SY5Y cells were analyzed. The BDNF expression in the SH-SY5Y cell extracts treated with herbs was significantly higher than that in the control

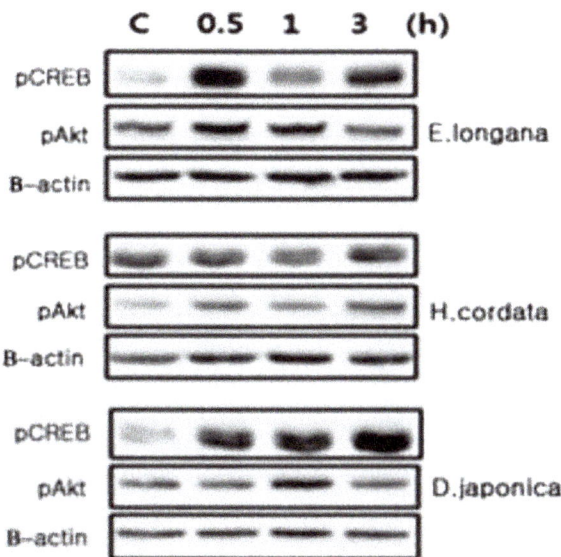

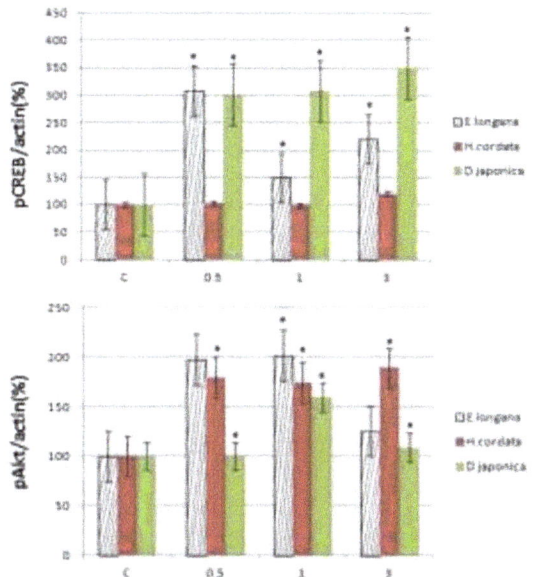

Figure 3 Time course of expression of pCREB and pAkt in neuroblastoma SH-SY5Y cells. To evaluate the protein level of pCREB and pAkt expression, cells were incubated with 30 μg/ml herb. For the control, nonincubated cells were analyzed. The level of pCREB and pAkt in cell lysates was measured by immunoblotting. Data are presented as means ± SEM of three determinations. *P < 0.05 vs. control.

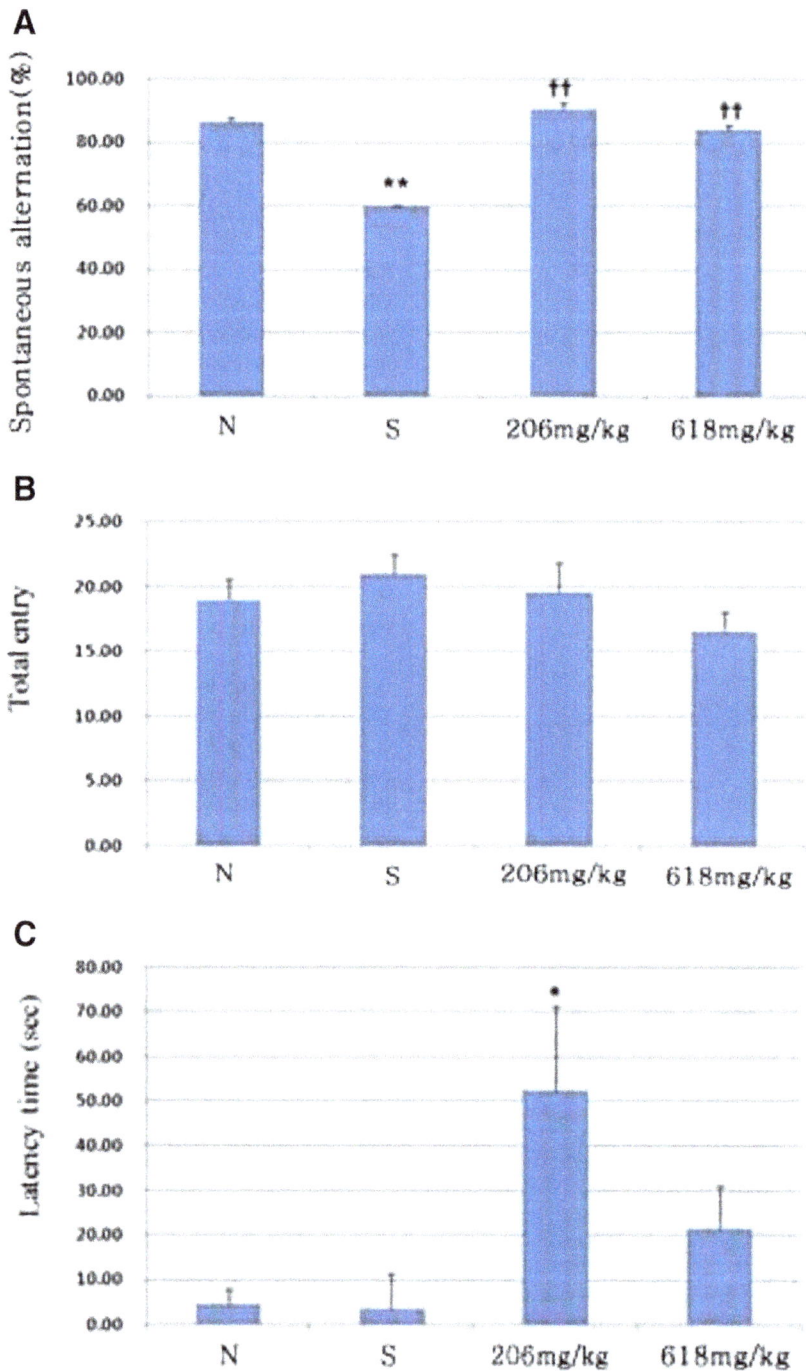

Figure 4 Attenuated effect of herb mixture on stress induced impairment of the Y-maze task and passive avoidance task in mice.
Spontaneous alternation in behavior **(A)** and the number of arm entries **(B)** were measured. **(C)** Mice were subjected to the training trial and the step-through latency time was measured. Data are presented as means ± SEM of three determinations. $^{*}P < 0.05$ vs. stress, $^{**}P < 0.01$ vs. normal, $^{††}P < 0.01$ vs. normal.

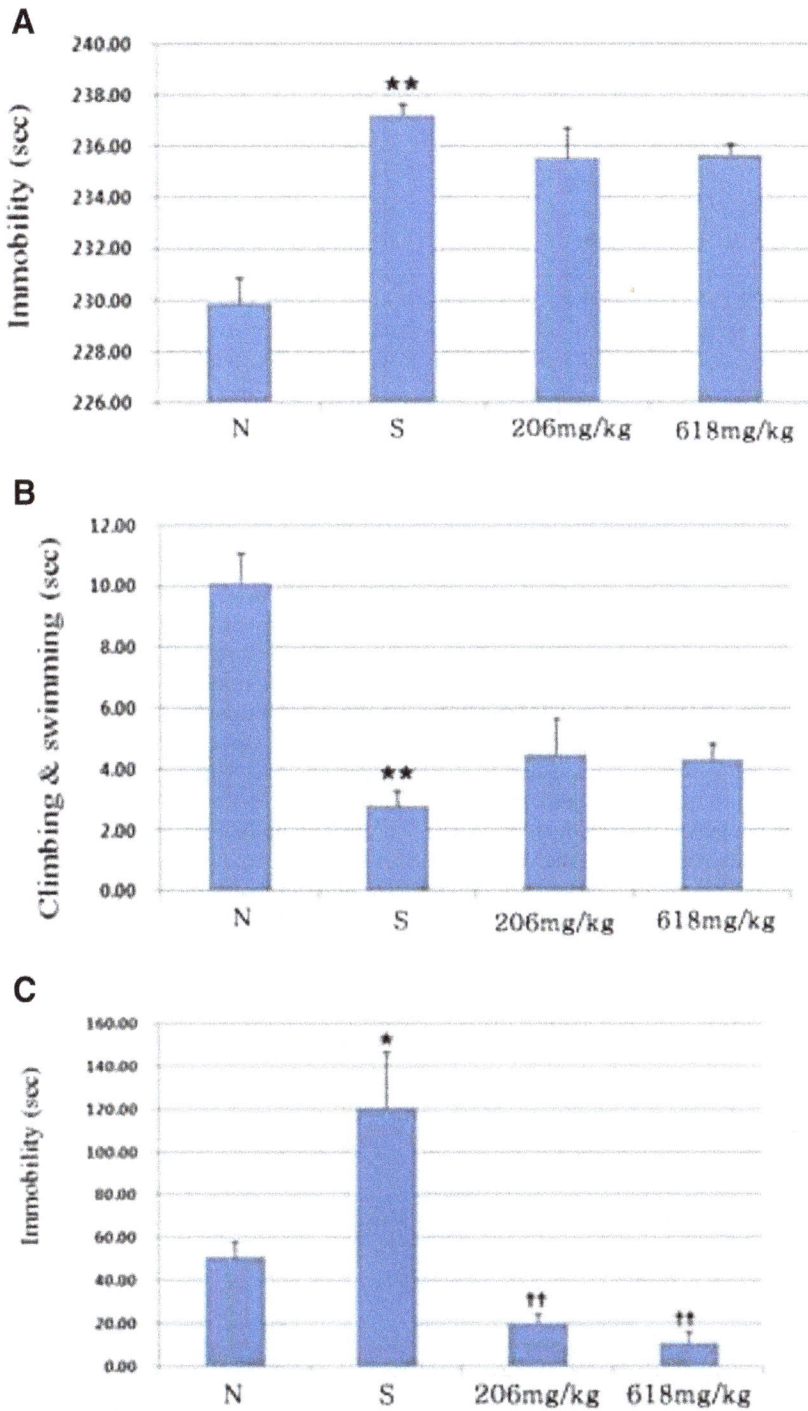

Figure 5 Effect of herbal mixture on duration of immobility (A), swimming and climbing (B) behaviors in mice when sampled during the 5 min swim test. (C) Effect of herbal mixture on the amount of immobility in mice during the tail suspension test. Behavior was observed during the 6 min test period and scored as mobile or immobile. Data are presented as means ± SEM of three determinations. [*]$P < 0.05$ vs. normal, [**]$P < .01$ vs. normal, [††]$P < 0.01$ vs. stress.

cells (Figure 2). Immunoblotting analysis confirmed these results (figure not shown). To determine the expression of pCREB and pAkt, the cultures were harvested at 30 min, 1 h and 3 h and immunoblotting was performed on the cell extracts (Figure 3). Compared to the control, the expression of pCREB treated with 30 µg/ml of *E. longana* was $308 \pm 8\%$, $150 \pm 11\%$ and $220 \pm 10\%$ at 30 min, 1 h and 3 h, respectively. For *H. cordata*, it was $102 \pm 11\%$, $98 \pm 15\%$ and $120 \pm 12\%$ at 30 min, 1 h and 3 h, respectively. In the case of *D. japonica*, it was $302 \pm 11\%$, $308 \pm 15\%$ and $350 \pm 14\%$ at 30 min, 1 h and 3 h, respectively. The pAkt expression in the cell extracts that were incubated with 30 µg/ml of *E. longana* was $198 \pm 11\%$, $202 \pm 15\%$ and $126 \pm 16\%$ at 30 min, 1 h and 3 h, respectively. For *H. cordata*, it was $180 \pm 11\%$, $175 \pm 10\%$ and $190 \pm 9\%$ at 30 min, 1 h and 3 h, respectively. In the case of *D. japonica*, it was $100 \pm 10\%$, $160 \pm 12\%$ and $109 \pm 17\%$ at 30 min, 1 h and 3 h, respectively. Overall each herb was able to induce the expression of pCREB and pAkt regardless of time course.

Antidepressant effect of herbal mixture

We examined whether herbal mixture attenuated depression in mice under stress conditions. We first performed the Y-maze test for spatial working memory. Only the stress mice displayed a reduced level of spontaneous alternation in the Y-maze test compared to that of the normal control group ($p < 0.01$, Figure 4A). However, mice in the experimental group, which were fed herbal mixture for 3 weeks, exhibited an increased level of spontaneous alternation ($p < 0.01$, Figure 4A). In addition, the total number of maze arm entries was not different among the groups (Figure 4B). We then examined the effects of herbal mixture on learning and memory using a passive avoidance test. Administration of low dose herbal mixture attenuated the learning memory impairment

induced by stress ($p < 0.05$, Figure 4C). This finding indicates that herbal mixture improved the stress induced memory impairment under stress conditions. We further examined the effect of herbal mixture on the forced swim test. In 5 min swim test, normal mice were immobile for 229.91 ± 1.0 sec and stress mice were immobile for 237.20 ± 0.4 sec ($p < 0.01$, Figure 5A). The immobility was the sum of the durations of floating, twitching and kicking behaviors. We observed that herbal mixture administration did not induce any significant change in immobility when compared to the stress group. But it trended in favor of herbal mixture. When climbing and swimming behaviors were combined, stress mice were less active with 2.80 ± 0.4 sec than those in normal group with 10.09 ± 1.0 ($p < 0.01$, Figure 5B). Herbal mixture caused improvement of activity compared with stress group but as a nonsignificant trend. The effects on immobility and swimming observed after the administration of high dose of herbal mixture were similar to those observed after the administration of low dose of herbal mixture. On the other hand, herbal mixture produced highly significant reduction in the immobility time in the tail suspension test ($p < 0.01$, Figure 5C). Figure 6 illustrates the serum corticosterone concentration among groups. Mice in the herbal mixture groups demonstrated lower serum corticosterone concentration than those in the stress group ($p < 0.05$). As expected, mice exposed to the chronic stress paradigm had elevated corticosterone level compared to those in the normal group ($p < 0.05$). Effects of the oral administration of herbal mixture on protein levels of BDNF in the hippocampi and cortices are shown in Figure 7. Statistical analysis indicated a significant effect of administration with herbal mixture. There were 54.55% ($p < 0.01$) and 52.15% ($p < 0.01$) increase in the levels of BDNF in the hippocampal tissues after administration with 206 and 618 mg/kg herbal mixture as compared with stress group,

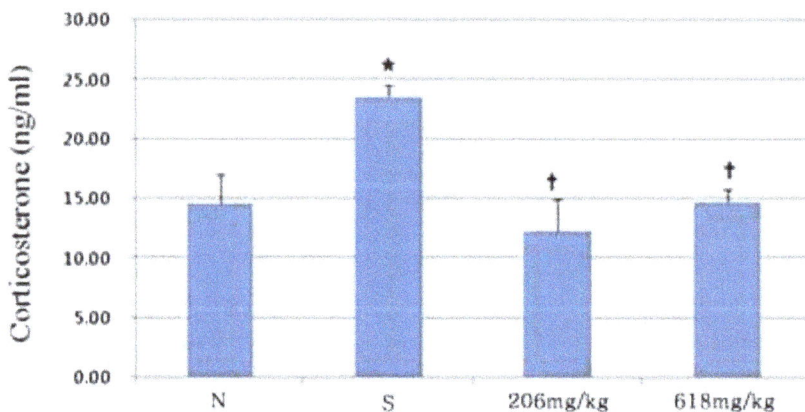

Figure 6 Effects of exposure to chronic stress and herbal mixture on corticosterone levels. Data are presented as means ± SEM of ten mice per group. $^*P < 0.05$ vs. normal, $^\dagger P < 0.05$ vs. stress.

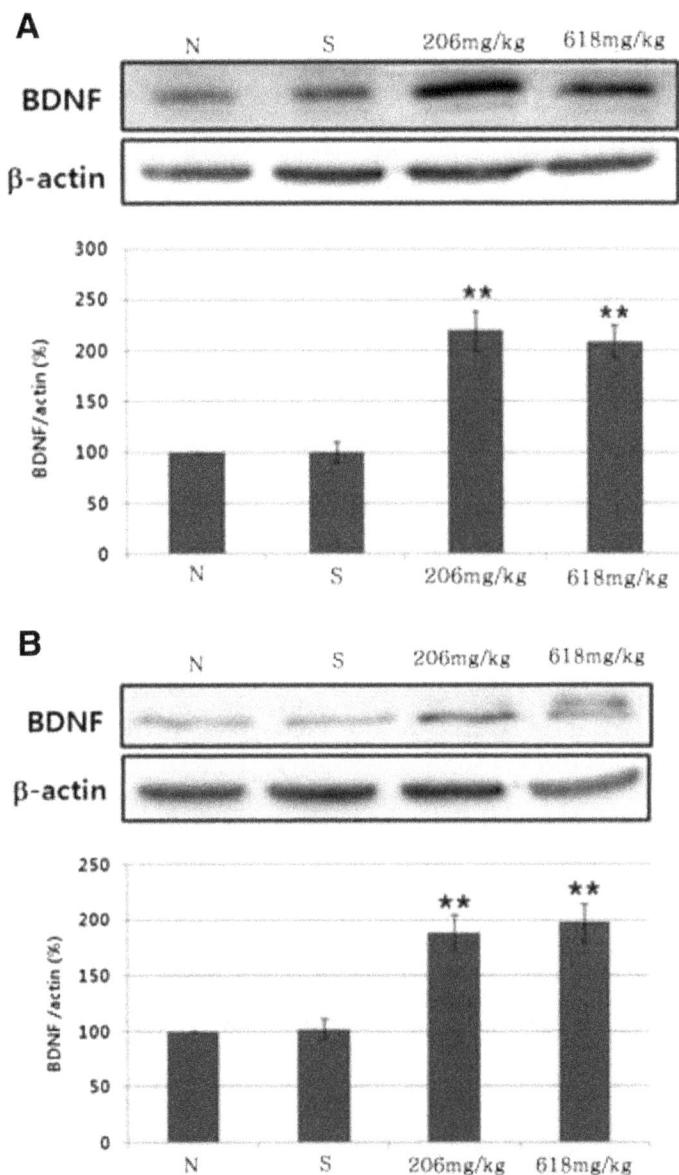

Figure 7 Effects of the oral administration of herbal mixture on protein levels of BDNF in the hippocampi (A) and cortices (B). Data are presented as means ± SEM of three determinations. $^{**}P < 0.01$ vs. stress.

respectively. In the cortical tissues, 206 mg/kg herbal mixture significantly increased the BDNF level (46.03%, p < 0.01 vs. stress) similar to that of 618 mg/kg herbal mixture (48.49%, p < 0.01 vs. stress).

Discussion

Numerous medicinal herbs have been employed as a form of mixture or decoction since their effects can be manifested after total and final reaction by their constituent compounds when administered to humans. The herbal mixture used in the present study consists of *E. longana*, *H. cordata* and *D. japonica* which demonstrated an inductive effect on the expression of BDNF, pCREB and pAkt. These herbs have been used as a therapeutic agent for cerebral disease especially in Korea in conjunction with Sasang Constitutional Medicine which takes a typological constitution approach to holistic medicine by balancing an individual's psychological, social and physical aspects to achieve wellness and increased longevity.

The present study demonstrated that oral administration of herbal mixture in both doses (206 and 618 mg/kg) alleviated stress induced learning and memory deficits for mice by remaining in the well-lit side of a two compartment apparatus and not entering the dark where it received the electrical stimulus. Since mouse innately gravitates to darkness, the animal has to suppress this instinct through pairing the aversive stimulus (electrical stimulus) with the desired compartment (dark chamber). Animals that do not remember the aversive stimulus will cross over earlier than animals that remember. In addition, it was clear that the level of exploratory activities was not affected by the spatial working memory of mice. Herbal mixture treatment also decreased the immobility time in the tail suspension test. In order to understand the molecular mechanism of herbal mixture induced antidepressant effects in the brain, the present study investigated BDNF protein levels in hippocampus and cortex of mice under stress and compared values with herbal mixture fed mice under stress. Treatment with herbal mixture showed a significant increase in BDNF translation level.

Chronic stress may lead to psychotic symptoms including depression and suicide [18]. Studies have shown that the hippocampus is affected by stress. Depression invoked by stress has been associated with neuronal atrophy and decreased volume of hippocampus [19-21]. Several clinical reports have shown depression-induced deregulation of serum BDNF concentration. Depressed patients were characterized by low serum BDNF levels [6,22,23], implying an inverse relationship between serum BDNF levels and the severity of depression. Support for this comes from a number of studies demonstrating that treatment with antidepressants has been shown to increase BDNF levels in serum [6,23,24] and plasma [25]. It is speculated that lower BDNF levels may be caused by dysregulation of BDNF expression. This was evidenced with decreased BDNF mRNA and protein levels in postmortem hippocampus and frontal cortex of suicide victims [26]. Recent reports further support the speculation that antidepressant treatment increased BDNF protein levels in serum [27] and in both prefrontal cortex and hippocampus [28]. In the current study, herbal mixture administration with low and high dose increased the BDNF protein levels in hippocampus and cortex compared to the stress group. Herbal mixture might have significantly increased the BDNF transcript levels as well although they were not evaluated in our study.

Several types of stressors have been known to disrupt BDNF expression. For example, single (one day) or repeated (7 days) immobilization for 2 hours per day markedly reduced BDNF mRNA levels in the dentate gyrus and hippocampus [29]. This was later confirmed by other investigators who used the same stress paradigm [30]. Other types of stressors such as footshock [31], early maternal deprivation [32], social defeat [33] and chronic unpredictable stress before pregnancy [34] were correlated with decreased BDNF expression. In our study using immobilization as a stressor, no significant changes in BDNF protein level were observed in hippocampus and cortex. It can be proposed that stress induced changes in BDNF protein level may be involved in other brain regions. The other hypothesis is that immobilization stress duration was too long enough to neutralize the downregulation of BDNF expression. Interestingly, brief immobilization stress can induce BDNF expression as part of a compensatory response to preserve hippocampal homeostasis to cope with new stress [35].

Our study provides further data that herbal mixture is able to modulate serum corticosterone level in mice under stress conditions. This effect could be either of peripheral origin through a direct action of herbal mixture on adrenal glands, or of central origin via the hypothalamic-pituitary-adrenal axis. The inverse relationship between memory performance and corticosterone level in stress conditions from our study confirms the past report that chronic stress in rodents has mostly impairing effects on memory [36]. Moreover, a long term immobilization stress has been shown to affect spatial memory [37] which is in accordance with our data of short term immobilization paradigm.

Conclusions
In conclusion, our study showed that herbal mixture administration has antidepressant effects in mice. Each herb induced the expression of BDNF, pCREB and pAkt. The administration of herbal mixture significantly increased BDNF protein expression in mouse hippocampus and cortex.

Competing interests
The authors declare that they have no competing interests.

Authors' contributions
SJ and CL designed the study. QFL and GWK carried out the experiment. BK and SCP drafted the manuscript. All authors read and approved the final manuscript.

Author details
[1]Dongguk University Research Institute of Biotechnology, Seoul 100-715, Republic of Korea. [2]Department of Neuropsychiatry, Graduate School of Oriental Medicine, Dongguk University, Gyeongju, Republic of Korea. [3]Department of Korean Neuropsychiatry, Dongguk University Bundang Oriental Hospital, Sungnam, Republic of Korea. [4]Department of Korean Neuropsychiatry, Dongguk University Ilsan Oriental Hospital, Goyang, Republic of Korea. [5]School of Biomedical Sciences, Charles Sturt University, Bathurst, NSW 2795, Australia.

References
1.   Baxter AJ, Ferrari AJ, Erskine HE, Charlson FJ, Degenhardt L, Whiteford HA: The global burden of mental and substance use disorders: changes in estimating burden between GBD1990 and GBD2010. *Epidemiol Psychiatr Sci* 2014, 23:1–11.

2. Bryant K, Wicks MN, Willis N: Recruitment of older African American males for depression research: lessons learned. *Arch Psychiatr Nurs* 2014, **28**:17–20.

3. Hung CJ, Wu CC, Chen WY, Chang CY, Kuan YH, Pan HC, Liao SL, Chen CJ: Depression-like effect of prenatal buprenorphine exposure in rats. *PLoS One* 2013, **8**:e82262.

4. Davies AM: The role of neurotrophins in the developing nervous system. *Neurobiol* 1994, **25**:1334–1348.

5. Duman RS, Monteggia LM: A neurotrophic model for stress-related mood disorders. *Biol Psychiatry* 2006, **59**:1116–1127.

6. Shimizu E, Hashimoto K, Okamura N, Koike K, Komatsu N, Kumakiri C, Nakazato M, Watanabe H, Shinoda N, Okada S, Iyo M: Alterations of serum levels of brain-derived neurotrophic factor (BDNF) in depressed patients with or without antidepressants. *Biol Psychiatry* 2003, **54**:70–75.

7. Tao X, Finkbeiner S, Arnold DB, Shaywitz AJ, Greenberg ME: Ca2+ influx regulates BDNF transcription by a CREB family transcription factor-dependent mechanism. *Neuron* 1998, **20**:709–726.

8. Crawford AA, Lewis S, Nutt D, Peters TJ, Cowen P, O'Donovan MC, Wiles N, Lewis G: Adverse effects from antidepressant treatment: randomised controlled trial of 601 depressed individuals. *Psychopharmacol (Berl)* 2014, **231**:2921–2931.

9. Ferguson JM: SSRI antidepressant medications: adverse effects and tolerability. *Prim Care Companion J Clin Psychiatry* 2001, **3**:22–27.

10. Rangkadilok N, Worasuttayangkurn L, Bennett RN, Satayavivad J: Identification and quantification of polyphenolic compounds in Longan (Euphoria longana Lam.) fruit. *J Agric Food Chem* 2005, **53**:1387–1392.

11. Panyathep A, Chewonarin T, Taneyhill K, Vinitketkumnuen U, Surh YJ: Inhibitory effects of dried longan (Euphoria longana Lam.) seed extract on invasion and matrix metalloproteinases of colon cancer cells. *J Agric Food Chem* 2013, **61**:3631–3641.

12. Kumar M, Prasad SK, Krishnamurthy S, Hemalatha S: Antihyperglycemic activity of Houttuynia cordata Thunb. in streptozotocin-induced diabetic rats. *Adv Pharmacol Sci* 2014, **2014**:809438.

13. Kim SK, Ryu SY, No J, Choi SU, Kim YS: Cytotoxic alkaloids from Houttuynia cordata. *Arch Pharm Res* 2001, **24**:518–521.

14. Cho EJ, Yokozawa T, Rhyu DY, Kim SC, Shibahara N, Park JC: Study on the inhibitory effects of Korean medicinal plants and their main compounds on the 1,1-diphenyl-2-picrylhydrazyl radical. *Phytomedicine* 2003, **10**:544–551.

15. Wu JN: Chinese Materia Medica. New York: Oxford University Press; 2005:264.

16. Kim KH, Choi SU, Choi SZ, Son MW, Lee KR: Withanolides from the rhizomes of Dioscorea japonica and their cytotoxicity. *J Agric Food Chem* 2011, **59**:6980–6984.

17. Saleem AM, Taufik Hidayat M, Mat Jais AM, Fakurazi S, Moklas M, Sulaiman MR, Amom Z: Antidepressant-like effect of aqueous extract of Channa striatus fillet in mice models of depression. *Eur Rev Med Pharmacol Sci* 2011, **15**:795–802.

18. Dwivedi Y: Brain-derived neurotrophic factor: role in depression and suicide. *Neuropsychiatr Dis Treat* 2009, **5**:433–449.

19. Sala M, Perez J, Soloff P, Ucelli di Nemi S, Caverzasi E, Soares JC, Brambilla P: Stress and hippocampal abnormalities in psychiatric disorders. *Eur Neuropsychopharmacol* 2004, **14**:393–405.

20. Campbell S, Marriott M, Nahmias C, MacQueen GM: Lower hippocampal volume in patients suffering from depression: a meta-analysis. *Am J Psychiatry* 2004, **161**:598–607.

21. Frodl T, Schaub A, Banac S, Charypar M, Jäger M, Kümmler P, Bottlender R, Zetzsche T, Born C, Leinsinger G, Reiser M, Möller HJ, Meisenzahl EM: Reduced hippocampal volume correlates with executive dysfunctioning in major depression. *J Psychiatry Neurosci* 2006, **31**:316–323.

22. Karege F, Perret G, Bondolfi G, Schwald M, Bertschy G, Aubry JM: Decreased serum brain-derived neurotrophic factor levels in major depressed patients. *Psychiatry Res* 2002, **109**:143–148.

23. Gonul AS, Akdeniz F, Taneli F, Donat O, Eker C, Vahip S: Effect of treatment on serum brain-derived neurotrophic factor levels in depressed patients. *Eur Arch Psychiatry Clin Neurosci* 2005, **255**:381–386.

24. Yoshimura R, Mitoma M, Sugita A, Hori H, Okamoto T, Umene W, Ueda N, Nakamura J: Effects of paroxetine or milnacipran on serum brain-derived neurotrophic factor in depressed patients. *Prog Neuropsychopharmacol Biol Psychiatry* 2007, **31**:1034–1037.

25. Lee HY, Kim YK: Plasma brain-derived neurotrophic factor as a peripheral marker for the action mechanism of antidepressants. *Neuropsychobiology* 2008, **57**:194–199.

26. Dwivedi Y, Rizavi HS, Conley RR, Roberts RC, Tamminga CA, Pandey GN: Altered gene expression of brain-derived neurotrophic factor and receptor tyrosine kinase B in postmortem brain of suicide subjects. *Arch Gen Psychiatry* 2003, **60**:804–815.

27. Huang TL, Lee CT, Liu YL: Serum brain-derived neurotrophic factor levels in patients with major depression: effects of antidepressants. *J Psychiatr Res* 2008, **42**:521–525.

28. Réus GZ, Stringari RB, Ribeiro KF, Ferraro AK, Vitto MF, Cesconetto P, Souza CT, Quevedo J: Ketamine plus imipramine treatment induces antidepressant-like behavior and increases CREB and BDNF protein levels and PKA and PKC phosphorylation in rat brain. *Behav Brain Res* 2011, **221**:166–171.

29. Smith MA, Makino S, Kvetnansky R, Post RM: Stress and glucocorticoids affect the expression of brain-derived neurotrophic factor and neurotrophin-3 mRNAs in the hippocampus. *J Neurosci* 1995, **15**:1768–1777.

30. Ueyama T, Kawai Y, Nemoto K, Sekimoto M, Toné S, Senba E: Immobilization stress reduced the expression of neurotrophins and their receptors in the rat brain. *Neurosci Res* 1997, **28**:103–110.

31. Rasmusson AM, Shi L, Duman R: Downregulation of BDNF mRNA in the hippocampal dentate gyrus after re-exposure to cues previously associated with footshock. *Neuropsychopharmacology* 2002, **27**:133–142.

32. Roceri M, Hendriks W, Racagni G, Ellenbroek BA, Riva MA: Early maternal deprivation reduces the expression of BDNF and NMDA receptor subunits in rat hippocampus. *Mol Psychiatry* 2002, **7**:609–616.

33. Pizarro JM, Lumley LA, Medina W, Robison CL, Chang WE, Alagappan A, Bah MJ, Dawood MY, Shah JD, Mark B, Kendall N, Smith MA, Saviolakis GA, Meyerhoff JL: Acute social defeat reduces neurotrophin expression in brain cortical and subcortical areas in mice. *Brain Res* 2004, **1025**:10–20.

34. Huang Y, Shi X, Xu H, Yang H, Chen T, Chen S, Chen X: Chronic unpredictable stress before pregnancy reduce the expression of brain-derived neurotrophic factor and N-methyl-D-aspartate receptor in hippocampus of offspring rats associated with impairment of memory. *Neurochem Res* 2010, **35**:1038–1049.

35. Marmigère F, Givalois L, Rage F, Arancibia S, Tapia-Arancibia L: Rapid induction of BDNF expression in the hippocampus during immobilization stress challenge in adult rats. *Hippocampus* 2003, **13**:646–655.

36. Wolf OT: HPA axis and memory. *Best Pract Res Clin Endocrinol Metab* 2003, **17**:287–299.

37. Kitraki E, Kremmyda O, Youlatos D, Alexis M, Kittas C: Spatial performance and corticosteroid receptor status in the 21-day restraint stress paradigm. *Ann N Y Acad Sci* 2004, **1018**:323–327.

3

Drug-drug interactions in inpatient and outpatient settings in Iran: a systematic review of the literature

Ehsan Nabovati[1,2], Hasan Vakili-Arki[1], Zhila Taherzadeh[3,4], Mohammad Reza Hasibian[6], Ameen Abu-Hanna[7] and Saeid Eslami[5,6,7]*

Abstract

Drug-drug interactions (DDIs) are an important type of adverse drug events. Yet overall incidence and pattern of DDIs in Iran has not been well documented and little information is available about the strategies that have been used for their prevention. The purpose of this study was to systematically review the literature on the incidence and pattern of DDIs in Iran as well as the used strategies for their prevention. PubMed, Scopus, electronic Persian databases, and Google Scholar were searched to identify published studies on DDIs in Iran. Additionally, the reference lists of all retrieved articles were reviewed to identify additional relevant articles. Eligible studies were those that analyzed original data on the incidence of DDIs in inpatient or outpatient settings in Iran. Articles about one specific DDI and drug interactions with herbs, diseases, and nutrients were excluded. The quality of included studies was assessed using quality assessment criteria. Database searches yielded 1053 potentially eligible citations. After removing duplicates, screening titles and abstracts, and reading full texts, 34 articles were found to be relevant. The quality assessment of the included studies showed a relatively poor quality. In terms of study setting, 18 and 16 studies have been conducted in inpatient and outpatient settings, respectively. All studies focused on potential DDIs while no study assessed actual DDIs. The median incidence of potential DDIs in outpatient settings was 8.5% per prescription while it was 19.2% in inpatient settings. The most indicated factor influencing DDIs incidence was patient age. The most involved drug classes in DDIs were beta blockers, angiotensin-converting-enzyme inhibitors (ACEIs), diuretic agents, and non-steroidal anti-inflammatory drugs (NSAIDs). Thirty-one studies were observational and three were experimental in which the strategies to reduce DDIs were applied. Although almost all studies concluded that the incidence of potential DDIs in Iran in both inpatient and outpatient settings was relatively high, there is still no evidence of the incidence of actual DDIs. More extensive research is needed to identify and minimize factors associated with incidence of DDIs, and to evaluate the effects of preventive interventions especially those that utilize information technology.

Keywords: Adverse drug events, Developing countries, Drug-drug interaction, Medication errors, Incidence, Intervention, Iran

* Correspondence: EslamiS@mums.ac.ir
[5]Pharmaceutical Research Center, School of Pharmacy, Mashhad University of Medical Sciences, Mashhad, Iran
[6]Department of Medical Informatics, Faculty of Medicine, Mashhad University of Medical Sciences, Mashhad, Iran
Full list of author information is available at the end of the article

Introduction

Adverse drug events (ADE) are the most common complications related to medication therapy among patients [1-3]. ADEs are common, costly, and may have life-threatening consequences [4-6]. The high incidence of medication use in medical therapy and possibility of human errors increase the incidence risk of these adverse events.

Drug-drug interactions (DDIs) are an important subgroup of ADEs [7] which are highly prevalent in patients receiving multiple-drug treatment [8]. DDIs may lead to severe adverse events which can result in patient hospitalization. Some studies have estimated that up to 3% of hospital admissions are caused by DDIs [9-11].

Although it is widely recognized that DDIs may harm patients, their incidence is still high [12]. The majority of these interactions occurred because either prescribers do not consider them relevant [13] or prescribers' knowledge of DDIs is generally poor [14]. Hence, they could be prevented through applying proper interventions. This can improve the quality of drug therapy and increase patient safety. Interventions aimed at reducing DDIs are likely to be more effective, if before their development, the incidence and pattern of DDIs are determined accurately.

Estimates about the incidence of DDIs in different countries vary from 6% to 70% due to variability in methodologies and settings [12,15-18]. Because of this variation, it is important that the related evidence is aggregated and summarized in each country, separately. To our knowledge, three systematic reviews in the literature reviewed DDIs studies. Espinosa-Bosch et al. conducted a review on English and Spanish studies which had reported incidence of DDIs in hospital care [19]. They showed that around 20% of hospitalized patients were susceptible to DDIs and incidence was higher in patients with heart disease and the elderly. Another review has summarized and described findings from studies that assessed harmful DDIs in elderly patients [20]. It has been conclusively shown that significant harm is associated with DDIs in elderly patients. Also, Riechelmann and Giglio systematically reviewed the studies, published in English, Portuguese, and Spanish, on the frequency of DDIs in cancer patients [21]. They estimated that about one-third of cancer patients are at the risk of DDIs.

None of the DDIs systematic reviews were conducted in a developing country. In Iran, several DDIs studies have been conducted, but there is uncertainty about their overall incidence, pattern of the most involved medication classes, and the possible interventions and their effectiveness.

The objective of this systematic review is to identify and summarize all evidence concerning DDIs in Iran as an example of a developing country. In this study we address four questions: (1) what is the incidence and pattern of DDIs?; (2) which factors are associated to incidence of DDIs?; (3) what interventions have been used to prevent this type of medication errors?; (4) which interventions have been effective in reducing DDIs?

Methods

Search strategy and data sources

A comprehensive search strategy for original articles was developed using terms related to drug interaction (drug interaction, adverse drug event, adverse drug reaction, medication error, prescription error) combined with terms related to Iran (Iran, Iranian).

The following electronic databases were searched for English articles using customized search strategies: MEDLINE/PubMed and Scopus. Persian Electronic databases including Scientific Information Database (SID), IranMedex, IranDoc, and MagIran were searched using Persian terms equivalent to the English terms mentioned above. The electronic databases were last searched on March 2013. To ensure that no article is missed, we also searched Google Scholar using both Persian and English search terms.

In a final search, the reference lists of all identified articles were also reviewed to identify additional relevant articles (snowball method).

Inclusion and exclusion criteria

All published studies on children, adults, and elderly patients that were conducted in either an outpatient or inpatient setting in Iran and published either in English or Persian were included. Various types of research designs including observational studies that reported the incidence of DDIs and interventional studies that evaluated an intervention on reduction of DDIs were included.

Articles about one specific DDI and drug interactions with herbs, diseases, and nutrients were excluded. Moreover, we excluded letters, opinions, conference papers, and dissertations.

Review procedure and data extraction

A reviewer conducted the search for the articles. Two reviewers (including the one conducting the literature search) considered the inclusion and exclusion criteria independently and screened the title and abstract of all potential relevant articles. Any discrepancies on the eligibility of the articles were resolved by discussion among the reviewers. After the inclusion process, the full text of eligible articles for the purposes of this review was retrieved. In the case of inaccessibility, the full text was requested from the authors by email. The full text of each eligible article was reviewed and abstracted into a prespecified form.

The data abstraction form was used to collect information on the following characteristics: objectives, setting, study period, type of study, sampling, data source, DDIs reference, main findings, details of reported DDIs, most frequent DDIs, factors associated with incidence of DDIs, interventions and their outcomes, and other relevant information.

Quality assessment of the included studies

There is no tool that assesses the quality of DDIs studies. A twelve-item quality assessment tool (Table 1) was developed based on the criteria taken from the tools for assessing the quality of medication error studies [22,23]. Overall quality scores ranged from 0 to 12 (0 to 6 points = poor, 7 to 9 points = moderate, 10 to 12 points = high). Two reviewers independently scored the quality criteria for each included study and a third reviewer resolved any discrepancies.

Due to variations in the methods used to report on DDI statistics, we mainly reported qualitative aggregate results.

Results

Literature search results

The flow diagram of literature search is shown in Figure 1. Electronic literature search on MEDLINE/PubMed, Scopus and Persian databases identified a total of 1053 records. 861 unique records remained after excluding duplicates. After reviewing titles and abstracts and applying inclusion and exclusion criteria, 54 articles were chosen for full text review. By hand-searching the references list, two additional relevant articles were also identified. Subsequently, the full texts of these potentially relevant articles were obtained except one [24] (even after contacting its authors by email). After detailed full text review of 55 articles, a further 21 articles were excluded, because they only assessed pattern of drug prescribing, only evaluated

Table 1 The tool used to rate the quality of the included studies

Quality assessment criteria	Score
1) Aims/objectives of the study clearly stated	1
2) Definition of what constitutes a DDI	1
3) DDI categories specified	1
4) DDI categories defined	1
5) Mention of DDI reference	1
6) Data collection method described clearly	1
7) Setting in which study was conducted described	1
8) Study subjects described	1
9) Sampling and calculation of sample size described (unit of measurement)	1
10) Potential or actual DDIs assessed	1
11) Measures in place to ensure that results are valid	1
12) Limitations of study listed	1
Maximum score	12 points

Each item is related to a quality assessment criterion with score 0 or 1.

quality of drug prescribing, or only estimated prescription errors without referring to DDIs. Finally, 34 relevant articles that met our specified criteria were included in this review.

General characteristics of the included studies

The oldest study was published in 1997 and the most recent one in 2013. Twenty-one studies (62%) had been written in Persian and 13 (38%) were in English. In terms of study setting, 15 (44%) and 19 (56%) studies have been conducted in inpatient and outpatient settings, respectively. In terms of study design, 31 studies (91%) were observational and three (9%) were experimental. The majority of studies, 20 out of 34, had used Drug Interaction Facts as their DDI compendia. Table 2 shows the general characteristics of the included studies.

Quality of the included studies

After the quality assessment of individual studies, none of them fulfilled all the quality criteria. Three studies (9%) were of higher quality (10 points), 16 studies (47%) were of moderate quality (7 to 9 points), and 15 studies (44%) were of poor quality (0 to 6 points). In terms of the quality assessment criteria, no study assessed actual DDIs, only four studies (12%) listed their limitations, and 15 studies (44%) defined DDIs categories.

Findings of the included studies

Twenty-five (73.5%) studies reported the overall incidence of potential DDIs in the study population (prescription or patient). Nine studies (26.5%) have not reported the overall incidence of DDIs. Among the studies performed in outpatient settings, nine studies assessed the overall incidence of potential DDIs in prescriptions in the population for all types of drugs. The median incidence of potential DDIs in prescriptions of these studies was 8.5% (Interquartile Range (IQR): 8.4-10.1). The other outpatient studies focused on the incidence of potential DDIs in cardiovascular drugs (DDIs percentage = 50%) [26], non-steroidal anti-inflammatory drugs (NSAIDs) (DDIs percentage = 49%) [30], antidepressant drugs (DDIs percentage =22%) [29], dental drugs (DDIs percentage =27%) [39], and elderly people (DDIs percentage =10% and 14%) [47,51].

Among the studies performed on inpatient prescriptions, four assessed the overall incidence of potential DDIs in prescriptions for all groups of patients in all departments and for all drug classes [24,25,52,53]. The median incidence of potential DDIs in these studies was 19.2% (IQR: 15.5-22). The focus of one study in inpatient setting was on pediatric patients (DDIs percentage = 21%) [37]. The two studies that focused on potential DDIs in hospitalized patients in the hematology and oncology departments reported the incidence of 38% and 63% [55,57].

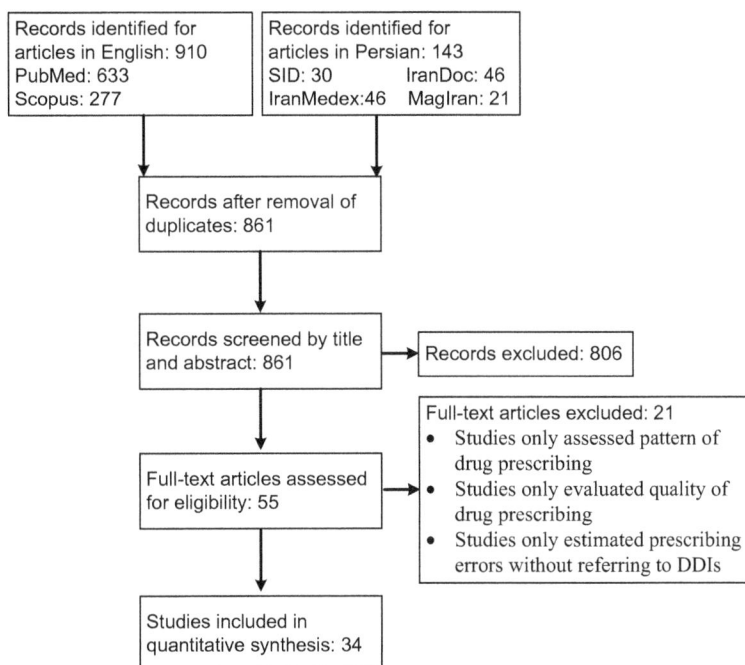

Figure 1 Flow diagram of the literature search and study selection. The search strategy focused on studies that analyzed original data on the incidence of DDIs in inpatient or outpatient settings in Iran.

More than half of the studies (21 studies, amounting to 62%) have grouped the identified DDIs in terms of severity and reported the percentage of major, moderate, and minor DDIs separately. The median percentage of major, moderate, and minor DDIs in these studies were 7.7% (IQR: 4.4-11.6), 67.4% (IQR: 51.3-75.3), and 24.2% (IQR: 16.4-41.9), respectively. Six additional studies (17.5%) have calculated the percentage of prescriptions with at least one DDI grouped by severity. The median percentage of prescriptions with major, moderate, and minor DDIs were 0.8% (IQR: 0.7-1.3), 10.2% (IQR: 5.6-11.2), and 9.6% (IQR: 3.6-22.8), respectively.

Fifteen studies (44%) have confirmed the association between the number of medications and the incidence of DDIs. The influence of other factors on incidence of DDIs was mentioned in 11 studies (32%). These factors are listed in Table 3.

Twenty three studies (67.6%) have determined the most frequent DDIs. Among them, eight studies have also classified the most frequent DDIs by severity. The most frequent major DDIs in the studies, which ranked in the first 10 identified DDIs, are listed in Table 4. As this table shows, five studies have ranked the major interaction between digoxin and furosemide among the most frequent interactions.

Names and classes of drugs which mostly contributed to DDIs have been reported by 14 studies (Table 5).

Beta blockers, angiotensin-converting-enzyme inhibitors (ACEIs), diuretic agents, and NSAIDs have been mentioned most often as drug classes. Digoxin contributed the most to major DDIs.

Interventional studies

Among the included studies, only three were interventional. All three were quasi experimental and have been conducted in outpatient settings. In the first study [34], the effects of face to face education, information feedback, and pamphlets designation were evaluated. The study shown that potential DDIs in general practitioners and specialists' prescriptions decreased (severe: 1.6% before vs. 0.24% after, moderate: 10.6% before vs. 2% after, minor: 5.1% before vs. 2.1% after, p-value < 0.001). In the second study [35], individualized feedback and workshop training programs were used. The study mentioned that potential DDIs with first significance degree (based on Drug Interactions Facts™) in general practitioners' prescriptions reduced significantly (0.4% before vs. 0.05% after interventions, p-value < 0.001). The third study [46] evaluated the effect of face-to-face training, audit feedback, and educational notes on the major DDIs in general practitioners and specialists' prescriptions. It demonstrated that severe DDIs diminished significantly (1.5% before vs. 0.4% after, p-value < 0.05).

Table 2 General characteristics of the included studies

Ref	Year	Language	Target population	Setting	Pathology/Drug type	Design	Duration	Sample Size/Unit of Analysis	Drug interaction database
[24]	1997	Persian	All	Outpatient	All	Observational (Retrospective)	2 months	3117 Prescriptions	-
[25]	1997	Persian	All	Inpatient (Internal, Surgery)	All	Observational (Retrospective)	3 months	1000 Prescriptions	-
[26]	1999	Persian	All	Outpatient	Cardiovascular drugs	Observational (Retrospective)	6 months	1038 Prescriptions	Drug Interaction Facts
[27]	2000	Persian	All	Outpatient	All	Observational (Retrospective)	12 Months	4750 Prescriptions	Drug Interaction Facts
[28]	2001	Persian	All	Outpatient	All	Observational (Retrospective)	3 months	1100 Prescriptions	Drug Interaction Facts
[29]	2000	Persian	All	Outpatient	Anti-Depression drugs	Observational (Retrospective)	6 months	3000 Prescriptions	Drug Interaction Facts
[30]	1999-2001	Persian	All	Outpatient	NSAID	Observational (Retrospective)	36 months	1927 Prescriptions	Hansten Drug Interactions
[31]	2000	Persian	All	Outpatient	All	Observational (Retrospective)	6 months	3000 Prescriptions	Drug Interaction Facts
[32]	2000	Persian	All	Outpatient	All	Observational (Retrospective)	12 months	1800 Prescriptions	Drug Interaction Facts
[33]	2001	Persian	All	Outpatient	All	Observational (Retrospective)	6 months	5300 Prescriptions	Drug Interaction Facts
[34]	2005-2006	Persian	All	Outpatient	All	Interventional (Quasi Experimental)	6 months	5300 Prescriptions – 43 Prescribers	Drug Interaction Facts
[35]	2002-2003	Persian	All	Outpatient	All	Interventional (Quasi Experimental)	12 months	6704 Prescriptions – 119 Prescribers	Drug Interaction Facts
[36]	2006	Persian	All	Inpatient	All	Observational (Retrospective)	1 month	6969 Prescriptions	-
[37]	2004	Persian	Pediatrics	Inpatient	All	Observational (Retrospective)	6 months	898 Medical Records	Drug Interaction Facts
[38]	2008	Persian	All	Outpatient	All	Observational (Retrospective)	6 months	167305 Prescriptions	-
[39]	2005 – 2006	Persian	All	Outpatient	Dental	Observational (Retrospective)	6 months	666 Prescriptions	-
[40]	2009	Persian	war-injured veterans with Psychiatric disorders	Outpatient	All	Observational (Retrospective)	3 months	150 Patients	Food and Drug Administration Package
[41]	2006 – 2007	Persian	All	Inpatient	All	Observational (Retrospective)	6 months	400 Medical Records	Hansten Drug Interactions

Table 2 General characteristics of the included studies *(Continued)*

Ref	Year	Language	Age	Setting	Population	Study design	Duration	Sample size	Tool
[42]	2009 – 2010	Persian	All	Inpatient (ICU)	All	Observational (Retrospective)	12 months	371 Medical Records	Drug Interaction Facts
[43]	2010	Persian	war-injured veterans with Psychiatric disorders	Inpatient	All	Observational (Retrospective)	4 months	1435 Patients	Food and Drug Administration Package
[44]	2009	Persian	Elderly	Inpatient (ICU)	All	Observational (Retrospective)	12 months	70 Patients	Drug Interaction Facts
[45]	2000	English	All	Inpatient (ICU, CCU, internal and infectious)	All	Observational (Retrospective)	6 months	3130 Prescriptions	Drug Interaction Facts
[46]	2002	English	All	Outpatient	All	Interventional (Quasi Experimental)	6 months	5600 Prescriptions	Drug Interaction Facts
[47]	2000	English	Elderly	Outpatient	All	Observational (Retrospective)	2 months	3000 Prescriptions	Drug-Reax (Micromedex)
[48]	2005	English	All	Inpatient (ICU)	All	Observational (Retrospective)	6 months	567 prescriptions	Drug Interaction Facts
[49]	2006 – 2008	English	All	Outpatient	All	Observational (Retrospective)	24 months	11,562,808 prescriptions	Drug Interaction Facts
[50]	2007 – 2009	English	All	Outpatient	All	Observational (Retrospective)	30 months	44,567,750 Prescriptions	Drug Interaction Facts
[51]	2005 – 2006	English	Elderly	Outpatient	All	Observational (Retrospective)	12 months	2041 Patients	Swedish Classification System
[52]	2001	English	All	Inpatient	All	Observational (Prospective)	3 months	519 Prescriptions	Drug Interaction Facts
[53]	2010	English	Adults	Inpatient	All	Observational (Retrospective)	12 months	1000 Prescriptions	A computerized DDI database system (Prescription Analyzer 2000, Sara Rayane Co., Iran)
[54]	2012	English	All	Inpatient (ICU)	All	Observational (Prospective)	20 days	101 patients	Drug Interaction Facts
[55]	2011 – 2012	English	All	Inpatient (hematology-oncology ward)	Cancer Patients/Anti-Cancer and Non-Anti-Cancer drugs	Observational (Prospective)	6 months	83 patients	On-Desktop Lexi-Interact
[56]	2011	English	All	Inpatient (Post-ICU)	All	Observational (Prospective)	6 months	203 patients	Online Lexi-Interact
[57]	2009 – 2010	English	All	Inpatient (hematology-oncology ward)	Cancer Patients	Observational (Retrospective)	12 months	224 patients	Drug Interaction Facts

Table 2 General characteristics of the included studies *(Continued)*

Range: 1997 – 2013	English: 13 Persian: 21	All Populations: 27	Outpatient: 19	Observational: 31	Minimum: 1 month	Prescription: 23	Prescriptions: Minimum: 519	FACT: 20
		Elderly: 3	Inpatient: 15	Interventional: 3	Maximum: 36 months	Patient: 11	Maximum: 44,564,650	Others: 9
		War-injured: 2	ICU: 6				Patients: Minimum: 70	
		Pediatrics: 1	All Dep.: 9		Mod: 6 months (38%)		Maximum: 2041	Not Stated: 5
		Adults: 1						

Table 3 Factors associated with incidence of DDIs

Factors		Description
Physician	Gender	The DDI incidence was significantly higher among male doctors [33,46].
	Age	Older physicians prescribed medications with more major DDIs than younger physicians (Not statistically significant) [46].
	Specialty	Major DDIs were higher in the prescriptions of specialist practitioners in comparison to general practitioners (cardiologists and internists ranked top on the list, while dermatologists ranked the lowest) [50].
		General practitioners had more prescriptions with major DDIs than specialists (statistically significant) [33].
		Significant level 1 DDIs[1] were higher in prescriptions of internal specialists and cardiologists than other practitioners [31].
		Significant level 2 DDIs[1] were higher in prescriptions of obstetrician and gynecologist than other practitioners [31].
		Significant level 3 DDIs[1] were higher in prescriptions of general physicians than specialists [31].
		General physicians prescribed more medications with major DDIs than specialists (Not statistically significant) [46].
	Number of Prescriptions	Physicians with 150 or more prescriptions in one month had more DDIs than the others (statistically significant) [33].
Patient	Gender	DDIs were significantly higher in female patients [53].
		DDIs were significantly higher in male patients [42].
	Age	Clinically relevant DDIs were more common for patients 75 years or above than other patients [51].
		DDIs were significantly higher in patients aged over 60 years than other patients [42,53,57].
	Disease	DDIs were significantly higher in cardiology patients than other patients [53].
		DDIs were higher in Hematologic cancer patients than patients suffer from other diseases [57].
		DDIs were higher in patients whose source of cancer was in different specific organs than other cancer patients [57].
	Length of Hospital Stay	DDIs were higher in patients with longer hospital stay than other patients [42,57].
	Department	DDIs occurred in surgery department more than the other departments [36].
	Drug	DDIs was significantly higher in patients who have been prescribed digoxin than other patients [53].

[1]Significance rating is based on Drug Interactions Facts™. The factors are related to physicians and patients' characteristics.

Discussion

This study aimed to provide an overview of the incidence and pattern of DDIs and associated factors in Iran, as an example of a developing country. This is the first review study that summarizes the available evidence of DDIs in Iran.

We identified and described the results of 34 relevant studies addressing the key questions of this review. The overall quality of DDIs studies in Iran was relatively poor, perhaps due to lack of a standard guideline for designing methodology and reporting results of medication error studies. The median incidence of potential DDIs in prescriptions in outpatient settings was 8.5%, while it was 19.2% in inpatient settings. Patient age was the most reported factor influencing the incidence of DDIs. Only three studies were interventional, and all showed significant reduction in potential DDIs.

Our results show that all DDIs studies in Iran assessed potential DDIs, while no study was performed on actual DDIs. Actual DDIs are interactions that actually lead to adverse clinical events in patients. Espinosa-Bosch et al. found a larger number of studies on potential DDIs than on actual DDIs in developed countries (42 vs. 5 studies) [19]. From eight studies included in the review of DDIs in oncology, six assessed potential DDIs while two reported actual DDIs [21]. Our findings in accordance with those from studies in developed countries confirm that there is little evidence of the incidence of actual DDIs in comparison to potential DDIs in the literature. The reason for this may be that identifying actual DDIs is much more complicated than potential DDIs. The majority of the included studies were retrospective which had used computerized programs to review physicians' orders and prescriptions and to identify potential DDIs. However, to identify actual DDIs, it is required to find the adverse events and confirm that they are a result of simultaneously administering two drugs in the patient regarding his/her condition. The adverse events from DDIs are either not identified or not documented accurately. It should be noted that due to inherent and recall biases and also ethical considerations, the conduction of study designs for assessing actual DDIs may be challenging.

We showed the overall incidence of DDIs in prescriptions in inpatient and outpatient settings reported by

Table 4 The most frequent major DDIs

The most frequent major DDIs	References
Digoxin + Furosemide	[25-27,50,53]
Captopril + Triamterene-H	[38,50]
Carvedilol + Salbutamol(Albuterol)	[56,57]
Aspirin + Clopidogrel	[56]
Clopidogrel + Omeprazole	[56]
Pantoprazole + Clopidogrel	[56]
Aspirin + Warfarin	[56]
Haloperidol + Propranolol	[50]
Amitriptyline + Clonidine	[50]
Chlorpromazine + Propranolol	[50]
Propranolol + Verapamil	[50]
Amiodaron + Digoxin	[50]
Gemfibrozil + Atorvastatin	[50]
Cyclosporine + Fluconazole	[55]
Cyclosporine + Phenytoin	[55]
Atorvastatin + Fluconazole	[55]
Lovastatin + Gemfibrozil	[55]
Arsenic Trioxide + Fluconazole	[55]
Aspirin + Ibuprofen	[32]
Theophylline + Propranolol	[32]
Pseudoephedrine + Furazolidone	[32]
Dextromethorphan + Furazolidone	[32]
Tranylcypromine + Levodopa	[29]
Clomipramine + Furazolidone	[29]
Clonazepam + Olanzapine	[43]
Digoxin + Verapamil	[46]
Rifampin + Isoniazid	[48]
Verapamil + Erythromycin	[53]

Iranian studies (inpatient: median = 8.5%, IQR: 8.4-10.1; outpatient: median = 19.2%, IQR: 15.5-22). The high incidence of DDIs may be associated with high number of drugs per prescription. The mean number of drugs per prescription in Iran is relatively high [58]. This mean number for the outpatient setting was 3.16 and 3.05 in 2010 and 2011, respectively, and 17% and 15% of these prescriptions involved more than four drugs in those years. No similar review aggregated the reported incidence of DDIs in the general population. The other review studies on DDIs have been conducted on either a specific group of patients, e.g. elderly, hospitalized patients, or specific types of drugs e.g. cardiovascular.

The aggregation and comparison of the results of the included studies showed a wide variability of DDIs incidence estimates in the Iranian healthcare community. Relatively few studies which were performed in the general population in developed countries also showed a wide variability of estimates on incidence of DDIs (i.e. 9.8% in Finland [59], 18.5% in Greece [17]). Moreover, a systematic review on incidence of medication errors in Iran showed a wide variability of estimates [60]. Different study methods, various drug interaction databases, diverse study populations, different sample sizes, and some other factors have caused this considerable variability; therefore, direct comparison between the studies is impossible. Maximum incidence of potential DDIs in prescriptions (50%) was reported in a study which assessed DDIs of cardiovascular drugs in outpatient prescriptions [26]. Similarly, the findings obtained in a study from a developed country showed that 80% of elderly hospitalized patients with heart diseases were susceptible to DDIs [61]. The high number of prescribed drugs and also frequent prescribing of some drugs with many possible DDIs may cause the high incidence of DDIs in this group of patients. One included study in our review reported the incidence of potential DDIs among cancer patients as 37.5% [57]. A study conducted in a developed country has shown that 27% of cancer patients were subject to DDIs [62]. Supporting the results of these studies, a review on DDIs among cancer patients reported that approximately one-third of cancer patients are susceptible to DDIs [21]. High growth in the number of new anti-cancer drugs may be one of the main reasons for this.

Incidence of DDIs may be associated with characteristics of patients, prescribers and pharmacists, or some barriers such as insufficient communication between these groups. Good communication between prescribers and pharmacists is crucial to reduce the risks of DDIs [63]. Among studies conducted in Iran, no study has assessed pharmacists' factors and communication between participants as determinants of DDIs. One review paper specified potential determinants of DDIs associated with pharmacists' characteristics [64]. In that review, the relationship between pharmacists and prescribers, quality of signals from surveillance programs, pharmacists' workload, and also availability, quality, and sensitivity of DDIs softwares have been mentioned as the main potential factors that contribute to the occurrence of DDIs. The Iranian studies showed that having heart disease, being old, and receiving digoxin were the main patient factors associated with high incidence of DDIs. Similarly, the findings from another review on the incidence of DDIs in a developed country highlighted these risk factors [19]. Many studies have emphasized that the high incidence of DDIs in the elderly is due to physiological changes related to age, suffering from multiple diseases, and a high rate of medication use. The results reported by Juurlink et al. [7], which show that digoxin toxicity due to DDIs leads to elderly hospitalization, is in line with the results of the Iranian studies. Concerning prescribers' factors, DDIs were higher in the prescriptions of male prescribers and physicians with greater

Table 5 The most common drugs contributing to DDIs

Names and classes of drugs	Percentage of identified DDIs	Reference
Beta Blockers	35.21%	[26]
Inotropic Drugs e.g. Digoxin	15.94%	
ACEIs[1] e.g. Captopril	15.35%	
Diuretics e.g. Furosemide	14.66%	
Calcium Channel Blockers e.g. Diltiazem	7.33%	
Nitrate e.g. Nitrocardin	4.18%	
Antihyperglycemic Drugs e.g. Clofibrate	4.09%	
Antiarrhythmic Drugs e.g. Amiodarone	2.64%	
Digoxin	50% of severe DDIs	[27]
Gentamicin	26.5% of moderate DDIs	
Diphenhydramine Compound	24.85%	[28]
Dextromethorphan-P	15.38%	
Pseudoephedrine	11.8%	
Antibiotics	7.1%	
Tricyclic Antidepressant	72.7%	[29]
MAOIs[4]	25.2%	
SRIs[3]	2.1%	
Antibiotics	Not specified	[24]
Central Nervous System Drugs	Not specified	
NSAIDs[2]	Not specified	
Antidepressant	52%	[40]
Anti Infectives	27.5%	[41]
Other Drugs	21.5%	
Antiarrhythmic	15.5%	
Antihypertensive	11.1%	
Anti-diabetic	5.6%	
Anticoagulant	5.6%	
Diuretics	3.7%	
Hormone	2.5%	
Salicylate	2.3%	
Anticonvulsant	1.8%	
Antidepressant	47.5%	[43]
Belladonna	4.4%	[49]
Phenytoin Compound	4.3%	
Cimetidine	3.8%	
Propranolol Hydrochloride	3.6%	
Gentamicin	3.5%	
Acetylsalicylic Acid	3.5%	
Aluminium MGS	3.4%	
Theophylline	3.3%	
Carbamazepine	2.8%	

Table 5 The most common drugs contributing to DDIs *(Continued)*

Contraceptive LD	2.7%	
Digoxin	Not specified	[50]
Diuretics	Not specified	
HMG CoA Reductase Inhibitors	Not specified	
Allopurinol	Not specified	
ACEIs	Not specified	
Warfarin	Not specified	
Gemfibrozil	Not specified	
Haloperidol	Not specified	
Amiodarone	Not specified	
Clonidine	Not specified	
Cardiovascular Drugs	Not specified	[52]
Digoxin	Most common in severe DDIs	[53]
ACEIs	Most common in severe and moderate DDIs	
Beta Blockers	Most common in moderate DDIs	
Fluoroquinolones	Most common in moderate DDIs	
Antacids	Most common in moderate DDIs	
Phenytoin	Not specified	[54]
Antimycotics for systemic use[5]	31.35%	[55]
Immunosuppressants	13.51%	
Sulfonamides and Trimethoprim	9.73%	
Antiepileptics	8.11%	
Antiemetics and Antinauseants	7.02%	
Antigout Preparations	4.05%	
Corticosteroids for Systemic Use, Plain	3.78%	
Other Antineoplastic Agents	2.43%	
Direct Acting Antivirals	2.43%	
Other Beta-lactam Antibacterials	2.16%	

Names and classes of drugs which mostly contributed to DDIs and percentage of identified DDIs by the relevant studies are shown.
[1]ACEIs: Angiotensin-Converting-Enzyme inhibitors.
[2]NSAIDs: Non-Steroidal Anti-Inflammatory Drugs.
[3]SSRIs: Selective Serotonin Reuptake Inhibitors.
[4]MAOIs: Monoamine Oxidase Inhibitors.
[5]Medication classes categorized by the Anatomical Therapeutic Chemical (ATC) classification system of the World Health Organization.

number of prescriptions in one month. This may be due to the fact that male and busy physicians may less consider the possibility of DDIs during the prescription phase. So far, no study has assessed pharmacological knowledge of prescribers specifically about DDIs.

Drugs most contributing to major DDIs were digoxin, followed by beta blockers, ACEIs, diuretic agents, and

NSAIDs. Digoxin, ACEIs, and diuretic agents are frequently prescribed to patients with heart diseases; therefore, this may be one of the reasons why DDIs are highly prevalent in these patients. These results are in the same line as two other reviews which mainly included studies from developed countries [19,20].

The included studies in this review have used various DDIs compendia, mostly (59%) Drug Interaction Facts. Studies have shown that there are discrepancies between DDI compendia [65,66]. In addition, other studies showed that the various performance measures used (such as accuracy, sensitivity, and specificity) of multiple DDI identifying software vary [67-69]. Therefore, one should consider these discrepancies in the resources when comparing the result of the DDI related studies. Clinical relevancy of DDIs is another important issue that should be considered when interpreting DDI related study results, as well as in practice.

Despite the high incidence of DDIs in Iran, only three studies implemented interventions to reduce them [34,35,46]. Two studies evaluated the effects of educational interventions on reduction of DDIs [34,46] and one study evaluated the effect of audit feedback on the quality of prescriptions [35]. The studies showed significant reduction of DDIs after the interventions. In recent years, computerized systems have been involved in medication error reduction strategies and shown to be effective [70]. Computerized physician order entry systems and drug interaction softwares linked to knowledge bases could detect potential DDIs and alert prescribers to prevent serious outcomes. These systems screen the drug list before finalizing an order. In case of a potential medication error, especially a DDI, alerts are displayed and changes in the prescription can be made. Although numerous studies in different countries mentioned the potential improvement of patient safety by computerized systems, there are no studies published on the evaluation of such systems in Iran.

It should be noted that the present review had several limitations. First, although the comprehensive searches were performed, we may have missed some relevant studies. It may be due to limitations of the Persian search engines. To overcome this limitation, we used several search strategies including searching bibliographies of included studies (snowball method). In addition, we searched Google Scholar using both Persian and English search terms. Second, the methodologies of the included studies in our review were heterogeneous. This made it difficult to aggregate their widely varying results. Therefore, no quantitative meta-analysis has been attempted. Third, we did not include results of the unpublished studies (e.g. dissertations and conference papers) in the review. This may affect our estimations. Finally, some of the included studies in our review had small sample sizes (Table 2)

that might have led to bias. These may have limited the generalizability of our results.

Due to the lack of studies addressing actual DDIs among Iranian patients, the incidence of adverse events caused by this type of medication errors remains unknown. It is recommended that future DDIs researches investigate the adverse events of DDIs through closely monitoring the patients who are provided with potentially interacting drugs. The prescribers should be aware of the high incidence of DDIs in their prescriptions. They also need to pay attention to patients who are frequently prescribed potentially interacting drugs (e.g. digoxin, beta blockers, NSAIDs, ACEIs, and diuretic agents). In the absence of studies assessing communication among the drug management team (physician, nurse, and pharmacist), it is suggested that future studies delve into aspects of this communication. Better communication between the team members could lead to a safe pharmacotherapy plan and reduce the risks of adverse events caused by DDIs. In recent years, information technology interventions have been employed to improve medication safety and shown to be effective in reducing the number of potential DDIs. We suggest designing and evaluation of such information technology interventions.

Conclusion

Although there is a large number of studies on the potential DDIs in Iran, there is still no evidence of the incidence of actual DDIs. The included studies in this review had relatively poor quality and were heterogeneous in their methodologies and reporting. However, almost all studies concluded that the incidence of DDIs in both inpatient and outpatient settings is high. Despite this high incidence, there is a limited number of interventional studies aimed at reducing DDIs incidence. Finally, more extensive research is needed to identify and minimize the factors associated with the incidence of DDIs, and to design and evaluate the effects of interventions especially those that utilize information technology to increase awareness about DDIs and decrease their incidence by the drug management team.

Abbreviations
DDI: Drug-drug interaction; ADE: Adverse drug event; NSAIDs: Non-steroidal anti-inflammatory drugs; ACEIs: Angiotensin-converting-enzyme inhibitors; MAOIs: Monoamine oxidase inhibitors; SSRIs: Selective serotonin reuptake inhibitors; ATC: Anatomical therapeutic chemical classification; IQR: Interquartile range.

Competing interests
The authors declare that they have no competing interests.

Authors' contributions
SE and EN conceived the study idea and design. SE, HV, and EN participated in the literature search, inclusion process, and data abstraction. SE, ZhT, and EN participated in the methodological quality assessment of the included studies and interpretation of data. EN drafted the manuscript. All authors

have been involved in critically revising the manuscript. All authors read and approved the final manuscript.

Acknowledgements
This study was a part of the first author's PhD thesis which was supported by a grant from Mashhad University of Medical Sciences Research Council.

Author details
[1]Student Research Committee, Department of Medical Informatics, Faculty of Medicine, Mashhad University of Medical Sciences, Mashhad, Iran. [2]Department of Health Information Management/Technology, School of Allied Health Professions, Kashan University of Medical Sciences, Kashan, Iran. [3]Neurogenic Inflammation Research Center, Faculty of Medicine, Mashhad University of Medical Sciences, Mashhad, Iran. [4]Targeted Drug Delivery Research Center, School of Pharmacy, Mashhad University of Medical Sciences, Mashhad, Iran. [5]Pharmaceutical Research Center, School of Pharmacy, Mashhad University of Medical Sciences, Mashhad, Iran. [6]Department of Medical Informatics, Faculty of Medicine, Mashhad University of Medical Sciences, Mashhad, Iran. [7]Department of Medical Informatics, Academic Medical Center, University of Amsterdam, Amsterdam, The Netherlands.

References
1. Gurwitz JH, Field TS, Harrold LR, Rothschild J, Debellis K, Seger AC, Cadoret C, Fish LS, Garber L, Kelleher M, Bates DW: **Incidence and preventability of adverse drug events among older persons in the ambulatory setting.** *JAMA* 2003, **289:**1107–1116.
2. Thomsen LA, Winterstein AG, Sondergaard B, Haugbolle LS, Melander A: **Systematic review of the incidence and characteristics of preventable adverse drug events in ambulatory care.** *Ann Pharmacother* 2007, **41:**1411–1426.
3. Tache SV, Sonnichsen A, Ashcroft DM: **Prevalence of adverse drug events in ambulatory care: a systematic review.** *Ann Pharmacother* 2011, **45:**977–989.
4. Lazarou J, Pomeranz BH, Corey PN: **Incidence of adverse drug reactions in hospitalized patients: a meta-analysis of prospective studies.** *JAMA* 1998, **279:**1200–1205.
5. Field TS, Gilman BH, Subramanian S, Fuller JC, Bates DW, Gurwitz JH: **The costs associated with adverse drug events among older adults in the ambulatory setting.** *Med Care* 2005, **43:**1171–1176.
6. Hug BL, Keohane C, Seger DL, Yoon C, Bates DW: **The costs of adverse drug events in community hospitals.** *Jt Comm J Qual Patient Saf* 2012, **38:**120–126.
7. Juurlink DN, Mamdani M, Kopp A, Laupacis A, Redelmeier DA: **Drug-drug interactions among elderly patients hospitalized for drug toxicity.** *JAMA* 2003, **289:**1652–1658.
8. Astrand E, Astrand B, Antonov K, Petersson G: **Potential drug interactions during a three-decade study period: a cross-sectional study of a prescription register.** *Eur J Clin Pharmacol* 2007, **63:**851–859.
9. Jankel CA, Fitterman LK: **Epidemiology of drug-drug interactions as a cause of hospital admissions.** *Drug Saf* 1993, **9:**51–59.
10. McDonnell PJ, Jacobs MR: **Hospital admissions resulting from preventable adverse drug reactions.** *Ann Pharmacother* 2002, **36:**1331–1336.
11. Peyriere H, Cassan S, Floutard E, Riviere S, Blayac JP, Hillaire-Buys D, Le Quellec A, Hansel S: **Adverse drug events associated with hospital admission.** *Ann Pharmacother* 2003, **37:**5–11.
12. Glintborg B, Andersen SE, Dalhoff K: **Drug-drug interactions among recently hospitalised patients–frequent but mostly clinically insignificant.** *Eur J Clin Pharmacol* 2005, **61:**675–681.
13. Askari M, Eslami S, Louws M, Dongelmans D, Wierenga P, Kuiper R, Abu-Hanna A: **Relevance of drug-drug interaction in the ICU - perceptions of intensivists and pharmacists.** *Stud Health Technol Inform* 2012, **180:**716–720.
14. Ko Y, Malone DC, Skrepnek GH, Armstrong EP, Murphy JE, Abarca J, Rehfeld RA, Reel SJ, Woosley RL: **Prescribers' knowledge of and sources of information for potential drug-drug interactions: a postal survey of US prescribers.** *Drug Saf* 2008, **31:**525–536.
15. Heininger-Rothbucher D, Bischinger S, Ulmer H, Pechlaner C, Speer G, Wiedermann CJ: **Incidence and risk of potential adverse drug interactions in the emergency room.** *Resuscitation* 2001, **49:**283–288.

16. Straubhaar B, Krahenbuhl S, Schlienger RG: **The prevalence of potential drug-drug interactions in patients with heart failure at hospital discharge.** *Drug Saf* 2006, **29:**79–90.
17. Chatsisvili A, Sapounidis I, Pavlidou G, Zoumpouridou E, Karakousis VA, Spanakis M, Teperikidis L, Niopas I: **Potential drug-drug interactions in prescriptions dispensed in community pharmacies in Greece.** *Pharm World Sci* 2010, **32:**187–193.
18. Marzolini C, Elzi L, Gibbons S, Weber R, Fux C, Furrer H, Chave JP, Cavassini M, Bernasconi E, Calmy A, Vernazza P, Khoo S, Ledergerber B, Back D, Battegay M: **Prevalence of comedications and effect of potential drug-drug interactions in the Swiss HIV Cohort Study.** *Antivir Ther* 2010, **15:**413–423.
19. Espinosa-Bosch M, Santos-Ramos B, Gil-Navarro MV, Santos-Rubio MD, Marin-Gil R, Villacorta-Linaza P: **Prevalence of drug interactions in hospital healthcare.** *Int J Clin Pharm* 2012, **34:**807–817.
20. Hines LE, Murphy JE: **Potentially harmful drug-drug interactions in the elderly: a review.** *Am J Geriatr Pharmacother* 2011, **9:**364–377.
21. Riechelmann RP, Del Giglio A: **Drug interactions in oncology: how common are they?** *Ann Oncol* 2009, **20:**1907–1912.
22. Alsulami Z, Conroy S, Choonara I: **Medication errors in the Middle East countries: a systematic review of the literature.** *Eur J Clin Pharmacol* 2013, **69:**995–1008.
23. Ghaleb MA, Barber N, Franklin BD, Yeung VW, Khaki ZF, Wong IC: **Systematic review of medication errors in pediatric patients.** *Ann Pharmacother* 2006, **40:**1766–1776.
24. Cheraghali AAM, Ali Dadi A, Panahi Y: **Evaluation of physicians prescriptions in hospitals affiliated to a medical science University in Tehran.** *Teb Va Tazkieh* 2002, **1:**30–36.
25. Rafeian M: **Drug interactions in internal and surgical wards of Kashani Hospital, Shahrekord, 1997.** *Tehran Univ Med J* 2001, **59:**86–91.
26. Morteza-Semnani K, Saeedi M, Gharipour O: **Evaluation of cardiovascular drugs interactions in insured prescriptions in Sari during the years 2000–2001.** *J Mazandaran Univ Med Sci* 2001, **11:**37–45.
27. Sobhani A, Shodjai H: **Prevalence of polypharmacy and correlations with sex, age and drug regimen in insurance prescription.** *J Guilan Univ Med Sci* 2001, **10:**90–96.
28. Nabavizadeh S, Khoshnevisan F: **Drug interactions in prescriptions of general practitioners in Yasuj city.** *J Armaghan Danesh* 2003, **7:**53–59.
29. Morteza-Semnani K, Saeidi M, Isazade Mashinchi M: **Evaluation of anti-depressant drugs interactions in insured prescriptions in Anzali in 1379.** *J Guilan Univ Med Sci* 2002, **11:**26–33.
30. Ebrahim Zadeh MA, Gholami K, Gharanjik U, Javadian PSM: **Evaluation of Drug Interactions of Non-Steroidal Anti-Inflammatory Drugs (Nsaids) in Sari insured prescriptions during 1999–2001.** *Razi J Med Sci* 2003, **10:**489–495.
31. Asgarirad H, Pourmorad F, Akbari K: **Pattern of prescription and drug interaction in prescriptions of Nowshahr and Chalous physicians (2001).** *Med J Hormozgan Univ* 2004, **7:**167–172.
32. Rashidi K, Senobar Tahaee SN: **Assessment of drug interactions in medical insurance prescriptions in Kurdistan province in 2000.** *Sci J Kurdistan Univ Med Sci* 2005, **10:**78–84.
33. Khouri V, Semnani S, Roushandel G: **Frequency distribution of drug interactions and some of related factors in prescriptions.** *Med J Tabriz Univ Med Sci Health Serv* 2006, **27:**29–32.
34. Ghorbani M, Hosseini M, KHouri V: **Evaluation of face to face training effects on reduction of drug interactions on insured prescription of physicians.** *Med Sci J Islamic Azad Univ Tehran Med Branch* 2007, **17:**171–175.
35. Zare N, Razmjoo M, Ghaeminia M, Zeighami B, Aghamaleki Z: **Effectiveness of the feedback and recalling education on quality of prescription by general practitioners in Shiraz.** *Zahedan J Res Med Sci* 2008, **9:**255–261.
36. Shayan Z, Shayan F: **Pattern of drug prescription in clinical ward of Motahari and Peimanie hospital in Khordad 1385.** *J Jahrom Univ Med Sci* 2007, **5:**44–50.
37. Valizadeh F, Ghasemi S, Nagafi S, Delfan B, Mohsenzadeh A: **Errors in medication orders and the nursing Staff's reports in medical notes of children.** *Iran J Pediatr* 2008, **18:**33–40.
38. Dolatabadi M, Jalili Rasti H: **Patterns of Physicians' drug prescription in Sabzevar Iran (2008).** *J Sabzevar Univ Med Sci* 2009, **16:**161–166.
39. Nezafati S, Maleki N, Golikhani R: **Quality assessment of health services insurance prescriptions among the dentists of Tabriz city in 2005–2006.** *Med J Tabriz Univ Med Sci* 2009, **31:**101–104.
40. Gorji A, Gharakhani M, Razeghi Jahromi S, Sadeghian H, Faghihzadeh S, Kazemi H, Arabkheradmand J, Koulivand P, Bayan L: **Multiple drug**

interactions in war-injured veterans. *Iran J War Public Health* 2010, **2**:23–28.

41. Alizadeh A, Rostamian A, Saeedpour K, Hemmati M, Khorasani Z, Mohagheghi M, Khatami Moghaddam M, Mousavi M: Drug interactions frequency in the bedridden patients in three hospitals of Tehran city. *Modern Care J* 2011, **7**:22–27.

42. Rafieii H, Arab M, Ranjbar H, Arab N, Sepehri G, Amiri M: The prevalence of potential drug interactions in Intensive Care Units. *Iran J Crit Care Nurs* 2012, **4**:191–196.

43. Esteghamat S, Esteghamat S, Bastani F, Kazemi H, Koulivand P, Bayan L, Gorji A: Potential drug interactions in war-injured veterans with psychaitric disorders. *Iran J War Public Health* 2012, **4**:24–31.

44. Rafiei H: The prevalence of potential drug interactions among critically ill elderly patients in the Intensive Care Unit (ICU). *Iran J Ageing* 2012, **6**:14–19.

45. Hajebi G, Mortazavi S: An Investigation of Drug Interactions in Hospital Pharmacy Prescriptions. *Iran J Pharm Res* 2002, **1**:15–19.

46. Khouri V, Abbasi A, Besharat S: The effect of active training in reducing severe drug interactions. *Iran J Med Edu* 2004, **6**:107–112.

47. Azoulay L, Zargarzadeh A, Salahshouri Z, Oraichi D, Berard A: Inappropriate medication prescribing in community-dwelling elderly people living in Iran. *Eur J Clin Pharmacol* 2005, **61**:913–919.

48. Abbasi Nazari M, Khanzadeh Moghadam N: Evaluation of Pharmacokinetic Drug Interactions in Prescriptions of Intensive Care Unit (ICU) in a Teaching Hospital. *Iran J Pharm Res* 2006, **5**:215–218.

49. Taheri E, Afshari R, Nazemian L: Population-based severity, onset and type of drug-drug interactions in prescriptions. *Methods Find Exp Clin Pharmacol* 2010, **32**:237–242.

50. Ahmadizar F, Soleymani F, Abdollahi M: Study of drug-drug interactions in prescriptions of general practitioners and specialists in Iran 2007–2009. *Iran J Pharm Res* 2011, **10**:921–931.

51. Ghadimi H, Esmaily HM, Wahlstrom R: General practitioners' prescribing patterns for the elderly in a province of Iran. *Pharmacoepidemiol Drug Saf* 2011, **20**:482–487.

52. Mortazavi S, Hajebi G: An investigation on the nature and extent of occurrence of errors of commission in hospital prescriptions. *Iran J Pharm Res* 2003, **2**:83–87.

53. Sepehri G, Khazaelli P, Dahooie FA, Sepehri E, Dehghani MR: Prevalence of potential drug interactions in an Iranian general hospital. *Indian J Pharm Sci* 2012, **74**:75–79.

54. Rafiei H, Esmaeli Abdar M, Amiri M, Ahmadinejad M: The study of harmful and beneficial drug interactions in intensive care, Kerman, Iran. *J Intensive Care Society* 2013, **14**:155–158.

55. Hadjibabaie M, Badri S, Ataei S, Moslehi AH, Karimzadeh I, Ghavamzadeh A: Potential drug-drug interactions at a referral hematology-oncology ward in Iran: a cross-sectional study. *Cancer Chemother Pharmacol* 2013, **71**:1619–1627.

56. Haji Aghajani M, Sistanizad M, Abbasinazari M, Abiar Ghamsari M, Ayazkhoo L, Safi O, Kazemi K, Kouchek M: Potential drug-drug interactions in post-CCU of a teaching hospital. *Iran J Pharm Res* 2013, **12**:243–248.

57. Tavakoli Ardakani M, Kazemian K, Salamzadeh J, Mehdizadeh M: Potential of drug interactions among hospitalized cancer patients in a developing country. *Iran J Pharm Res* 2013, **12**:175–182.

58. National indicators for drug prescription in Iran. http://fdo.behdasht.gov. ir/index.aspx?siteid=114&pageid=45999.

59. Heikkila T, Lekander T, Raunio H: Use of an online surveillance system for screening drug interactions in prescriptions in community pharmacies. *Eur J Clin Pharmacol* 2006, **62**:661–665.

60. Mansouri A, Ahmadvand A, Hadjibabaie M, Kargar M, Javadi M, Gholami K: Types and severity of medication errors in Iran; a review of the current literature. *Daru* 2013, **21**:49.

61. Kohler GI, Bode-Boger SM, Busse R, Hoopmann M, Welte T, Boger RH: Drug-drug interactions in medical patients: effects of in-hospital treatment and relation to multiple drug use. *Int J Clin Pharmacol Ther* 2000, **38**:504–513.

62. Sokol KC, Knudsen JF, Li MM: Polypharmacy in older oncology patients and the need for an interdisciplinary approach to side-effect management. *J Clin Pharm Ther* 2007, **32**:169–175.

63. Mallet L, Spinewine A, Huang A: The challenge of managing drug interactions in elderly people. *Lancet* 2007, **370**:185–191.

64. Becker ML, Kallewaard M, Caspers PW, Schalekamp T, Stricker BH: Potential determinants of drug-drug interaction associated dispensing in community pharmacies. *Drug Saf* 2005, **28**:371–378.

65. Fulda TR, Valuck RJ, Zanden JV, Parker S, Byrns PJ, The USPDURAP: Disagreement among drug compendia on inclusion and ratings of drug-drug interactions. *Curr Ther Res* 2000, **61**:540–548.

66. Vitry AI: Comparative assessment of four drug interaction compendia. *Br J Clin Pharmacol* 2007, **63**:709–714.

67. Barrons R: Evaluation of personal digital assistant software for drug interactions. *Am J Health Syst Pharm* 2004, **61**:380–385.

68. Reis AM, Cassiani SH: Evaluation of three brands of drug interaction software for use in intensive care units. *Pharm World Sci* 2010, **32**:822–828.

69. Vonbach P, Dubied A, Krahenbuhl S, Beer JH: Evaluation of frequently used drug interaction screening programs. *Pharm World Sci* 2008, **30**:367–374.

70. Eslami S, de Keizer NF, Abu-Hanna A: The impact of computerized physician medication order entry in hospitalized patients–a systematic review. *Int J Med Inform* 2008, **77**:365–376.

4

Isotretinoin-associated Sweet's syndrome

Jamileh Moghimi[1], Daryiush Pahlevan[2], Maryam Azizzadeh[2], Hamid Hamidi[3] and Mohsen Pourazizi[4*]

Abstract

Objective: Sweet's syndrome (SS) is characterized by various clinical symptoms, physical features, and pathological findings. Although cases of SS are very rare, there has been an increase in the incidence of drug-induced SS. Till date, there have been only few reported cases of isotretinoin-induced SS.

Case summary: In this report, we describe the case of a 19-year-old girl who developed SS after systemic treatment with oral isotretinoin for nodulocystic acne.

Conclusions: The findings of this report emphasize the importance of evaluating isotretinoin as a possible, though uncommon, cause of SS and replacing it with another treatment if its involvement is suspected.

Keyword: Sweet syndrome, Isotretinoin, Neutrophilic dermatosis, Drug reaction

Background

Sweet's syndrome (SS) is characterized by painful erythematous skin lesions due to neutrophil infiltration in the upper dermis, fever, leukocytosis with a predominance of neutrophils, and increased erythrocyte sedimentation rate (ESR) [1,2]. There are three clinical forms of SS: classical (idiopathic), malignancy associated, and drug induced [3]. Classical SS usually develops in women aged between 30 and 40 years and is often preceded by upper respiratory or gastrointestinal tract infection, inflammatory bowel disease, and pregnancy. Malignancy-associated SS can occur as a paraneoplastic syndrome. Drug-induced SS most commonly occurs in patients who have been treated with granulocyte colony-stimulating factor [3]. Although this form of SS is very rare, there has been an increase in the incidence of drug-induced SS [4]. Here we describe the case of a 19-year-old girl who developed drug-induced SS after systemic treatment with oral isotretinoin (13-cis-retinoic acid) for nodulocystic acne and emphasize the importance of evaluating isotretinoin as a possible, though uncommon, cause of SS.

Case presentation

A 19-year-old girl presented to the rheumatology clinic because of malaise, polyarthralgia, and weight loss (5 kg), which she experienced during six months before presentation to the clinic. She did not have any fever during presentation to the clinic. During two weeks before presentation to the clinic, she developed very painful and tender skin lesions on her legs and in the suprapubic area. Her medical history was insignificant. She had no history of inflammatory bowel disease or rheumatological disease. She did not have symptoms indicative of contact dermatitis or any history of drug intake, except for the use of isotretinoin for severe facial acne vulgaris, which was initiated one year ago at a dose of 20 mg twice daily and was tapered gradually to a dose of 20 mg weekly. A similar lesion appeared 1 month after the initiation of isotretinoin therapy. These lesions resolved without intervention. However, the lesions at the time of presentation to the clinic were more severe and painful, and the patient was admitted to the hospital for clinical evaluation. Physical examination showed that she was unnaturally thin and that she looked ill. Her vital signs were not remarkable, and she did not have fever, lymphadenopathy, hepatosplenomegaly, and other symptoms. Dermatological examination showed tender erythematous plaques with pustules and crust on the ventromedial aspects of her mid-thighs, suprapubic region, and right calf [Figure 1]. Initial laboratory examination determined leukocytosis (23100 cells/mm^3) and neutrophilia (65%).

* Correspondence: m.pourazizi@yahoo.com
[4]Students' Research Committee, Semnan University of Medical Sciences, Semnan, Iran
Full list of author information is available at the end of the article

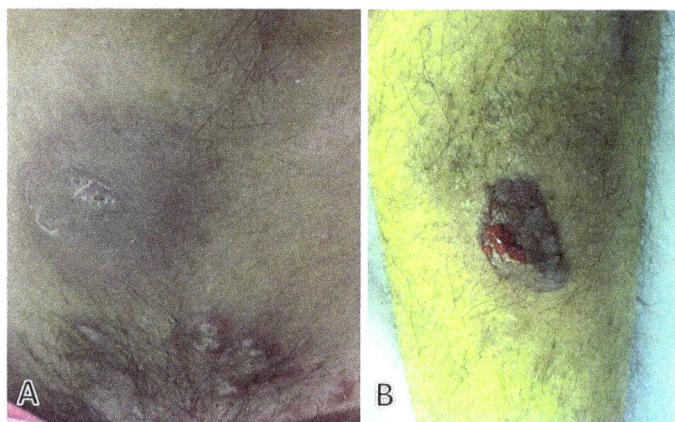

Figure 1 Isotretinoin-associated Sweet's Syndrome. Erythematous, edematous, painful plaques on suprapubic area **(A)** and right lower extremity **(B)**.

Group A streptococcal throat culture and anti-streptolysin O titers were negative. Her ESR was >100. Antineutrophil cytoplasmic antibody and antinuclear antibody titers and blood, wound, and urine cultures were negative. Tuberculosis skin test (PPD skin test) provided insignificant results. Kidney and liver function tests, urine analysis, echocardiography, chest radiography, and total abdominopelvic sonography yielded normal results. Bone marrow aspiration and biopsy yielded normal results. Therefore, hematological and solid organ malignancies were ruled out. Skin punch biopsy from a new, well-developed lesion showed spongiotic epidermis with mild dermal edema. Massive aggregates of neutrophils were observed in the upper and mid-dermis, but there was no obvious sign of vasculitis [Figure 2]. Thus, the patient was diagnosed as having drug-induced SS due to isotretinoin based on the above observations and criteria for SS. Isotretinoin therapy was stopped, and prednisolone therapy was initiated at a

dose of 60 mg/day (1 mg/kg). Dose tapering was initiated after 2 weeks; after 6 weeks, the dose was tapered to 5 mg/day. Complete resolution of the lesions was observed within 4 weeks. The patient was advised to avoid isotretinoin and asked to return for follow-ups.

Ethical approval
This is a report of rare case, however the report was approved by the Ethics Committee of Semnan University of Medical Sciences, Semnan, Iran.

Conclusions
Etiologically, SS may be associated with drugs, infections, and paraneoplastic or inflammatory conditions such as inflammatory bowel diseases and rheumatological diseases. When no triggering factor is detected, the disease is categorized as classic or idiopathic [4].

Only few cases of SS have been reported to be caused by drug reactions. Drug-induced SS is rare and probably represents <5% of all cases [5]. The clinical presentation and histology of drug-induced SS are similar to those of idiopathic SS [6]. Neutrophilia is often absent in drug-induced SS probably because many of these cases are caused by the use of hematopoietic growth factors that are used for reversing chemotherapy-induced neutropenia. Lesions in drug-induced SS usually develop approximately one week after the initiation of the drug [7]. After withdrawing the causative drug, fever abates in 1–3 days and lesions disappear within 3–30 days [5]. Systemic corticosteroids may be required in severe cases. Drugs associated with drug-induced SS include all-trans-retinoic acid and G-CSF or GM-CSF [5]. Some cases may be attributed to trimethoprim/sulfamethoxazole, norfloxacin, furosemide, celecoxib, tetracyclines, and antiepileptic drugs [4,7]. Other implicated drugs are summarized in Table 1 [4].

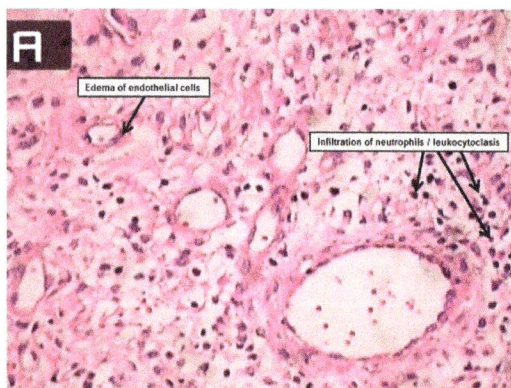

Figure 2 Isotretinoin-associated Sweet's Syndrome. Edema of dermis, infiltration of neutrophils and leukocytoclasis, edema of endothelial cells and no vasculitis.

Table 1 Drugs reported as inducing Sweet's syndrome

Granulocytes growth factors	G-CSF (granulocyte-colony stimulating factor); GM-CSF (granulocyte monocyte colony stimulating factor); All trans-retinoic acid
Vaccination	Calmette-Guérin; Influenza; Streptococcus pneumonia; Small-pox
Antibiotics	Doxycyclin; Cyclines (minocycline, tetracycline and doxycycline); Quinolones: norfloxacin, ofloxacin; Nitrofurantoin; Streptogramin (quinupristin/dalfopristin); Trimethoprim-sulphamethoxazole
Antivirals	Abacavir; Acyclovir
Anti-tumoural biotherapies	Proteasomes inhibitors (bortezomib); Tyrosine kinases inhibitors (imatinib)
Non-steroidal anti-inflammatory drugs	Diclofenac; Celecoxib; Rofecoxib
Psychotropes	Amoxapine; Clozapine; Diazepam; Lormetazepam
Miscellaneous	Azathioprine; Carbamazepine; Furosemide; Hydralazine; Isotretinoin; Lenalidomide; Oral contraceptive; Levonorgestrel/ethynil oestradiol; gestodene/ethynil oestradiol; Propylthiouracil

Drug-induced SS is uncommon. Because of the lack of useful and appropriate criteria for its diagnosis, Walker and Cohen proposed five specific diagnostic criteria in 1996 [7]. Thompson and Montarella performed a systematic review of literature on drug-induced SS and evaluated the degree of causal relationships in different case reports [4]. In our case, we used the modified Naranjo criteria to diagnose drug-induced SS [4]. The modified scale includes 10 criteria: presence of previous conclusive reports; temporary onset related to drug administration; temporary resolution of lesions after drug withdrawal or treatment with a specific antagonist; temporary recurrence of lesions due to drug readministration; presence of alternative causes (other than drugs) that could cause the reaction; appearance of lesions after placebo administration; drug detection in the blood (or other fluids) at concentrations known to be toxic; role of drug dosage in the worsening or improvement of the reaction; history of exposure to the same or similar drugs, followed by a similar reaction; and confirmation of an adverse event by any objective evidence [4]. The case reported here had a causality score of 4 based on the above criteria (Possible). This score was not higher because no rechallenge was performed due to the severity of the symptoms. There were no signs of any inflammatory disease, neoplasia, or pregnancy. To the best of our knowledge, this is the third case of SS caused by isotretinoin and the second case of SS caused by isotretinoin therapy for acne vulgaris.

The first case was reported by Gyorfy et al in 2003. They reported the cases of two children who developed SS due to isotretinoin administration. However, the children were administered this drug to prevent neuroblastoma recurrence and dysplastic colon re-emergence after bone marrow transplantation and not for acne treatment [8].

The other case of isotretinoin-induced SS was reported by Ammar et al. in 2007 in a 19-year-old man who received isotretinoin for severe acne vulgaris that was resistant to standard topical acne treatment. After one week of the treatment, the patient developed SS. His condition was improved by continuing isotretinoin and by initiating corticosteroids. However, he was diagnosed as having ulcerative colitis two years later [9].

In drug-induced SS, a pre-existing underlying condition associated with SS should be excluded. Clinical criteria can help in distinguishing drug-induced SS from underlying conditions. Based on the observation made in this case, we emphasize the importance of evaluating isotretinoin as a possible, though uncommon, cause of SS and replacing it with other treatments if its involvement is suspected.

Consent

Written informed consent was obtained from the patient for the publication of this report.

Abbreviations
SS: Sweet's syndrome; ESR: Erythrocyte sedimentation rate.

Competing interests
The authors declare that they have no competing interests.

Authors' contributions
JM and MP was managing the case.MP, DP and MA drafting the paper. JM and HH were managing the case and scientific editing of the manuscript. All authors read and approved the final manuscript.

Author details
[1]Department of Internal Medicine, School of Medicine, Semnan University of Medical Sciences, Semnan, Iran. [2]Research Center for Social Determinants of Health, Semnan University of Medical Sciences, Semnan, Iran. [3]Department of Dermatology, School of Medicine, Arak University of Medical Sciences, Arak, Iran. [4]Students' Research Committee, Semnan University of Medical Sciences, Semnan, Iran.

References
1. Cohen PR, Kurzrock R: Sweet's syndrome revisited: a review of disease concepts. *Int J Dermatol* 2003, **42**:761–778.
2. Neoh CY, Tan AWH, Ng SK: Sweet's syndrome: a spectrum of unusual clinical presentations and associations. *Br J Dermatol* 2007, **6**(3):480–485.
3. Bonamigo RR, Razera F, Olm GS: Neutrophilic dermatoses: part I. *An Bras Dermatol* 2011, **86**(1):11–25.
4. Thompson DF, Montarella KE: Drug-induced Sweet's syndrome. *Ann Pharmacother* 2007, **41**:802–811.
5. Roujeau JC: Neutrophilic drug eruptions. *Clin Dermatol* 2000, **18**:331–337.

6.   Saez M, Garcia-Bustinduy M, Noda A, Dorta S, Escoda M, Fagundo E, *et al*:
     Drug-induced Sweet's syndrome. *J Eur Acad Derm Venereol* 2004, **18**:233.
7.   Walker DC, Cohen PR: **Trimethoprim-sulfamethoxazole-associated acute
     febrile neutrophilic dermatosis: case report and review of drug-induced
     Sweet's syndrome.** *J Am Acad Dermatol* 1996, **34**:918–923.
8.   Gyorfy A, Kovács T, Szegedi I, Oláh E, Kiss C: **Sweet syndrome associated
     with 13-cis-retinoic acid (isotretinoin) therapy.** *Med Pediatr Oncol* 2003,
     40(2):135–136.
9.   Ammar D, Denguezli M, Ghariani N, Sriha B, Belajouza C, Nouira R: **Sweet's
     syndrome complicating isotretinoin therapy in acne.** *Ann Dermatol
     Venereol* 2007, **134**(2):151–154.

5

Osteogenic potential of *punica granatum* through matrix mineralization, cell cycle progression and runx2 gene expression in primary rat osteoblasts

Sahabjada Siddiqui and Mohammad Arshad[*]

Abstract

Background: Osteoporosis is one of the prevalent diseases in ageing populations. Due to side effects of many chemotherapeutic agents, there is always a need to search for herbal products to treat the disorder. *Punica granatum* (PG) represent a potent fruit-bearing medicinal herb which exerted valuable anti-osteoporotic activities. The present study was carried out to validate the *in vitro* osteogenic effects of the PG seed extract in primary calvarial osteoblast cultures harvested from neonatal rats.

Methods: The ethanolic extract of PG was subjected to evaluate cell proliferation, regeneration, mineralization and formation of collagen matrix using MTT, alkaline phosphatase, Alizarin Red-S staining and Sirius Red dye, respectively. Cell cycle progression and osteogenic gene Runx2 expression were carried out by flow cytometry and real time PCR, respectively.

Results: Exposure of different concentrations (10–100 μg/ml) of the extract on osteoblastic cells showed characteristic morphological changes and increment in cell number. A significant growth in cell proliferation, ALP activity, collagen contents and matrix mineralization of osteoblasts in a dose dependent manner ($p < 0.05$), suggested that PG has a stimulatory effect on osteoblastic bone formation or potential activity against osteoporosis. In addition, PG extract also enhanced DNA content in S phase of cell cycle and Runx2 gene expression level in osteoblasts.

Conclusion: The data clearly indicated that PG promoting bone cell proliferation and differentiation in primary osteoblasts might be due to elevating the osteogenic gene Runx2 expression. The present study provides an evidence for PG could be a promising herbal medicinal candidate that able to develop drugs for osteoporosis.

Keywords: Cell cycle, Osteoblast, Osteogenesis, *Punica granatum*, Runx2

Introduction

Osteoporosis is a metabolic bone disorders that afflicts about 200 million people worldwide. It is mainly prevalent in women (approximately 80%) and also older men [1]. The bone remodeling process is the alternative of this severe concern, and it's dependable for repair of damage or formation and resorption of bones to maintain the integrity of the skeleton. However, any abnormalities in remodeling that lead to fracture in the bones and osteoporosis.

Recently, several conventional and antiresorptive drugs are used to reduce fracture risk in osteoporosis including hormone replacement therapy (HRT), bisphosphonates,

selective estrogen receptor modulators (SERMs) and calcitonin [2]. However, these drugs and therapy have multiple side effects, which causes heart related issues, headache, dizziness, anorexia, cramping of legs and gastrointestinal related problem, particularly pain in stomach and heartburn [3]. The research still continues for the enhancement of such benefit to lower risk involved in human beings.

Anabolic or osteogenic therapies are preferred for pharmacological development to treat osteoporosis [4]. Parathyroid hormone (PTH 1–34) only anabolic agent for the treatment of postmenopausal osteoporosis that is also recommended by the FDA (Food and Drug Administration) which regulates the formation of bones by enhancing the cell proliferation of the osteoblastic lineage or inducing differentiation of osteoblast progenitor cells.

* Correspondence: molendolab@gmail.com
Molecular Endocrinology Laboratory, Department of Zoology, University of Lucknow, Lucknow 226007, India

Whilst, this therapy is also related to an increased risk of cancer, such as osteosarcoma [5,6].

In the recent time, several medicinal plants are used for health care treatments and management especially bone related diseases. Although compared with other drug treatments, herbal products create no/little side effects. *Punica granatum* (Pomegranate, PG) is one of the most potent fruit-bearing medicinal herbs widely distributed throughout the Mediterranean region of southern Europe, northern Africa and tropical Africa, Indian subcontinent, Central Asia and the drier parts of South-East Asia. PG seeds contain punicic acid, ellagic acid, steroidal estrogen and non-steroidal phytoestrogens, including comesten, coumoestrol and isoflavones genistein, daidzein and ascorbic acids. PG also contains estrogenic compound such as luteolin, quercetin, kaempferol, estrone and estradiol, which are responsible for bone formation and also inhibit the resorption process [7-12]. A non-isoflavone phytoestrogenic compounds such as quercetin, rutin, apigenin and coumestrol has also been reported in various legumes [13]. A crude PG extract and its seed oil enhance bone healing properties and prevent loss of bones because of the proliferation of osteoblast, inhibition of osteoclast cell and also decrease the inflammation. [14,15]. Recently, PG has been also utilized to inhibit acetyl cholinesterase activity as a new source for management of Alzheimer's disease [16].

Osteoblast differentiation and proliferation mediated by different growth factors such as bone morphogenetic proteins (BMPs), transforming growth factor beta (TGFβ) and core-binding factor alpha1 (Cbfα1) are known to be targeted the osteogenic Runt-related transcription factor2 (Runx2) gene [17]. Runx2 is the key transcription factor initiating and regulating the early osteogenesis and late mineralization of bone. Furthermore, Runx2 triggers the expression of major bone matrix genes during the early stages of osteoblast differentiation [18].

There is no evidence regarding the investigation of the PG seed extract on bone cell proliferation, differentiation, and collagen matrix formation in primary culture of osteoblasts. The present study also described the matrix mineralization activity along with osteogenic gene Runx2 expression by real time PCR and DNA content analysis in the S phase of the cell cycle in osteoblastic cells. The findings suggested that PG may be a potent osteogenic herbal drug that induces bone cells proliferation and regeneration following increased DNA contents and Runx2 gene expression which provide future prospects in the development of anti-osteoporotic drugs and therapy.

Materials and methods
Reagents and chemicals
Alpha modified minimum essential medium (α-MEM), fetal bovine serum (FBS), MTT (3-(4,5-dimethylthiazol-2-yl) -2,5-diphenyltetrazolium bromide) dye, *p*-nitrophenyl phosphate (pNPP), naphthol ASMX phosphate, fast blue BB salt, ascorbic acid and Sirius Red dye were purchased from Himedia, India. β-glycerophosphate, Ribonuclease (RNase) A and propidium iodide (PI) were purchased from Sigma-Aldrich, USA. RNAiso Plus reagent was procured from Takara, India. cDNA synthesis kit was purchased from Thermo Scientific, USA and SYBER green kit from Roche, USA. All the reagents used were of high purity grade.

Plant materials and extraction
The fresh cultivated PG plant was collected from nearby University of Lucknow, Lucknow, India. Plant materials were identified and authenticated from Department of Pharmacognosy, Faculty of Pharmacy, Integral University, Lucknow. A reference specimen (voucher No. IU/PHAR/HRB/14/08) has been deposited in the herbarium of Faculty of Pharmacy, Integral University, Lucknow. Seed parts of collecting plant were air dried in the shade and crushed to a powder in a mechanical grinder. The 95% ethanolic extract of PG was prepared with the help of Soxhlet apparatus (Borosil Glass Works Limited, India) at 60°C and Whatman No. 1 filter paper was used to obtain filtrate of extract. The filtrate was concentrated in vacuum at 40°C using a rotary evaporator (BUCHI Rotavapor R-205, Switzerland).

Primary culture of osteoblasts
Osteoblastic cells were isolated from neonatal rat pups calvaria using sequential digestion with slight modification [19]. Briefly, calvaria were dissected from four to five neonatal (1–2 days old) rat pups. After removal of sutures and adherent mesenchymal tissues, calvaria were subjected to five sequential (10–15 min) digestions at 37°C in shaking water bath at 120 rpm containing each of 0.1% dispase and collagenase type II enzymes. Supernatants were pooled from the second to fifth digestions in a tube containing 800 μl FBS. Cells were re-suspended in α-MEM containing 10% FBS with 1% penicillin/streptomycin solution and transfer in T-25 cm^2 culture flasks. The flasks were incubated at 37°C with 5% CO_2 in CO_2 incubator (Excella ECO-170, New Brunswick). The study was approved by the Institutional Animal Ethics Committee of Azad Institute of Pharmacy and Research, Lucknow (Ref. No.: AIPR/2013-14/1398).

Cell proliferation
The proliferative effect of PG extract was determined using MTT assay with some modification [20]. Calvarial osteoblasts were suspended in α-MEM medium and plated at a density of 2×10^3 cells/well in a 96 wells plate. After overnight incubation, the medium was replaced with a medium containing PG extract solution prepared in media with

different concentrations (0, 10, 25, 50 and 100 µg/ml) in triplicate for 48 h. 17β-estradiol (E2) at the concentration of 1 nM was used as a positive control. After exposure period, 10 µl of 5 mg/ml MTT solution was added to each wells and further incubated at 37°C. After 4 h, medium was discarded and 100 µl of dimethyl sulphoxide (DMSO) was added to solubilise the dark blue formazan crystals at 37°C for 10 min. Absorbance was recorded at 540 nm with microplate reader (BIORAD-680, USA) and the percentage viable cells were calculated using the formula:

$$\% \, \text{Cell viability} = [(\text{OD of treated}) / (\text{OD of control})] \times 100$$

The cellular morphology was also observed in other sets of PG treatment under trinocular inverted phase contrast microscopy (Nikon ECLIPSE Ti-S, Japan).

Alkaline phosphatase (ALP) activity

ALP assay is based on the hydrolysis of pNPP by ALP into a yellow colored product at alkaline pH. ALP activity of osteoblasts was determined with a slight modification [21]. A 100 µl of cell suspension containing 2×10^3 cells /well was seeded in 96-well plates using α-MEM supplemented with 10% FBS, 10 mM β-glycerophosphate, 50 µg/ ml ascorbic acid and 1% penicillin/streptomycin (osteoblast differentiation medium) and treated with different concentrations (10–100 µg/ml) of the extract for 48 h. E2 at the concentration of 1 nM was used as a positive control. After completion of incubation period, osteoblast cultures were fixed in 4% paraformaldehyde and stained with a solution containing 0.1 mg/ml naphthol ASMX phosphate, 0.5% N, N- dimethylformamide, 2 mM MgCl2, and 0.6 mg/ml of fast blue BB salt in 0.1 mM Tris–HCl (pH 8.5) for 20 min. The formation of color was examined and images were taken under an inverted phase contrast microscope. For the quantitative estimation of ALP, the plate was fixed and kept in –70°C for 20 min, and then brought to 37°C for freeze fracture. Next, 50 µl of chilled *p*-nitrophenyl phosphate (pNPP) substrate was added to each wells and incubated at 37°C for 30 min for color development. The absorbance was measured at 405 nM using an ELISA reader.

Assessment of collagen deposition

Sirius Red is an anionic dye that binds strongly to collagen molecules. Collagen deposition was quantified using Sirius Red dye following slightly modification [22]. Treated cells were washed with PBS and dried at 37°C in 96-wells plate for overnight incubation and then stained with 20 µl of Sirius Red dye (0.1% in saturated picric acid) for 1 h with mild shaking. Sirius Red dye solution (pH 3.5) was prepared in saturated aqueous picric acid (1.3% in H_2O) at a concentration of 0.1 mg/ml. The stained cell layers were extensively washed with 0.01 N HCl to remove all non-

bounded dye. After rinsing, photographs were taken under inverted phase contrast microscope. For quantitative analysis, the stained cells were dissolved in 0.2 ml 0.1 N NaOH at shaker for 30 min. Next, absorbance was measured colorimetrically at 550 nm against 0.1 N NaOH serve as a blank.

Mineralization assay

Alizarin Red S, an anthraquinone derivative, was used to identify calcium content in osteoblasts according to a method reported previously [23]. Approximately, 2×10^4 cells/well were seeded in 12-wells culture plate in osteoblast differentiation medium with 10^{-7} M dexamethasone. Cells were treated with PG extract at various concentrations (10–100 µg/ml) for 21 days and the medium was changed every alternate day. At the end of the experiment, cells were washed with PBS and fixed with 4% paraformaldehyde in PBS for 15 min. The fixed cells were stained with 40 mM Alizarin Red-S (pH 4.5) for 30 min followed by washing with distilled water. Calcified nodules appearing as bright red color were photographed under inverted phase contrast microscopy. For quantification of staining, 100 mM cetylpyridinium chloride solution was added for 1 h in each well to solubilise and to release calciumbound alizarin red into solution. A 100 µl of the supernatant from each well were transferred in 96 well plate in triplicate and the absorbance was recorded at 570 nm by a microplate reader.

Cellular DNA content

Cell cycle phase distribution with cellular DNA content was analyzed using flow cytometry with some modification [24]. Osteoblasts were planted in 6-wells plate at a density 1×10^6 cells/well and treated with different concentrations (10–100 µg/ml) of extract for 48 h. E2 at the concentration of 10 nM was used as a positive control. Cultured cells were washed with cold PBS and fixed in 70% ethanol at −20°C for 2 h. Fixed cells were treated with RNase A (10 mg/ml) and stained with PI dye in the dark for 30 min at room temperature. The PI dye fluorescence of individual nuclei was measured by using a flow cytometer (BD FACS Calibur, Becton Dickinson, USA) and data were analyzed using Cell Quest Pro V 3.2.1 software (Becton Dickinson, USA).

Quantitative real-time PCR (qPCR)

The total RNA was isolated from cultured osteoblasts treated with PG extract using RNAiso Plus reagent. Aliquots of 2.0 µg of total RNA in a 10 µl reaction volume were subjected to PCR using a cDNA synthesis kit. Quantitative real-time PCR was performed in light cycler PCR system (LightCycler 480, Roche, USA) using SYBER green kit following manufacturer's instruction. Runx2 gene expression in calvarial osteoblasts was determined by qPCR using an optimized protocol [25]. Sequence of primer pairs of the genes used in the present study were; runx2- CCACAGAGCTATTAAAGTGACAGTG (F), AACAAACTAGGTTTAGAGTCATCAAGC (R) and GAPDH (housekeeping gene) - CAGCAAGGATACTGA GAGCAAGAG (F), GGATGGAATTGTGAGGGAGATG (R). All the data were normalized to GAPDH expression to study the relative expression of the targeted gene.

Statistics

All results were represented as the means ± SEM of results from all replicates and statistically significance was determined by one-way analysis of variance (ANOVA) followed by Dunnett's multiple comparison tests. Probability values of $p < 0.05$ were considered to be statistically significant. All analysis was conducted using the Graph Pad Prism (Ver. 5.1) software.

Results and discussion

Microscopic observation of osteoblastic cells

The morphological changes of untreated (control) and treated osteoblasts with different concentrations of PG extract at 48 h are shown in Figure 1A. The typical spindle shaped with fibroblastic appearance was observed in control under inverted phase contrast microscope. The concentrations 10 and 25 µg/ml of extract enhanced the cell proliferation, moreover, 50 and 100 µg/ml of PG showed the more dense appearance with increased number of cells as compared to control that attributed differentiation of osteoblastic cells. The results revealed that cells exposed to PG extract induce differentiation of osteoblasts as a function of dose due to their morphological alterations and number of cells increment [26].

Effect of PG on the cell proliferation of osteoblasts

The effect of different doses (10–100 µg/ml) of PG extract on osteoblastic cell proliferation was tested at 48 h (Figure 1B). As compared to control group (cells without extract treatment), PG significantly increased the cell proliferation to 13.03 ($p < 0.05$) and 24.28% ($p < 0.001$) at 10 and 25 µg/ml, respectively. Moreover, 50 and 100 µg/ml of PG extract induced cell proliferation to 39.64 and 62.59% ($p < 0.001$) respectively. The results revealed that PG extract induced the significant cell proliferation in a dose dependent manner. Exposure of cells to 1 nM of 17β-estradiol as a positive control, increased the cell proliferation to 41.72% ($p < 0.001$) as compared to control. The proliferative effects of PG extract might be due to their estrogenic nature of its contents, including quercetin, kaempferol, estrone and estradiol, which promote bone cell proliferation [11]. A study has shown that PG promoted osteoblast MC3T3-E1 cell proliferation up to approximately 2-fold at 250 µg/ml of plant extracts [7]. Both osteoblast and MCF-7 (human breast adenocarcinoma) cells are an estrogen receptor positive (ER$^+$) cells. A similar study has also revealed that MCF-7 cells exposed to legume extracts containing quercetin, daidzein, genistein and kaempferol glycosides at various concentrations (1–1000 µg/ml) showed a maximum cell proliferation at 100 µg/ml of the extracts [27].

Effect of PG on ALP activity of osteoblasts

Quantitative estimation of alkaline phosphatase activity is one of the biochemical methods, which described the early cell differentiation of osteoblastic cells [28]. Fast blue BB salt-ASMX-phosphate complex acted on ALP activity which appeared to be blue in color. The qualitative data showed that PG extract stimulated ALP stain by increasing the rate of osteoblast cell differentiation in a dose dependent manner (Figure 2A). As observed from numerical data (Figure 2B), concentrations 10 and 25 µg/ml of extract induced ALP level to 9.66% ($p < 0.05$) and 22.49% ($p < 0.01$) significantly as compared to control. Also, 50 and 100 µg/ml of extract induced the significant ALP level to 34.67 and 43.95% ($p < 0.01$) respectively as compared to control. Exposure of cells to 1 nM of E2 increased ALP activity to 36.66% ($p < 0.01$) as compared to control. Results of ALP assay were the consistent with

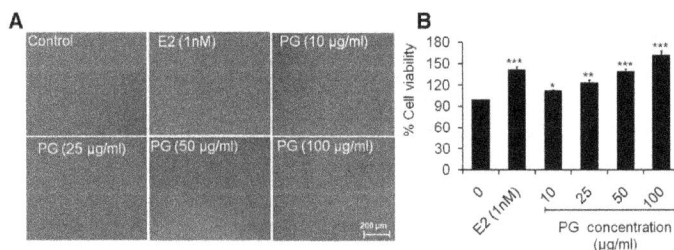

Figure 1 Percent cell proliferation of primary osteoblasts. (A) Morphology of osteoblasts under inverted phase contrast microscope treated with different concentrations of PG extract at 48 h **(B)** Percent cell proliferation of osteoblasts treated with 10–100 µg/ml of PG extract. Values were obtained from three independent experiments and expressed as mean ± SEM. $^*p < 0.05$, $^{**}p < 0.01$ and $^{***}p < 0.001$ as compared with control.

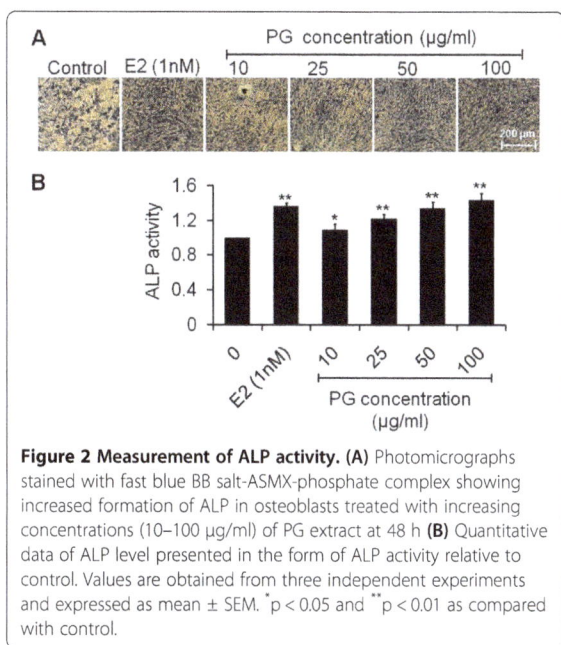

Figure 2 Measurement of ALP activity. (A) Photomicrographs stained with fast blue BB salt-ASMX-phosphate complex showing increased formation of ALP in osteoblasts treated with increasing concentrations (10–100 µg/ml) of PG extract at 48 h **(B)** Quantitative data of ALP level presented in the form of ALP activity relative to control. Values are obtained from three independent experiments and expressed as mean ± SEM. *p < 0.05 and **p < 0.01 as compared with control.

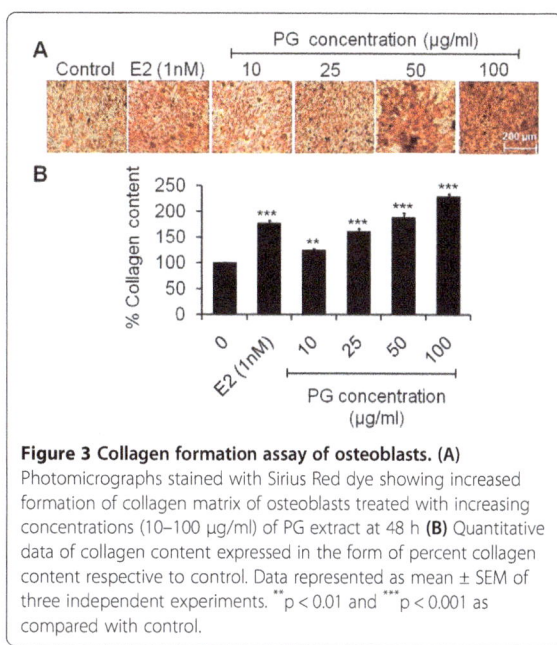

Figure 3 Collagen formation assay of osteoblasts. (A) Photomicrographs stained with Sirius Red dye showing increased formation of collagen matrix of osteoblasts treated with increasing concentrations (10–100 µg/ml) of PG extract at 48 h **(B)** Quantitative data of collagen content expressed in the form of percent collagen content respective to control. Data represented as mean ± SEM of three independent experiments. **p < 0.01 and ***p < 0.001 as compared with control.

MTT assay data which suggested that cell proliferation also correlate with cell differentiation. These results indicate that PG extract induces regeneration of osteoblasts as a function of dose might be due to the presence of estrogenic compounds. PG containing estrogenic compounds daidzein and genistein has been reported to possess stimulatory effects synthesizing alkaline phosphatase by osteoblasts *in vitro* [29].

Effect of PG on collagen deposition by osteoblasts

Sirius Red stain was used to assess the extent of collagen (predominantly collagen type I and III fibers) deposited by osteoblasts which developed dense and cross-linked collagen. Collagen comprises 85-90% of the total organic bone matrix [30]. Histological analysis showed that PG extract increases collagen content in osteoblasts in a dose dependent manner as compared to control. PG extract exposed on cells was able to enhance in the collagen density significantly as evident by dark red clusters of collagen evenly distributed throughout the stimulated region (Figure 3A). Further, quantitative measurement of the Sirius Red staining intensity in osteoblasts culture showed a significant increment of 24.96 (p < 0.01), 62.40, 89.37 and 129.84% (p < 0.001) of collagen secretion at 10, 25, 50 and 100 µg/ml of PG exposure, respectively as compared to control (Figure 3B). Exposure of osteoblasts to 1 nM of E2 increased the collagen content to only 77.95% (p < 0.001) as compared to control. Bone shows a variety of structural organizations which is related to the balance between the amount of collagen

and mineral [31]. However, not only mineral matrix deposition is essential to ensure a healthy bone, giving strength and rigidity in the skeletal system, but also the adequate deposition of organic matrix (collagen) contributes to bone architecture. Therefore, experiments were conducted to determine whether PG extract exposure enhances the organic matrix deposition. PG treated osteoblasts progressively deposited more collagen (Figure 3A and B) suggesting the collagen deposition induced by PG is a function of dose. A study has reported that ascorbic acid stimulates the formation of collagen matrix at multiple levels, including gene expression, hydroxylation of proline and lysine in collagen during post-translational modification [32].

Effect of PG on osteoblast mineralization

Mineralized nodule formation describes the final stages of osteoblastic differentiation at 21 days. As observed from photomicrographs, osteoblastic cells in proliferation period exhibited a fibroblastic morphology monolayer in control cells. As the progress in mineralization, the cells continued growing slowly and formed a mosaic like multiple layers which was greater at 100 µg/ml of PG extract (Figure 4A). The percent calcification data of Alizarin stain showed that treatment of osteoblasts at 10, 25, 50 and 100 µg/ml of extract significantly increased mineralized nodule formation that signifying by 26.15 (p < 0.01), 44.55, 65.64 and 82.81% (p < 0.001), respectively as compared to control (Figure 4B). Exposure of

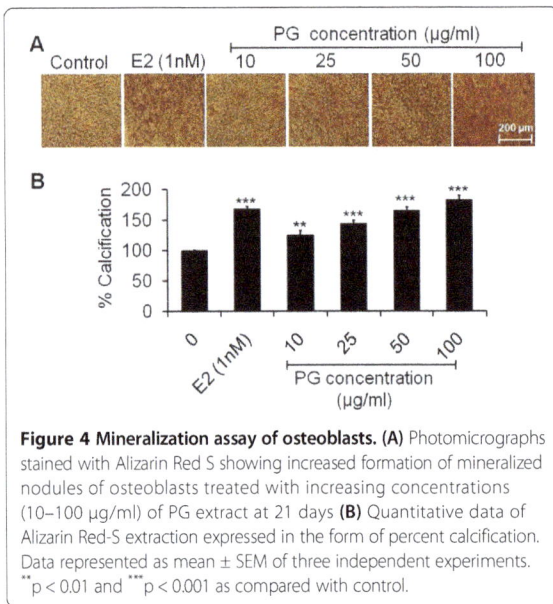

Figure 4 Mineralization assay of osteoblasts. (A) Photomicrographs stained with Alizarin Red S showing increased formation of mineralized nodules of osteoblasts treated with increasing concentrations (10–100 µg/ml) of PG extract at 21 days **(B)** Quantitative data of Alizarin Red-S extraction expressed in the form of percent calcification. Data represented as mean ± SEM of three independent experiments. $^{**}p < 0.01$ and $^{***}p < 0.001$ as compared with control.

Effect of PG on cellular DNA content and cell cycle distribution of osteoblasts

The cellular DNA content and proportion of cells in different phases of the cell cycle was analyzed by using flow cytometry. Osteoblastic cells were treated with one lower (25 µg/ml) and one higher concentration (100 µg/ml) of the PG extract for 48 h and observed the different phases of the cell cycle. As evident from the results (Figure 5), a normal distribution of cell cycle was observed in the control group. At 25 µg/ml of PG extract, the accumulation of cells (DNA content) in S phase was sharply increased from 12.67 to 31.54% as compared to control. Moreover, 100 µg/ml concentration of the extract resulted to an incredible increment of DNA content in S phase by 78.72% as compared to control. Exposure of osteoblasts to 1 nM of E2 increased the DNA content in S phase by 44.08% greater at 25 µg/ml of PG treatment. These data indicate that the PG extract induce the cell proliferation by accumulating the DNA content in S phase of the cell cycle. A similar study has reported that estradiol induced the expression of estrogen receptor by promoting S phase of cell cycle in human osteosarcoma cell lines and pilose antler polypeptides promoted chondrocytes proliferation by accelerating cell cycle progression in S phase [35,24].

Effect of PG on osteogenic gene runx2 expression

To determine these results could be extended to another protein present in the organic bone matrix and effect of PG on the expression of Runx2 gene. Runx2 is a noncollagenous, highly conserved transcription factor involved in the regulation of mineralized matrix of bone. Increased expression of osteogenic gene was observed by qPCR in osteoblasts treated with PG extract at 48 h. As cleared from results (Figure 6), 10 µg/ml of PG extract significantly elevated the Runx2 expression as compared to

osteoblasts to 1 nM of E2 increased the mineralization content to 68.85% (p < 0.001) as compared to control. Increased mineralization is synonymous to increased calcium deposition. The ability to form an extracellular matrix that can undergo regulated mineralization is the ultimate phenotypic expression of an osteogenic tissue [33]. PG treatment increased the calcium content notably in the mineralized matrix at 21 days of osteoblasts when compared with untreated cells. In this context, the phytoestrogen genistein has been previously found to stimulate bone mineralization *in vitro* [34].

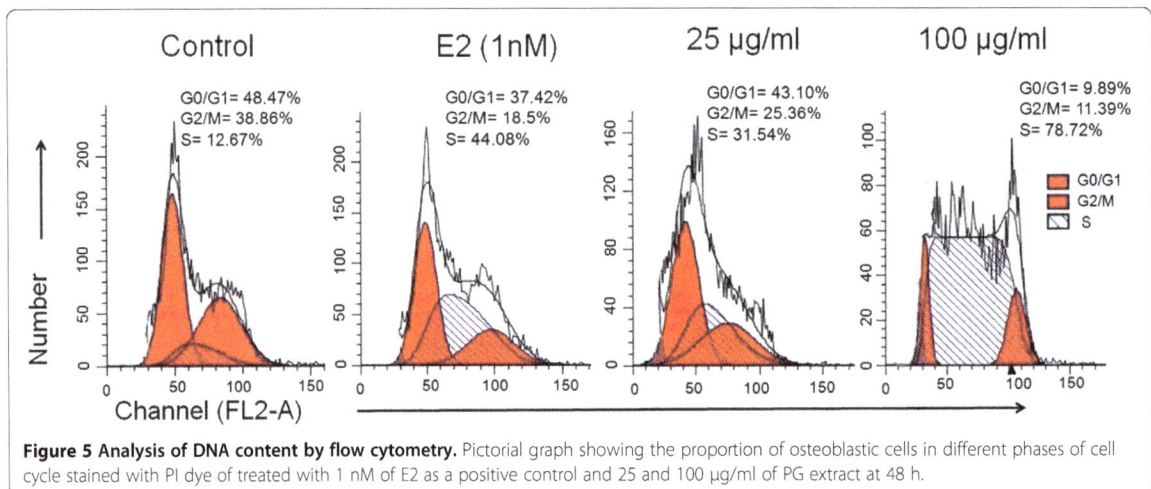

Figure 5 Analysis of DNA content by flow cytometry. Pictorial graph showing the proportion of osteoblastic cells in different phases of cell cycle stained with PI dye of treated with 1 nM of E2 as a positive control and 25 and 100 µg/ml of PG extract at 48 h.

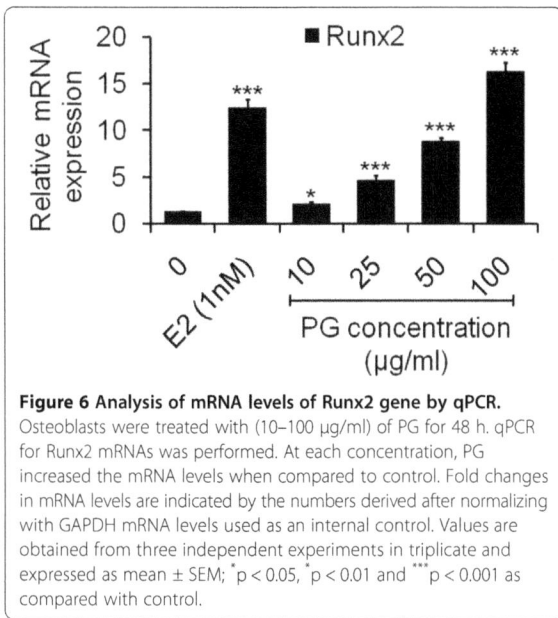

Figure 6 Analysis of mRNA levels of Runx2 gene by qPCR.
Osteoblasts were treated with (10–100 µg/ml) of PG for 48 h. qPCR for Runx2 mRNAs was performed. At each concentration, PG increased the mRNA levels when compared to control. Fold changes in mRNA levels are indicated by the numbers derived after normalizing with GAPDH mRNA levels used as an internal control. Values are obtained from three independent experiments in triplicate and expressed as mean ± SEM; $^*p < 0.05$, $^{**}p < 0.01$ and $^{***}p < 0.001$ as compared with control.

control ($p < 0.05$). Moreover, concentrations 25, 50 and 100 µg/ml of PG increased the remarkable Runx2 level in a dose dependent manner ($p < 0.001$) as compared to control. It has been reported that Runx2 bonds to the osteoblast specific cis acting element which is found in the promoter region of all major osteoblast specific genes like osteocalcin, type-I collagen, BSP, OPN, ALP and control their expression [36]. Hence, it is reasonable to speculate that the estrogenic compounds such as β-sitosterol present in PG could have acted in a manner to induce mRNA expression of ALP, collagen and their protein levels and consequently increased Runx2 gene expression in osteoblastic cells. Furthermore, flavonoids have also been shown to increase the expression of Runx2 [37,38]. Thus, β-sitosterol and flavonoids present in PG might be responsible for the increased expression and transcriptional activity of Runx2.

Conclusion

The present study showed that osteogenic potential of PG extract in primary calvaria osteoblasts is based on two salient features. (1) Cytochemical studies including cell proliferation, ALP stain, collagenation, matrix mineralization and DNA content in the S phase of the cell cycle in osteoblasts are the key parameters, which favor the osteogenic potential of PG. (2) A molecular marker Runx2 is a highly conserved osteogenic transcription factor involved in the regulation of bone cells proliferation and differentiation, which is also favors the osteogenic nature of PG.

Even though E2 used as a positive control shows the slightly higher effect on the proliferation, differentiation, collagenation, mineralization, DNA content and Runx2 gene expression of osteoblasts than lower doses, however, the side effects of the long-term use of estrogen, such as a higher incidence of endometrial cancer, cardiovascular disease and breast carcinoma, could not be ignored.

Thus, the results from this study suggest that PG promotes the function of osteoblasts and plays an important role in remodeling of the bone, which indicated that it may be one of anti-osteoporotic herbal candidate free from side effects. Accordingly, PG might be useful for alternative pharmacological agent of osteoporosis and skeletal tissues may benefit from the consumption of PG.

Abbreviations

ALP: Alkaline phosphatase; α-MEM: Alpha modified minimum essential medium; E2: 17β-estradiol; BMPs: Bone morphogenetic proteins; Cbfα1: Core-binding factor alpha-1; DMSO: Dimethyl sulfoxide; ELISA: Enzyme linked immunosorbent assay; FBS: Fetal bovine serum; FDA: Food and drug administration; HRT: Hormone replacement therapy; MTT: (3-(4,5-dimethylthiazol-2-yl)-2,5-diphenyltetrazolium bromide); PBS: Phosphate buffered saline; PG: *Punica granatum*; pNPP: *p*-nitrophenyl phosphate; PTH: Parathyroid hormone; PI: Propidium iodide; qPCR: Quantitative real-time PCR; Runx2: Runt-related transcription factor 2; SEM: Standard error mean; SERMs: Selective estrogen receptor modulators; TGFβ: Transforming growth factors.

Competing interests

The authors declare that they have no competing interests.

Authors' contributions

SS and MA participated in the design of the study. SS performed the experimental work and data interpretation. SS and MA involved in review of the paper. Both authors read and approved the final version of the manuscript.

Authors' information

Sahabjada Siddiqui, M.Sc. in Biotechnology; Md Arshad, Ph.D. in Endocrinology, CDRI, Lucknow and Assistant Professor at University of Lucknow.

Acknowledgments

Authors are thankful to UGC Major Research Project File No. 37-436/2009 (SR), New Delhi, India for financial support. Author Sahabjada Siddiqui is thankful to ICMR, New Delhi, India for the award of Senior Research Fellowship (No. 45/26/2013/BMS/TRM). Authors are thankful to the Director, Azad Institute of Pharmacy and Research, Lucknow for providing research facilities for animal experiment.

References

1. Kaunitz AM, Mcclung MR, Feldman RG: Post menopausal osteoporosis: fracture risk and prevention. *J Fam Pract* 2009, **58**:S1–S6.
2. Maclaughlin EJ, Sleeper RB, McNatty D, Raehl CL: Management of age-related osteoporosis and prevention of associated fractures. *Ther Clin Risk Manag* 2006, **2**:281–295.
3. Rizzoli R, Reginster JY, Boonen S, Bréart G, Diez-Perez A, Felsenberg D, Kaufman JM, Kanis JA, Cooper C: Adverse reactions and drug-drug interactions in the management of women with postmenopausal osteoporosis. *Calcif Tissue Int* 2011, **89**:91–104.
4. Dixit P, Khan MP, Swarnkar G, Chattopadhyay N, Maurya R: Osteogenic constituents from *pterospermum acerifolium* willd. Flowers. *Bioorg Med Chem Lett* 2011, **21**:4617–4621.

5. John MR, Arai M, Rubin DA, Jonsson KB, Jüppner H: Identification and characterization of the murine and human gene encoding the tuberoinfundibular peptide of 39 residues. Endocrinology 2002, 143:1047–1057.

6. Wang W, Olson D, Cheng B, Guo X, Wang K: Sanguis Draconis resin stimulates osteoblast alkaline phosphatase activity and mineralization in MC3T3-E1 cells. J Ethnopharmacol 2012, 142:168–174.

7. Kim YH, Choi EM: Stimulation of osteoblastic differentiation and inhibition of interleukin-6 and nitric oxide in MC3T3-E1 cells by pomegranate ethanol extract. Phytother Res 2009, 23:737–739.

8. van Elswijk DA, Schobel UP, Lansky EP, Irth H, van der Greef J: Rapid dereplication of estrogenic compounds in pomegranate (punica granatum) using on-line biochemical detection coupled to mass spectrometry. Phytochemistry 2004, 65:233–241.

9. Trivedi R, Kumar A, Gupta V, Kumar S, Nagar GK, Romero JR, Dwivedi AK, Chattopadhyay N: Effects of Egb 761 on bone mineral density, bone microstructure, and osteoblast function: Possible roles of quercetin and kaempferol. Mol Cell Endocrinol 2009, 302:86–91.

10. Heftmann E, Ko ST, Bennett RD: Identification of estrone in pomegranate seeds. Phytochemistry 1966, 5:1337–1339.

11. Jurenka J: Therapeutic applications of pomegranate (punica granatum L.): a review. Alterm Med Rev 2008, 13:128–144.

12. Pérez-Vicente A, Gil-Izquierdo A, García-Viguera C: In vitro gastrointestinal digestion study of pomegranate juice phenolic compounds, anthocyanins, and vitamin C. J Agric Food Chem 2002, 50:2308–2312.

13. Konar N: Non-isoflavone phytoestrogenic compound contents of various legumes. Eur Food Res Technol 2013, 236:523–530.

14. Spilmont M, Léotoing L, Davicco MJ, Lebecque P, Mercier S, Miot-Noirault E, Pilet P, Rios L, Wittrant Y, Coxam V: Pomegranate seed oil prevents bone loss in a mice model of osteoporosis, through osteoblastic stimulation, osteoclastic inhibition and decreased inflammatory status. J Nutr Biochem 2013, 24:1840–1848.

15. Mori-Okamoto J, Otawara-Hamamoto Y, Yamato H, Yoshimura H: Pomegranate extract improves a depressive state and bone properties in menopausal syndrome model ovariectomized mice. J Ethnopharmacol 2004, 92:93–101.

16. Jazayeri SB, Amanlou A, Ghanadian N, Pasalar P, Amanlou M: A preliminary investigation of anticholinesterase activity of some Iranian medicinal plants commonly used in traditional medicine. Daru 2014, 22:17.

17. Yamaguchi A, Komori T, Suda T: Regulation of osteoblast differentiation mediated by bone morphogenetic proteins, hedgehogs, and Cbfa1. Endocr Rev 2000, 21:393–411.

18. Komori T: Regulation of osteoblast differentiation by Runx2. Adv Exp Med Biol 2010, 658:43–49.

19. Orriss IR, Taylor SE, Arnett TR: Rat osteoblast cultures. Methods Mol Biol 2012, 816:31–41.

20. Ashfaq M, Singh S, Sharma A, Verma N: Cytotoxic evaluation of the hierarchal web of carbon micro-nanofibers. Ind Eng Chem Res 2013, 52:4672–4682.

21. Moutahir-Belqasmi F, Balmain N, Lieberrher M, Borzeix S, Berland S, Barthelemy M, Peduzzi J, Milet C, Lopez E: Effect of water soluble extract of nacre (pinctada maxima) on alkaline phosphatase activity and Bcl-2 expression in primary cultured osteoblasts from neonatal rat calvaria. J Mater Sci Mater Med 2001, 12:1–6.

22. Tullberg-Reinert H, Jundt G: In situ measurement of collagen synthesis by human bone cells with a sirius red-based colorimetric microassay: effects of transforming growth factor beta2 and ascorbic acid 2-phosphate. Histochem Cell Biol 1999, 112:271–276.

23. Weivoda MM, Hohl RJ: Effects of farnesyl pyrophosphate accumulation on calvarial osteoblast differentiation. Endocrinology 2011, 152:3113–3122.

24. Lin JH, Deng LX, Wu ZY, Chen L, Zhang L: Pilose antler polypeptides promote chondrocyte proliferation via the tyrosine kinase signaling pathway. J Occup Med Toxicol 2011, 6:27.

25. Dixit P, Chand K, Khan MP, Siddiqui JA, Tewari D, Ngueguim FT, Chattopadhyay N, Maurya R: Phytoceramides and acylated phytosterol glucosides from pterospermum acerifolium willd. Seed coat and their osteogenic activity. Phytochemistry 2012, 81:117–125.

26. Abiramasundari G, Sumalatha KR, Sreepriya M: Effects of tinospora cordifolia (menispermaceae) on the proliferation, osteogenic differentiation and mineralization of osteoblast model systems in vitro. J Ethnopharmacol 2012, 141:474–480.

27. Zhao QW, Li B, Weber N, Lou YJ: Estrogen-like effects of ethanol extracts from several Chinese legumes on MCF-7 cell. Eur Food Res Technol 2005, 221:828–833.

28. Bhargavan B, Gautam AK, Singh D, Kumar A, Chaurasia S, Tyagi AM, Yadav DK, Mishra JS, Singh AB, Sanyal S, Goel A, Maurya R, Chattopadhyay N: Methoxylated isoflavones, cajanin and isoformononetin, have non-estrogenic bone forming effect via differential mitogen activated protein kinase (MAPK) signalling. J Cell Biochem 2009, 108:388–399.

29. Sugimoto E, Yamaguchi M: Stimulatory effect of daidzein in osteoblastic MC3T3-E1 cells. Biochem Pharmacol 2000, 259:471–475.

30. Sasano Y, Li HC, Zhu JX, Imanaka-Yoshida K, Mizoguchi I, Kagayama M: Immunohistochemical localization of type I collagen, fibronectin and tenascin C during embryonic osteogenesis in the dentary of mandibles and tibias in rats. Histochem J 2000, 32:591–598.

31. Landis WJ: The strength of a calcified tissue depends in part on the molecular structure and organization of its constituent mineral crystals in their organic matrix. Bone 1995, 16:533–544.

32. Franceschi RT, Iyer BS, Cui Y: Effects of ascorbic acid on collagen matrix formation and osteoblast differentiation in murine MC3T3-E1 cells. J Bone Miner Res 1994, 9:843–854.

33. Muthusami S, Senthilkumar K, Vignesh C, Ilangovan R, Stanley J, Selvamurugan N, Srinivasan N: Effects of cissus quadrangularis on the proliferation, differentiation and matrix mineralization of human osteoblast like SaOS-2 cells. J Cell Bioch 2011, 112:1035–1045.

34. Morris C, Thorpe J, Ambrosio L, Santin M: The soybean isoflavone genistein induces differentiation of MG63 human osteosarcoma osteoblasts. J Nutr 2006, 136:1166–1170.

35. Ikegami A, Inoue S, Hosoi T, Kaneki M, Mizuno Y, Akedo Y, Ouchi Y, Orimo H: Cell cycle-dependent expression of estrogen receptor and effect of estrogen on proliferation of synchronized human osteoblast-like osteosarcoma cells. Endocrinology 1994, 135:782–789.

36. Ducy P, Starbuck M, Priemel M, Shen J, Pinero G, Geoffroy V, Amling M, Karsenty G: A Cbfa1-dependent genetic pathway controls bone formation beyond embryonic development. Genes Dev 1999, 13:1025–1036.

37. Chen CH, Ho ML, Chang JK, Hung SH, Wang GJ: Green tea catechin enhances osteogenesis in a bone marrow mesenchymal stem cell line. Osteoporos Int 2005, 16:2039–2045.

38. Qian G, Zhang X, Lu L, Wu X, Li S, Meng J: Regulation of Cbfa1 expression by total flavonoids of Herba epimedii. Endocr J 2006, 53:87–94.

6

Modified Gadonanotubes as a promising novel MRI contrasting agent

Rouzbeh Jahanbakhsh[1], Fatemeh Atyabi[1,2*], Saeed Shanehsazzadeh[3], Zahra Sobhani[1], Mohsen Adeli[4,5] and Rassoul Dinarvand[1,2]

Abstract

Background and purpose of the study: Carbon nanotubes (CNTs) are emerging drug and imaging carrier systems which show significant versatility. One of the extraordinary characteristics of CNTs as Magnetic Resonance Imaging (MRI) contrasting agent is the extremely large proton relaxivities when loaded with gadolinium ion (Gd_n^{3+}) clusters.

Methods: In this study equated Gd_n^{3+} clusters were loaded in the sidewall defects of oxidized multiwalled (MW) CNTs. The amount of loaded gadolinium ion into the MWCNTs was quantified by inductively coupled plasma (ICP) method. To improve water solubility and biocompatibility of the system, the complexes were functionalized using diamine-terminated oligomeric poly (ethylene glycol) via a thermal reaction method.

Results: Gd_n^{3+} loaded PEGylated oxidized CNTs (Gd_n^{3+}@CNTs-PEG) is freely soluble in water and stable in phosphate buffer saline having particle size of about 200 nm. Transmission electron microscopy (TEM) images clearly showed formation of PEGylated CNTs. MRI analysis showed that the prepared solution represents 10% more signal intensity even in half concentration of Gd^{3+} in comparison with commerciality available contrasting agent Magnevist®. In addition hydrophilic layer of PEG at the surface of CNTs could prepare stealth nanoparticles to escape RES.

Conclusion: It was shown that Gd_n^{3+}@CNTs-PEG was capable to accumulate in tumors through enhanced permeability and retention effect. Moreover this system has a potential for early detection of diseases or tumors at the initial stages.

Keywords: Carbon nanotubes, Contrast agent, MRI, Functionalization, Gadolinium, Pegylation

Introduction

Carbon nanotubes (CNTs) have unique physicochemical properties in biomedical and biological applications; hence have attracted attentions in different fields of nanotechnology [1-3]. Large specific surface area, efficient thermal and electrical conductivities, high mechanical strength, heat release in a radiofrequency field and capability of carrying therapeutics and imaging agents are some of these multifunctional features [4,5]. One of the extraordinary characteristics of CNTs loaded with gadolinium is their extremely large proton relaxivities which potentially could be used as magnetic resonance imaging (MRI) contrast agents (CA).

MRI is a powerful noninvasive imaging technique based on the differences between proton relaxation rates of water [6]. To enhance the contrast between different tissues and to detect disease states, using MRI CAs is inevitable [7,8]. Gadolinium (Gd^{3+}) with seven unpaired electrons and large magnetic moment is a suitable agent for this purpose. Although the equated Gd^{3+} ion is toxic, the most contrast enhancements are based on Gd^{3+}. Chelation or encapsulation of Gd^{3+}, decreases the toxicity of this ion for medical applications [7,9]. One of the most commercially used CA is gadolinium-diethylene triamine penta acetic acid, (Gd^{3+}-DTPA) commercially available as Magnevist®. Due to lack of specificity and sensitivity, this product is not very effective in early detection of the disease, so it has been classified as a traditional CAs [8].

Sitharaman et al. developed the first CNT-based contrast agent. They demonstrated that Gd@Ultra-short single-walled carbon nanotubes (gadonanotubes) drastically

* Correspondence: atyabifa@tums.ac.ir
[1]Department of Pharmaceutics, Faculty of Pharmacy, Tehran University of Medical Sciences, Tehran 14174, Iran
[2]Nanotechnology Research Centre, Faculty of Pharmacy, Tehran University of Medical Sciences, Tehran 14174, Iran
Full list of author information is available at the end of the article

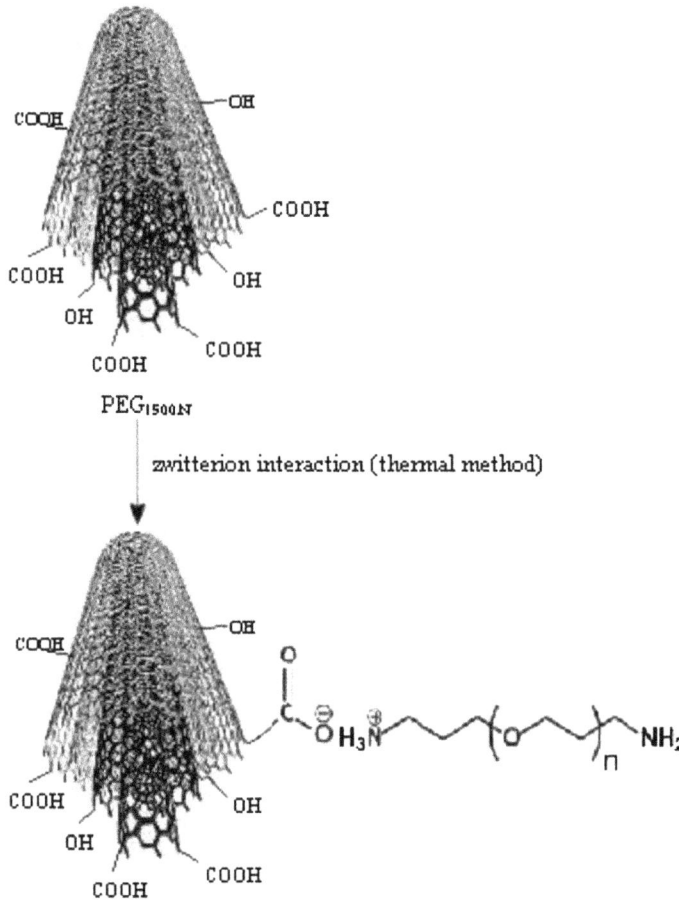

Figure 1 Schematic diagram of functionalization of oxidized CNTs loaded with Gd^{3+} (Gd_n^{3+}@CNTs) with diamine-terminated PEG via zwitterion interactions.

increase MRI efficacy compared to the traditional CAs [9]. However, the most challenging part of using CNTs in biological system is lack of solubility and hence its toxicity. Even though oxidation of CNTs improve their dispersibility, but it`s still not enough to call them as a suitable carriers. Wrapping biocompatible and biodegradable polyethylene glycol (PEG) onto the CNTs makes them soluble and helping them to escape reticuloendothelial system (RES) uptake. This modification causes longer blood circulation of CNTs and facilitates the passive targeting to the cancer cells

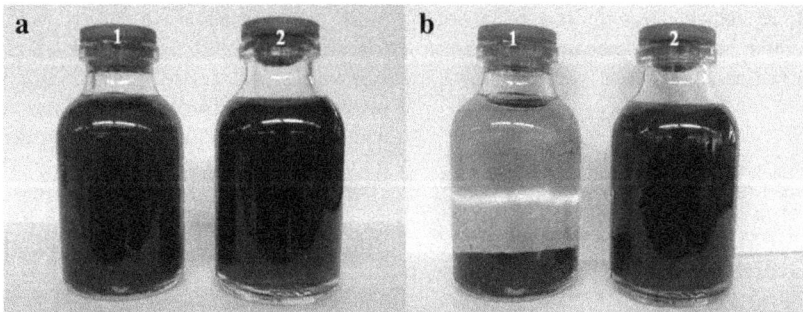

Figure 2 Dispersion of Gd_n^{3+}@CNTs (1) and Gd_n^{3+}@CNTs-PEG (2) immediately after sonication in PBS (a) and 2 months later (b).

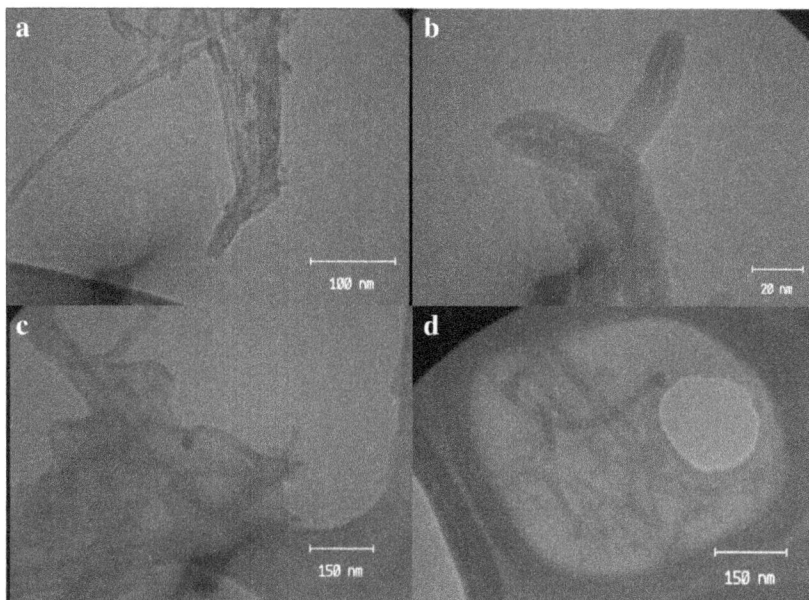

Figure 3 TEM images of Gd_n^{3+}@CNTs (a-b) and Gd_n^{3+}@CNTs-PEG (c-d).

through the enhanced permeability and retention (EPR) effect of tumor blood vessels [10-12]. Accordingly these particles can be applied for detection of tumors at the early stages.

In this work multi walled CNTs were functionalized by PEGylation and loaded with Gd_n^{3+} enhance contrast effect of commercial Gd. T_1/T_2 measurements revealed that signal intensity of Gd_n^{3+}@CNTs-PEG was more than commercial Magnevist®.

Methods and materials
Oxidation of MWCNTs
MWCNTs (number of walls 3–15, outer diameter 5–20 nm, and length 1–10 μm) were purchased from Plasmachem (GmbH, Berlin, Germany). CNTs were oxidized according to the procedure reported before [13]. Briefly, 20 ml of sulfuric acid and nitric acid mixture (3:1 v/v) were added to 1 g of MWCNTs in a reaction flask and the mixture was sonicated for 30 min. Reaction medium was refluxed for 21 h at 120°C. The mixture was cooled and diluted with 1 L of distilled water, filtered, and washed with deionized water to adjust pH to ≈ 6. The product was dried by vacuum oven.

Loading of GdCl₃ (H₂O)₆ into the oxidized MWCNTs
100 mg of oxidized MWCNTs (O-MWCNTs) and 100 mg of $GdCl_3.6H_2O$ (REacton®, 99.9%) were stirred together in 100 ml deionized water and sonicated in a bath sonicator for 60 min. The solution was left undisturbed overnight whereupon the Gd^{3+}-loaded oxidized CNTs (Gd_n^{3+}@CNTs)

flocculated from the solution. The supernatant was then decanted off. To remove any unabsorbed $GdCl_3$, remained sediment was dispersed in 25 ml of fresh deionized water with batch sonication and again, the Gd_n^{3+}@CNTs flocculated from solution was collected by decantation. This procedure was repeated 3 times. The final product was dried by vacuum oven.

Functionalization of Gd_n^{3+}@CNTs with PEG_{1500N}
28 mg of Gd_n^{3+}@CNTs was mixed with 474 mg Poly (ethylene glycol) bis (3-aminopropyl) terminated (M_n~1,500, Aldrich) and the mixture was stirred at ≈ 120°C under nitrogen atmosphere for 6 days. Upon the addition of deionized water to the mixture, the suspension was placed in a membrane tube (molecular weight cutoff ~12000) for dialysis against fresh deionized water for 3 days to remove free PEG. Dialysis phases were also collected for the confirmation of absence of free Gd^{3+} ion by ICP. To removing large nanotube bundles the suspension was centrifuged three times at 13000 rpm for 15 min and the supernatant was freeze-dried.

Determination of size and morphology
Dynamic light scattering (DLS) (Malvern Zetasizer ZS, Malvern UK) was used to determine the dynamic diameter and size distributions of Gd_n^{3+}@CNTs-PEG.

Transmission electron microscopy (TEM) and Thermal gravimetric analyses (TGA) (Shimadzu, Japan) was applied for characterization of preparation.

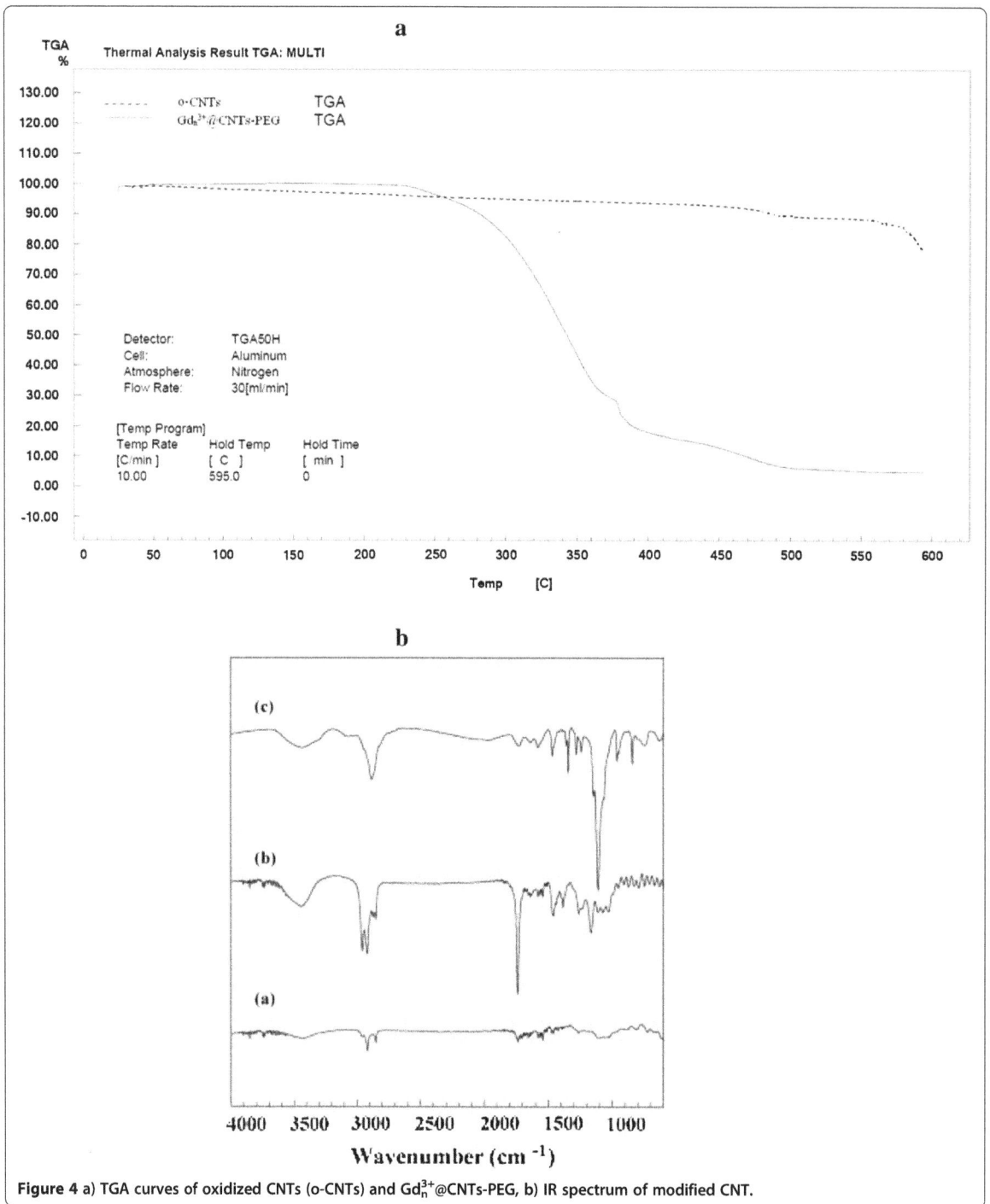

Figure 4 a) TGA curves of oxidized CNTs (o-CNTs) and Gd_n^{3+}@CNTs-PEG, b) IR spectrum of modified CNT.

ICP sample preparation

For ICP (Inductively Coupled Plasma) analysis, samples should digest with strong oxidizing agents like HNO3 or concentrated H2O2. As this harsh condition is not enough for digesting MWCNTs, in this study the nanotubes were first heated in oven at 650°C for 5 h. Fallowing cooling the sample, the solid residue was dissolved in the solution of HNO_3(2%) and the Gd content was

Table 1 T1 values (msec) derived from equations 1 and 2 for Gdn3+@CNTs-PEG with different Gd3+ concentration and Magnevist®

TR (Sec)	Concentration of Gd mM/mL					Magnevist®	Water
	0.1818	0.1	0.05	0.025	0.0125	0.1818	
T1	190.69	328.95	572.74	926.78	1385.23	405.35	3076.92
1/T1	0.005244	0.00304	0.001746	0.001079	0.0007219	0.002467	0.000325
R^2 value	0.98	0.99	0.99	0.99	0.99	0.99	0.99

determined by ICP-Optical Emission Spectrometer (Varian 720-ES).

In vitro T1/T2 measurement

The T1- and T2-weighted spin echo images at 1.5 Tesla (repetition time/echo time 250/16 msec and repetition time/echo time 4000/64 msec) were analyzed qualitatively. The signal intensities of vials with contrast medium in solution and contrast medium in cells with the corresponding Gd concentrations were visually compared.

For quantitative data analysis, the obtained MR images were transferred as digital imaging and communication in medicine (DICOM) images to a Dicom Works version 1.3.5 (DicomWorks, Lyon, France) [14,15]). For each concentration, three samplings and the maximum regions of interest were considered. Five concentrations of the carbon nanotubes (0.1818, 0.1, 0.05, 0.025 mM Gd or 0.1818, 0.1, 0.05, 0.025, 0.0125 mM/mL Gd) were prepared in sodium chloride 0.9%.

The imaging parameters were as follows: Standard Spin Echo, # of Echoes =1, TE=15 ms, TR=100, 200, 400, 600,1000, 2000 ms, Matrix=512*384, Slice Thickness=4 mm ,FOV=25 cm, NEX=3, Pixel Band width: 130 for T1 measurements and Standard Spin Echo, # of Echoes =4, TE=15/30/45/60 ms, TR=3000 ms, Matrix=512*384, Slice Thickness=4 mm, FOV=25 cm, NEX=3, Pixel Band width: 130 for T2 measurements.

T1 and T2 maps were calculated assuming mono exponential signal decay. T1 maps were calculated from four SE images with a fixed TE of 11 ms at 1.5T and variable TR values of 100, 200, 400, 600, 1000 and 2000 ms using a nonlinear function least-square curve fitting on a pixel-by-pixel basis. The signal intensity for each pixel as a function of time was expressed as follows (Equation 1) [16]:

$$Signal_{SE1}(TR, T_1) = S_{01}\left(1 - e^{-\frac{TR}{T_1}}\right)$$

T2 maps were calculated accordingly from four SE images with a fixed TR of 3000 ms and TE values of 15, 30, 45, and 60 ms on the 1.5T MR scanner. The signal intensity for each pixel as a function of time was expressed as follows (Equation 2):

$$Signal_{SE4}(TE, T_2) = S_0 e^{-\frac{TE}{T_2}} \Rightarrow ln(Signal_{SE4})$$
$$= ln(S_0) - \frac{TE}{T_2}$$

Care was taken to analyze only data points with signal intensities significantly above the noise level.

Statistical analysis

One-way analysis of variance was used for comparison of the results. P values of 0.05 or less were considered as significant.

Results and discussion

Loading of Gd_n^{3+} into the CNTs

In the presence study, MWCNTs were oxidized with harsh acid condition and then loaded with Gd_n^{3+}. Oxidizing occurred with the mixture of sulfuric and nitric acid (3:1). This procedure removes metal catalysts impurity and creates an open end termini in the structure and also sidewall defects that are stabilized by –COOH and –OH groups [12,17-19]. These hydrophilic holes are the very well place for accumulation of hydrophilic metal ions (e.g. Gd^{3+}) on the surface or inside of the interior of a CNT [18,20]. Besides the –COOH group could be coupled to different chemical or biochemical groups [18-21].

Table 2 T2 values (msec) derived from equations 1 and 2 for Gd_n^{3+}@CNTs-PEG with different Gd^{3+} concentration and Magnevist®

TE (Sec)	Concentration of Gd mM/mL					Magnevist®	
	0.1818	0.1	0.05	0.025	0.0125	0.1818	Water
1/T2	19.95	15.29	12.36	10.90	9.85	6.42	8.80
T2	0.0501	0.0654	0.0809	0.0917	0.1015	0.1558	0.1136
R^2 value	0.99	0.99	0.99	0.98	0.97	0.99	96

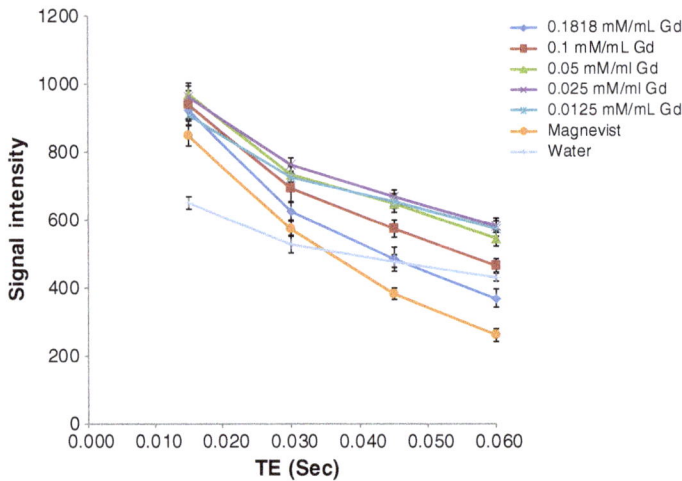

Figure 5 Signal changes based on echo time variation.

The oxidized MWCNTs were loaded by soaking and sonicating them in double distilled water containing aqueous GdCl$_3$. After sedimentation and dialysis to remove unloaded Gd^{3+} into the oxidized MWCNTs, Gd$_n^{3+}$@CNTs was functionalized with PEG. ICP analysis showed the Gd$_n^{3+}$ content of Gd$_n^{3+}$@CNTs and Gd$_n^{3+}$@CNTs-PEG to be 4.328% and 0.02% (w/w) respectively. The absence of free Gd^{3+} ion in the sample was confirmed by analysis the final dialysis medium through ICP, no detectable Gd^{3+} was shown.

Solubilization and stabilization of Gd$_n^{3+}$@CNTs with PEG

Carbon nanotubes have a rigid structure and presence in bundles, so they are essentially insoluble in any solvents. As a result, solubilization of CNTs via chemical functionalization has been attracted much recent attentions [1,5,10,17,18]. Among the possible hydrophilic polymers, with regard to biocompatibility, PEG is attractive for use with CNTs because of being nontoxic, properly stable and having a low immunogenicity [1,10,11,21]. Gd$_n^{3+}$@CNTs was functionalized with PEG$_{1500N}$ (Gd$_n^{3+}$@CNTs-PEG). As reported by other researches, the attachment of diamine-terminated poly(ethylene glycol) with Gd$_n^{3+}$@CNTs were done via thermal reaction and zwitterion interaction between terminated amines of PEG and carboxylic groups of oxidized CNTs as shown in Figure 1 [21].

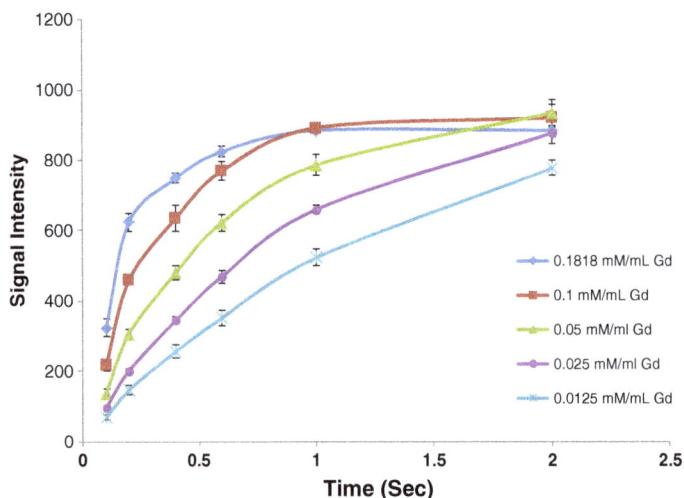

Figure 6 Signal changes based on repetition time variation.

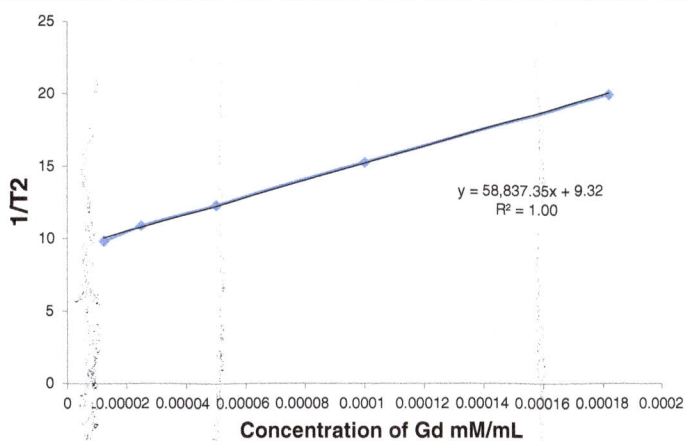

Figure 7 1/T2 values at different Gd^{3+} concentrations. The line slope represents the r_1 value.

As expected, the solution of the Gd_n^{3+}@CNTs-PEG was more stable than Gd_n^{3+}@CNTs in PBS. The Gd_n^{3+}@CNTs-PEG remained homogeneous over 2 months of observation time whereas in the Gd_n^{3+}@CNTs black precipitation appeared after a few days (Figure 2).

Characterization of Gd_n^{3+}@CNTs-PEG

The particle size of Gd_n^{3+}@CNTs-PEG in water evaluated by Dynamic Light Scattering technique was about 200 nm with narrow poly dispersity index (PDI : 0.361). This particle size is appropriate for IV administration of solubilized gadonanotubes as a contrasting agent.

Typical transmission electron microscopy (TEM) images of the functionalized MWCNTs loaded Gd^{3+} ions are shown in Figure 3. In the Gd_n^{3+}@CNTs-PEG image, wrapping PEG is can be clearly found around the nanotubes and the outer layer of polymer phase is discontinuous. Additionally nanotubes are dispersed either individually or in small bundles whereas in the image of Gd_n^{3+}@CNTs, tight bundles of nanotubes can be seen.

Thermo gravimetric analysis (TGA) and IR spectroscopy was employed to determine either the tube is wrapped by polymer chains. Thermograms and IR spectrum of Gd_n^{3+}@CNTs-PEG and oxidized MWCNTs are shown in Figure 4. Wrapped PEG started to thermally degrade in the temperature range of 312°C. When the temperature reached to 450°C, PEG had essentially decomposed completely. According to the weight loss of PEG in Gd_n^{3+}@CNTs-PEG (about 95%), content of MWCNT in this compound is low. TEM images and ICP results also confirmed this low content of MWCNT in the Gd_n^{3+}@CNTs-PEG.

For oxidized MWCNTs, a weight loss was detected at 470°C, which can be attributed to the thermally unstable functional groups, e.g. –COOH and –OH on MWCNTs, formed during oxidation. These results indicate that PEG chains have successfully wrapped onto the MWCNT surfaces.

T1/T2 measurement

T1/T2 measurements were performed in vitro, using magnetic resonance imaging apparatus. The analysis investigated that Gd_n^{3+}@CNTs-PEG solution in almost same and half concentration of Gd^{3+} compare to Magnevist® showed 29% and 9% more signal intensity respectively.

The results of T1/T2 relaxation time (derived from equations 1 and 2) are shown in Tables 1 and 2 and Figures 5 and 6.

Gd_n^{3+}@CNTs-PEG clearly caused a significant decrease in both T1 and T2 relaxation time compared with Magnevist®. As shown in Table 1, the T1 values at the same concentration of Gd^{3+} in the Gd_n^{3+}@CNTs-PEG and Magnevist® were 190.7 msec and 405.4 msec, respectively. If we depicted the 1/T1 value at different Gd^{3+} concentration the r_1 value will be obtained 26.6 $(mMol^{-1}.sec^{-1})$ as shown in Figure 7, while other studies show that the r_1 value for Magnevist® was only 13.4 $(mMol^{-1}.sec^{-1})$ [22].

Table 2 shows the T2 values for Gd_n^{3+}@CNTs-PEG at different Gd^{3+} concentrations. The r_2 value for Gd_n^{3+}@CNTs-PEG was 58.8 $(mMol^{-1}.sec^{-1})$ which was greater than Magnevist®. Data in tables and T1/T2 weighted images (Figure 8) showed that the signal increments of Gd_n^{3+}@CNTs-PEG were much higher even with half

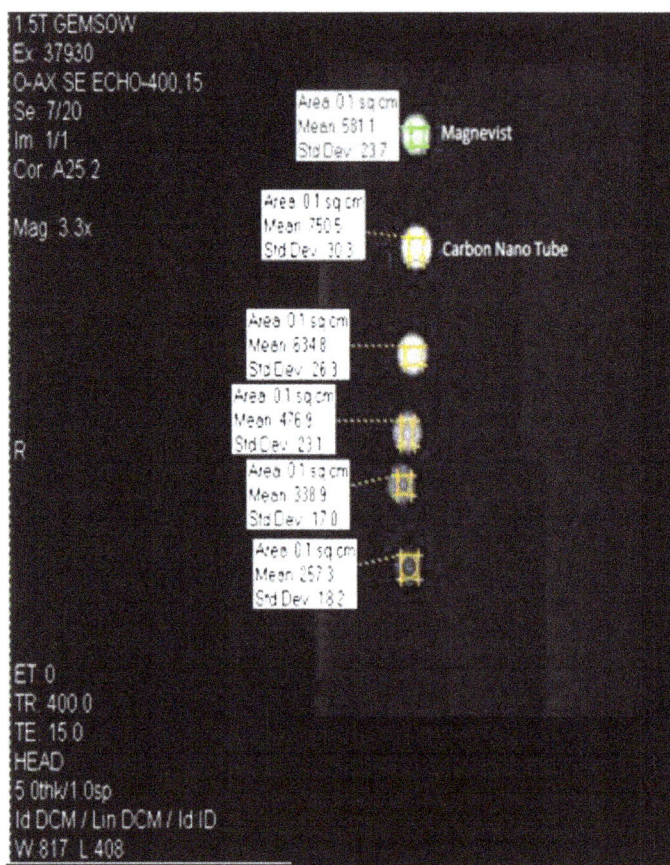

Figure 8 The discrepancies among different concentrations of Gd^{3+} in the Gd_n^{3+}@CNTs-PEG and Magnevist® at T1 weighted image. Five concentrations of the Gd_n^{3+}@CNTs-PEG (0.1818, 0.1, 0.05, 0.025 mMolarGd) were sorted, respectively from top to bottom by diluting with sodium chloride 0.9%.

concentration of Gd^{3+} compare with the conventional contrast agent Magnevist®.

MR imaging of the samples (in test tubes) was performed using a 1.5T MR scanner (Signa, GE Medical Systems, Milwaukee, WI, USA) and a standard circularly polarized head coil (Clinical MR Solutions, Brookfield, WI, USA). All probes were placed in a water-containing plastic container (as shown in Figure 8) at room temperature (25°C) to avoid susceptibility artifacts from the surrounding air in the scans.

As shown in Figure 8 the signal intensity of Magnevist® and Gd_n^{3+}@CNTs-PEG at the same image condition, same protocol, same region of interest (ROI) area, and same Gd^{3+} concentration was 581.1 and 750.5, respectively. Therefore the signal intensity of Gd_n^{3+}@CNTs-PEG PEG was 29% and 9% more than Magnevist®, at equal or half of Gd^{3+} concentration, respectively.

Conclusions

In order to increase proton relaxivity characteristics of gadolinium ion (Gd $_n^{3+}$ -ion) clusters, carbon nanotubes have been proven to be a good candidate. Addition of polyethylene glycol to this complex could improve the expected properties of the preparation as far as its solubility, stability and more over MRI contrasting ability of them. This could be the basis for further study to reach ideal goal which is detection of any abnormal tissues or tumors at the early stages.

Competing interest
The authors declare that they have no competing interests regarding present work.

Authors' contributions
RJ conducted the experimental work and help in drafting the manuscript, FA conceived the study supervised the work and is the corresponding author of the work, SS performed the MRI experiments and ZS helped with the interpretation of the data analysis, MA helped with synthesis part of the work, RD reviewed and edited the manuscript. All authors read and approved the final manuscript.

Acknowledgments

The author would like to thanks the kind help of Dr. Keith B Hartman for his useful suggestions.

Author details

[1]Department of Pharmaceutics, Faculty of Pharmacy, Tehran University of Medical Sciences, Tehran 14174, Iran. [2]Nanotechnology Research Centre, Faculty of Pharmacy, Tehran University of Medical Sciences, Tehran 14174, Iran. [3]Department of Biomedical Physics and Engineering, School of Medicine, Tehran University of Medical Sciences, Tehran, Iran. [4]Department of Chemistry, Sharif University of Technology, Tehran, Iran. [5]Department of Chemistry, Faculty of Science, Lorestan University, Khoramabad, Iran.

References

1. Liu Z, Tabakman S, Welsher K, Dai H: **Carbon nanotubes in biology and medicine: In vitro and in vivo detection, imaging and drug delivery.** *Nano Research* 2009, **2**:85–120.
2. Hartman KB, Wilson LJ, Rosenblum MG: **Detecting and Treating Cancer with Nanotechnology.** *Mol Diag Ther* 2008, **12**:1–14.
3. Sobhani Z, Dinarvand R, Atyabi F, Ghahremani M, Adeli M: **Increased paclitaxel cytotoxicity against cancer cell lines using a novel functionalized carbon nanotube.** *Int J Nanomedicine* 2011, **6**:705–719.
4. Gannon CJ, Cherukuri P, Yakobson BI, Cognet L, Kanzius JS, Kittrell C, Weisman RB, Pasquali M, Schmidt HK, Smalley RE, Curley SA: **Carbon nanotube-enhanced thermal destruction of cancer cells in a noninvasive radiofrequency field.** *Cancer* 2007, **110**:2654–2665.
5. Kam NWS, O'Connell M, Wisdom JA, Dai HJ: **Carbon nanotubes as multifunctional biological transporters and near-infrared agents for selective cancer cell destruction.** *P Natl Acad Sci USA* 2005, **102**:11600–11605.
6. Geraldes CF, Laurent S: **Classification and basic properties of contrast agents for magnetic resonance imaging.** *Contrast Media Mol Imaging* 2009, **4**:1–23.
7. Sitharaman B, Wilson LJ: **Gadofullerenes and gadonanotubes: A new paradigm for high-performance magnetic resonance imaging contrast agent probes.** *J Biomed Nanotechnol* 2007, **3**:342–352.
8. Mody VV, Nounou MI, Bikram M: **Novel nanomedicine-based MRI contrast agents for gynecological malignancies.** *Adv Drug Deliv Rev* 2009, **61**:795–807.
9. Sitharaman B, Kissell KR, Hartman KB, Tran LA, Baikalov A, Rusakova I, Sun Y, Khant HA, Ludtke SJ, Chiu W: **Superparamagnetic gadonanotubes are high-performance MRI contrast agents.** *Chem Commun* 2005, **31**:3915–3917.
10. Foldvari M, Bagonluri M: **Carbon nanotubes as functional excipients for nanomedicines: II. Drug delivery and biocompatibility issues.** *Nanomedicine: Nanotechnology, Biology, and Medicine* 2008, **4**:183–200.
11. Yang ST, Fernando KA, Liu JH, Wang J, Sun HF, Liu Y, Chen M, Huang Y, Wang X, Wang H, Sun YP: **Covalently PEGylated carbon nanotubes with stealth character in vivo.** *Small* 2008, **4**:940–944.
12. Firme CP III, Bandaru PR: **Toxicity issues in the application of carbon nanotubes to biological systems.** *Nanomedicine: Nanotechnology, Biology and Medicine* 2010, **6**:245–256.
13. Tsang SC, Chen YK, Harris PJF, Green MLH: **A Simple Chemical Method of Opening and Filling Carbon Nanotubes.** *Nature* 1994, **372**:159–162.
14. Puech PA, Boussel L, Belfkih S, Lemaitre L, Douek P, Beuscart R: **DicomWorks: software for reviewing DICOM studies and promoting low-cost teleradiology.** *J Digit Imaging* 2007, **20**:122–130.
15. Jabr-Milane LS, van Vlerken LE, Yadav S, Amiji MM: **Multi-functional nanocarriers to overcome tumor drug resistance.** *Cancer Treat Rev* 2008, **34**:592–602.
16. Engström M, Klasson A, Pedersen H, Vahlberg C, Käll PO, Uvdal K: **High proton relaxivity for gadolinium oxide nanoparticles.** *Magnetic Resonance Materials in Physics, Biology and Medicine* 2006, **19**:180–186.
17. Klumpp C, Kostarelos K, Prato M, Bianco A: **Functionalized carbon nanotubes as emerging nanovectors for the delivery of therapeutics.** *Biochim Biophys Acta* 2006, **1758**:404–412.
18. Prato M, Kostarelos K, Bianco A: **Functionalized carbon nanotubes in drug design and discovery.** *Accounts of chemical research* 2007, **41**:60–68.
19. Cai SY, Kong JL: **Advance in Research on Carbon Nanotubes as Diagnostic and Therapeutic Agents for Tumor.** *Chin J Anal Chem* 2009, **37**:1240–1246.
20. Hashimoto A, Yorimitsu H, Ajima K, Suenaga K, Isobe H, Miyawaki J, Yudasaka M, Iijima S, Nakamura E: **Selective deposition of a gadolinium(III) cluster in a hole opening of single-wall carbon nanohorn.** *Proc Natl Acad Sci USA* 2004, **101**:8527–8530.
21. Huang W, Fernando S, Allard LF, Sun YP: **Solubilization of single-walled carbon nanotubes with diamine-terminated oligomeric poly (ethylene glycol) in different functionalization reactions.** *Nano Lett* 2003, **3**:565–568.
22. Svenson S, Prud'homme RK: **Polymer modified nanoparticles as targeted MR imaging agents.** In *Multifunctional nanoparticles for drug delivery applications: imaging, targeting, and delivery.* New York: Springer; 2012:186.

7

Presence of phthalate derivatives in the essential oils of a medicinal plant *Achillea tenuifolia*

Azadeh Manayi[1], Mahdieh Kurepaz-mahmoodabadi[1], Ahmad R Gohari[1], Yousef Ajani[2] and Soodabeh Saeidnia[1*]

Abstract

Background: Phthalate, esters of phthalic acid, are mainly applied as plasticizers and cause several human health and environment hazards. The essential oils of *Achillea* species have attracted a great concern, since several biological activities have been reported from varieties of these medicinal species. On the other side, due to the problems regarding the waste disposal in developing countries, phthalate derivatives can easily release from waste disposal to the water and soil resulting in probable absorption and accumulation by medicinal and dietary plants. As a matter of fact, although the toxicity of phthalate derivatives in human is well-known, food crops and medicinal plants have been exposing to phthalates that can be detected in their extracts and essential oils. *Achillea tenuifolia* (Compositea) is one of these herbaceous plants with traditional applications which widely growing in Iran.

Finding: The plant root was subjected to hydro-distillation for 4 h using Clevenger type apparatus to obtain its essential oil before and after acid treatment. Both of the hydro-distilled essential oils were analysed by GC-MS method resulted in recognition of their constituent. Phthalate contamination as (1, 2-benzenedicarboxylic acid, bis (2-methylpropyl) ester (5.4%) and phthalic acid (4.5%), were identified in the first and second extracted oils, respectively.

Conclusion: As a warning, due to the potential role of phthalates to cause reproductive toxicity, disturb of endocrine system and causing cancers, medicinal plants have to be considered through quality control for detection of these compounds.

Keywords: *Achillea tenuifolia*, Compositae, Phthalate contamination, Acid treatment

Findings

Regarding the recent published articles on probable pollution of medicinal plants and other natural medicines like marine algae to phthalate [1,2], finding a detection and even quantification method for phthalates, which can be accurate, fast and cost effective, is a considerable challenge particularly in standardization of herbal extracts and phytopharmaceuticals.

In fact, phthalates are the esters of phthalic acid and mainly used as plasticizers. They are manufactured by reacting phthalic anhydride with alcohols (ranged from methanol (C1) to tridecyl alcohol (C13)) in both straight and branching chains. Due to the toxicity concerns related to lower molecular weight phthalates (3–6 C), they are now being slowly replaced in the US, Canada, and European Union by high molecular weight phthalates (>6 C). The reason might be

behind their higher permanency and durability in nature [2]. It is assumed that six million tonnes plasticizers are consumed every year, of which phthalates used in a large number of products including enteric coated pharmaceutical pills and supplements (as viscosity control agents), gelling agents, film formers, stabilizers, dispersants, lubricants, binders, emulsifying agents, and suspending agents [3]. These compounds interfere with endocrine systems in humans specially sex hormones and thyroids [4]. In addition, induction of inflammation, early puberty in girls, oxidative stress, asthma, and allergic symptoms were reported because of these compounds [5-7]. Literature review showed that these compounds could exhibit toxicity in liver, kidney, lung and testis in both animal and human [2,5]. Accumulation of phthalates may occur in a variety of herbal medicines especially those are growing up in water and rivers due to the exposure of plants' roots to the polluted wastewater. Consequent exposure of animals and humans to phthalate by using polluted herbs, crops

* Correspondence: saeidnia_s@tums.ac.ir
[1]Medicinal Plants Research Center, Faculty of Pharmacy, Tehran University of Medical Sciences, P.O. Box 14155–6451, Tehran, Iran
Full list of author information is available at the end of the article

and vegetables is possible, since phthalates accumulate in plants [1].

Achillea tenuifolia is distributed in the north and north-west of Iran with small yellow flowers, woody based and several stems [8]. This plant has been used as traditional herbal remedies against sweating and bleeding along with regulation of menstrual cycle and reduction of heavy bleeding and pain [9]. The previous study revealed that the oil of the plant compromised of several monoterpenes and sesquiterpenes [9-12]. There is also a report on the phytochemical content of the root extract demonstrating the presence of tannins, sterols and terpenoids [13].

Recently, we reported high percentage of phthalate in a medicinal plant, *Lythrum salicaria* [14]. In continuing our research on detection of phthalate in medicinal and food plants, here we focused on detection of these compounds in the root oil of *A. tenuifolia*.

Methods

Plant material and isolation of essential oils

The roots of *A. tenuifolia* were collected from Qazvin province (1500 m above the sea level) in June 2011(No. 1624) deposited at the Herbarium of Institute of Medicinal Plants, Jahade-Daneshgahi (ACECR), Karaj, Iran.

Air-dried roots (200 g) were submitted to hydro-distillation in a Clevenger-type apparatus for 4 h, subsequently, 10 mL hydrochloric acid (Merck, Darmstadt, Germany) (1 N) was added to the residue of the root over night at room temperature and hydro-distilled again for 4 h. As a result of acid attendance in the mixture, hydrolysing procedure of glycosidic components was successfully facilitated. The oils after extraction were separately collected in screw capped glass vials and dried over anhydrous sodium sulphate (Merck, Darmstadt, Germany) and stored at 4°C until analyses.

GC-MS analysis

The essential oil was analysed by GC-MS method on a Thermoquest-Finnigan Trace GC-MS instrument (ThermoQuest, Manchester, UK) equipped with a DB-5 fused silica column (60 m × 0.25 mm i.d., film thickness 0.25 μm). The oven temperature was raised from 60°C to 250°C at a rate of 5°C/min and held for 10 min; transfer line temperature was 250°C. Helium was used as a carrier gas at a flow rate of 1.1 mL/min with a split ratio equal to 1/50. The quadrupole mass spectrometer was scanned over the 35–465 amu with an ionizing voltage of 70 eV and an ionization current of 150 μA. The compounds were identified by comparison of retention indices (RI, DB-5) with those reported in the literature and libraries [15-23].

Results and discussion

The hydro-distillation of the root of *A. tenuifolia* resulted in extraction of the essential oils before and after acidic hydrolysis in extremely scarce amounts of colourless oils. In order to make sure about the sources of phthalate compounds in this study, no plastic container was used all through the procedure, and no solvent was used during extraction process except for hydrochloric acid that was purchased by analytical grade with no phthalate pollution. In addition, the solvents, used for injection of the samples to GC-MS, were injected alone to the chromatograph just before sample injection in order to detect probable contamination peaks. Taking together, any phthalate peaks detected in this study would highly unlikely be originated from storage, extraction and analysis procedure. GC-MS analysis of the volatile oils revealed the presence of 24 and 29 volatile components in the oils before and after acid treatment, representing 95.3% and 94.2% of the total oils, respectively (Table 1). Palmitic acid (36.9%), 5-dodecyldihydro-2(3H)-furanone (14.9%) and pentadecanoic acid (5.7%) were detected as the major constituents of the untreated essential oil, while the major volatile aglycones were identified as isovaleric acid (24.9%), palmitic acid (15.8%), cyclohexane (13.3%), cyclohexadecanolide (7.2%) and 5-dodecyldihydro-2(3H)-furanone (6.1%) in the hydrolysed oil. Chemical structures of the identified compounds are illustrated in the Figure 1. However, in the previous study on the aerial parts of this plant, monoterpenes were characterized as the major constituents of the oil [5,6]. Regarding the present results, palmitic acid and 5-dodecyldihydro-2(3H)-furanone were dominant in both volatile oils. The most considerable point found among the identified compounds is the presence of phthalate contaminations (compounds 31 and 32 in Figure 1) in both oils identifying as 1,2-benzenedicarboxylic acid, bis (2-methylpropyl) ester (5.4%) in the oil before acid treatment and phthalic acid (4.5%) in the oil after acid treatment. Presence of phthalic acid in the oil after acid treatment probably attributed to the hydrolysis of its derivatives during acid treatment.

Detection of the mentioned compounds in the oils revealed that these contaminations are able to absorb from water and soil into the plant root. The plant, employed in this study, was gathered from a mountainous region near a seasonal river, which was surrounded by lots of disposed plastics and water bottles. Therefore, the source of contamination would most probably be polluted water particularly, regarding the point that we reduced the probable external contamination during storage, extraction and analysis procedure. Actually, these phthalate derivatives are widely used in plastic items, medical and pharmaceutical products, health care products, food containers, toys and paints. It seems that in Iran, the major sources of these compounds might be disposal plastics and chemical factories. Phthalate contaminations have previously been reported from the essential oils of the plants in several studies reported phthalate contaminations in the plants oils [14,24-27]. Exposure to phthalates during pregnancy

Table 1 Percentage composition of the essential oils obtained from *A. tenuifolia* root before and after acidic hydrolysis

No.	Identified compounds	KI	RT	Percentage (%)	
				Content[a]	Content[b]
1	Cyclohexane	752	5.12	-	13.3
2	n-octane	900	6.68	-	0.4
3	Iso-valeric acid	976	8.15	-	24.9
4	2-methyl butanoic acid	978	8.19	-	0.6
5	n-decane	1098	11.16	0.6	1.2
6	Benzene-acetaldehyde	1146	12.43	-	0.2
7	Linalool oxide (cis) furanoid	1176	13.3	-	0.4
8	Linalool oxide (trans) pyranoid	1191	13.73	-	0.3
9	Camphor	1245	15.23	0.3	-
10	Terpinene-4-ol	1273	16.15	0.5	-
11	Alpha-terpineal	1289	16.54	0.6	-
12	Dodecane	1297	16.8	-	0.5
13	Eugenol	1453	21.28	1	2.7
14	Methyl eugenol	1490	22.07	0.4	-
15	n-dodecanol	1493	22.15	0.4	-
16	n-tetradecane	1497	22.27	-	0.3
17	Pentadecane	1597	24.81	-	0.1
18	Dodecanoic acid	1649	26.04	2.6	-
19	Spatulenol	1687	26.99	2	-
20	Caryophyllene oxide	1690	27.07	2	-
21	Hexadecane	1697	27.23	-	0.4
22	Tetradecanal (myristaldehyde)	1763	27.54	3.9	1.8
23	Dill apiol	1771	28.91	-	0.1
24	Apiol	1788	29.3	0.5	-
25	Tetradecanoic acid (myristic acid)	1842	30.95	4	1.9
26	Cyclocolorenone	1855	30.8	0.5	-
27	Octadecanal	1895	31.3	-	0.3
28	Hexadecanal	1897	31.7	0.3	0.4
29	Pentadecanoic acid	1902	32.28	5.7	4.5
30	6,10,14-trimethyl, 2-pentadecanone	1928	32.38	0.9	-
31[c]	Phthalic acid	1944	32.7	-	4.5
32[c]	1,2-benzenedicarboxylic acid, bis (2-methylpropyl) ester	1955	32.93	5.4	-
33	Hexadecanoic acid (palmitic acid)	2027	34.32	36.6	15.8
34	9-octadecanoic acid (oleic acid)	2048	34.38	9.7	-
35	Cyclohexadecanolide	2053	34.9	-	7.2
36	Ethyl stearate	2079	35.41	0.9	-
37	Docosane	2087	35.57	0.5	0.2
38	Ethylhexadecanoate	2091	35.65	-	0.4
39	Heneicosane	2145	37.72	-	0.5
40	5-dodecyldihydro-2(3H)-furanone	2150	37.92	14.9	6
41	Ethyl linoleate	2177	38.95	1.3	2.5
42	Nonadecanal	2226	40.3	-	2
43	Tricosane	2322	42.63	-	0.8

Table 1 Percentage composition of the essential oils obtained from _A. tenuifolia_ root before and after acidic hydrolysis
(Continued)

Hemiterpenoids	-	24.9
Monoterpenes	2.8	3.4
Sesquiterpenes	4.5	-
Phenylpropanoids	0.5	0.1
C_xH_y	1.3	17.8
$C_xH_yO_z$	86.4	48
Phthalate contamination	5.4	4.5
Total	95.5	94.2

_KI_: Kovats Index on DB-5 with reference to n-alkanes injected after the oil at the same chromatographic conditions, _RT_: Retention Time, a: values of the percentages before acidic hydrolysis, b: values of percentage after acidic hydrolysis, c: phthalate derivatives contaminations.

produced serious adverse effects like miscarriage, low birth weight, and preterm birth trough induction of inflammation and oxidative stress [6]. Moreover, fetal exposure to phthalate is associated with behavioral and mental ability; for instance in the third trimester of pregnancy they caused neurogical problems in children even until 4–9 years [28]. Although finding such a toxic manmade group of compounds is not a new concern and they are now replaced in the USA, Canada, and European Union by other plasticizers, but there is a complicated situation in developing countries. In fact, U.S. Environmental Protection Agency (EPA) has current management plan that includes the following eight phthalates: dibutyl phthalate (DBP), diisobutyl phthalate (DIBP), butyl benzyl phthalate

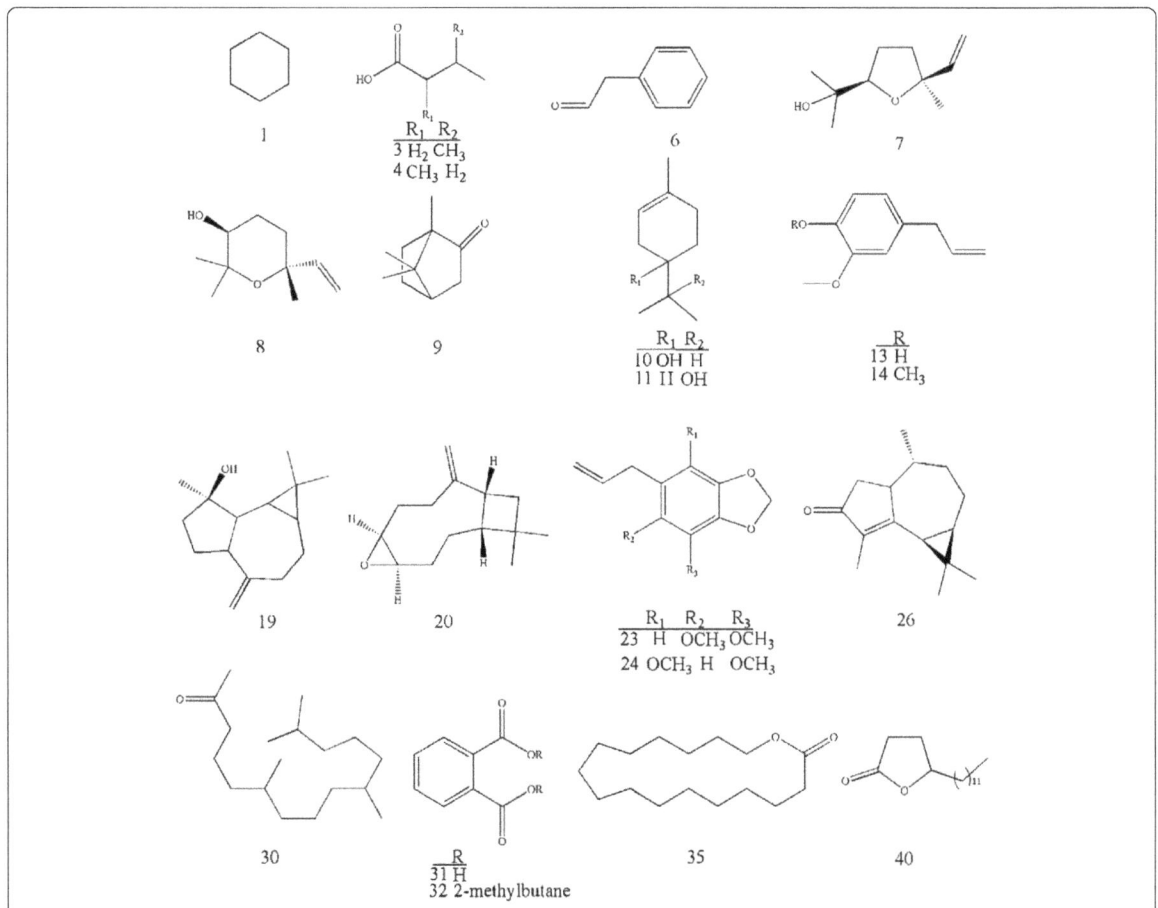

Figure 1 Chemical structures of some identified components and phthalates (31 and 32) from the essential oils of _A. tenuifolia_ root.

(BBP), di-n-pentyl phthalate (DnPP), di(2-ethylhexyl) phthalate (DEHP), di-n-octyl phthalate (DnOP), diisononyl phthalate (DINP), and diisodecyl phthalate (DIDP), of which, BBP, DEHP, and DBP cause the most toxicity to terrestrial organisms, fish, and aquatic invertebrates. Medical device assessments for DEHP have been developed by Food and Drug Administration (FDA), Health Canada Medical Devices Bureau and the European Union Scientific Committee on Medicinal Products and Medical Devices. They concluded that premature infants are the population most highly exposed to phthalates via these uses. Furthermore, The European Commission (2005) banned DEHP, DBP and BBP in all toys and childcare articles. Encouraging industry to move away from phthalates is future plan of EPA [29].

Conclusion

Finding the phthalate esters in the essential oil of *A. tenuifolia* indicated that these toxic compounds, which have been used as the plasticizers in chemical and pharmaceutical industries, are able to be simply released into the water and soil and accumulate in the plants even in the medicinal species that are growing wildly in mountainous areas surrounded by lots of municipal solid wastes, disposed plastics and water bottles. Derivatives of phthalate esters are able to cause reproductive and developmental toxicity [1,26] regarding their chemical structures. The toxicity of phthalate esters have been well-documented demonstrating that different organisms and tissues of the human and animal bodies could be affected by them including kidney, liver, thyroid and testes [1,2,30]. Besides, they could sensitize eye, skin and mucus membranes in human [2]. Taken together, pollution of medicinal plants to phthalate esters in developing countries seems cause a major problem in human health area, which needs more attention in both quality control and standardization of herbal medicines as well as Food and Drug policies or strategies by Ministry of Health.

Competing interests

The authors declare that they have no competing interests.

Authors' contributions

AM: GC analysis and drafting the article; MKM: Essential oil extraction and preparation; ARG: Plant gathering and GC/MS analysis; YA: Identification of the plant's scientific name; SS: Conception and designing the study and editing the article; All the authors have read and approved the final version of the article.

Acknowledgements

This paper is the result of an in-house study and no grants or funds have been received.

Author details

[1]Medicinal Plants Research Center, Faculty of Pharmacy, Tehran University of Medical Sciences, P.O. Box 14155-6451, Tehran, Iran. [2]Institute of Medicinal Plants (IMP), Iranian Academic Centre for Education, Culture and Research (ACECR), Karaj, Iran.

References

1. Saeidnia S, Abdollahi M: Are medicinal plants polluted with phthalates? *Daru J Fac Pharm Tehran Univ Med Sci* 2013, 21:43.
2. Saeidnia S: Phthalate. In *Encyclopedia of Toxicology. Volume 3.* 3rd edition. Edited by Wexler P. London: Elsevier Inc., Academic Press; 2014:928–933.
3. Rudel RA, Perovich LJ: Endocrine disrupting chemicals in indoor and outdoor air. *Atmos Environ* 2009, 43:170–181.
4. Schecter A: Phthalates: human exposure and related health effects. In *Dioxins and Health: Including Other Persistent Organic Pollutants and Endocrine Disruptors.* 3rd edition. Edited by Meeker JD, Ferguson KK. Hoboken: John Wiley & Sons, Inc; 2012.
5. The Lowell Center for Sustainable Production at the University of Massachusetts: *Phthalates and Their Alternatives: Health and Environmental Concerns,* Massachusetts; 2011. http://www.sustainableproduction.org/downloads/PhthalateAlternatives-January2011.pdf [Last access: Nov 22, 2014]
6. Ferguson KK, Cantonwine DE, Rivera-González LO, Loch-Caruso R, Mukherjee B, Anzalota Del Toro LV, Jiménez-Vélez B, Calafat AM, Ye X, Alshawabkeh AN, Cordero JF, Meeker JD: Urinary phthalate metabolite associations with biomarkers of inflammation and oxidative stress across pregnancy in puerto rico. *Environ Sci Technol* 2014, 48:7018–7025.
7. Swan SH: Environmental phthalate exposure in relation to reproductive outcomes and other health endpoints in humans. *Environ Res* 2008, 108:177–184.
8. Ghahreman A: *Flore de l' Irane en couleurs naturelles.* Tehran: Institute of Forests and Rangelands (Iran) and Tehran university; 1996.
9. Shafaghat A: Composition and antibacterial activity of the volatile oils from different parts of *Achillea tenuifolia* Lam. from Iran. *J Med Plants* 2009, 8:93–98.
10. Aghjani Z, Masoudi S, Rustaiyan A: Composition of the essential oil from flowers of *Achillea tenuifolia* lam. *J Essent Oil Res* 2000, 12:723–724.
11. Maffei M, Mucciarelli M, Scannerini S: Essential oils from *Achillea* species of different geographic origin. *Biochem Sys Ecol* 1994, 22:679–687.
12. Rahimmalek M, Tabatabaei BES, Etemadi N, Goli SAH, Arzani A, Zeinali H: Essential oil variation among and within six *Achillea* species transferred from different ecological regions in Iran to the field conditions. *Ind Crop Prod* 2009, 29:348–355.
13. Manayi A, Mirnezami T, Saeidnia S, Ajani Y: Pharmacognostical evaluation, phytochemical analysis and antioxidant activity of the roots of *Achillea tenuifolia* LAM. *Pharmacogn J* 2012, 4:14–19.
14. Manayi A, Saeidnia S, Shekarchi M, Hadjiakhoondi A, Shams Ardekani MR, Khanavi M: Comparative study of the essential oil and hydrolate composition of *Lythrum salicaria* L. obtained by hydro-distillation and microwave distillation methods. *Res J Pharmacogn* 2012, 1:37–42.
15. Marques FA, McElfresh JS, Millar JG: Kováts retention indexes of monounsaturated C12, C14, and C16 alcohols, acetates and aldehydes commonly found in lepidopteran pheromone blends. *J Braz Chem Soc* 2000, 11:592–599.
16. Alberts AC, Sharp TR, Werner DI, Weldon PJ: Seasonal variation of lipids in femoral gland secretions of male green iguanas (*Iguana iguana*). *J Chem Ecol* 1992, 18:703–712.
17. Chen H, Yang Y, Xue J, Wei J, Zhang Z, Chen H: Comparison of compositions and antimicrobial activities of essential oils from chemically stimulated agarwood, wild agarwood and healthy *Aquilaria sinensis* (Lour.) gilg trees. *Molecules (Basel, Switzerland)* 2011, 16:4884–4896.
18. Nixon LN, Wong E, Johnson CB, Birch EJ: Nonacidic constituents of volatiles from cooked mutton. *J Agri Food Chem* 1979, 27:355–359.
19. Yayli N, Gulec C, Ucuncu O, Yasar A, Ulker S, Cuskuncelebi K, Terzioglu S: Composition and antimicrobial activities of volatile components of *Minuartia meyeri.* *Turk J Chem* 2006, 30:71–76.
20. MacLeod G, Ames JM: Gas chromatography–mass spectrometry of the volatile components of cooked scorzonera. *Phytochemistry* 1991, 30:883–888.
21. Valim MF, Rouseff RL, Lin J: Gas chromatographic-olfactometric characterization of aroma compounds in two types of cashew apple nectar. *J Agric Food Chem* 2003, 51:1010–1015.
22. Beaulieu JC, Grimm CC: Identification of volatile compounds in cantaloupe at various developmental stages using solid phase microextraction. *J Agric Food Chem* 2001, 49:1345–1352.

23. Adams RP: *Identification of Essential oil Components by gas Chromatography/ Mass Spectorscopy. 4th edn.* Carol Stream, Ill USA: Allured Publishing Corporation; 1995.
24. Srinivasan GV, Sharanappa P, Leela NK, Sadashiva GT, Vijayan KK: **Chemical composition and antimicrobial activity of the essential oil of *Leea indica* (Burm.f.).** *Merr flowers Nat Prod Radiance* 2009, **8:**488–493.
25. Muthuchelian K, Ramalakshmi S: **Analysis of bioactive constituents from the leaves of *Mallotus tetracoccus* (Roxb.) Kurz, by gas chromatography–mass spectrometry.** *Int J Pharm Sci Res* 2011, **2:**1449–1454.
26. Nadaf M, Halimi-khalilabad M, Monfaredi L, Neyestani M: **Chemical composition of the essential oil of *Stachys lavandulifolia* (after flowering) growing wild in darkesh protected area (North Khorassan province Iran).** *Asian J Plant Sci Res* 2011, **1:**1–4.
27. Di -Bella G, Saitta M, Pellegrino M, Salvo F, Dugo G: **Contamination of Italian citrus essential oils: presence of phthalate esters.** *J Agric Food Chem* 1999, **47:**1009–1012.
28. Walter J, Crinnion ND: **Toxic effects of the easily avoidable phthalates and parabens.** *Alt Med Rev* 2012, **15:**190–196.
29. U.S. Environmental Protection Agency: Phthalates action plan. 2012, file:/// C:/Users/soodabeh/AppData/Local/Temp/ phthalates_actionplan_revised_2012-03-14.pdf [Last accessed: Oct 6, 2014]
30. Turner A, Rawling MC: **The behaviour of di-(2-ethylhexyl) phthalate in estuaries.** *Mar Chem* 2000, **68:**203–217.

8

Fungal transformation of androsta-1,4-diene-3, 17-dione by *Aspergillus brasiliensis*

Tahereh Hosseinabadi[1], Hossein Vahidi[1], Bahman Nickavar[1] and Farzad Kobarfard[2*]

Abstract

Background: The biotransformation of steroids by fungal biocatalysts has been recognized for many years. There are numerous fungi of the genus *Aspergillus* which have been shown to transform different steroid substances. The possibility of using filamentous fungi *Aspergillus brasiliensis* cells in the biotransformation of androsta-1,4-diene-3,17-dione, was evaluated.

Methods: The fungal strain was inoculated into the transformation medium which supplemented with androstadienedione as a substrate and fermentation continued for 5 days. The metabolites were extracted and isolated by thin layer chromatography. The structures of these metabolites were elucidated using ^{1}H-NMR, broadband decoupled ^{13}C-NMR, EI Mass and IR spectroscopies.

Results: The fermentation yielded one reduced product: 17β-hydroxyandrost-1,4-dien-3-one and two hydroxylated metabolites: 11α-hydroxyandrost-1,4-diene-3,17-dione and 12β-hydroxyandrost-1,4-diene-3,17-dione.

Conclusions: The results obtained in this study show that *A. brasiliendsis* could be considered as a biocatalyst for producing important derivatives from androstadienedione.

Keywords: *Aspergillus brasiliensis*, Fungi, Androsta-1, 4-diene-3, 17-dione, Steroid, Biotransformation

Background

Microbial biotransformation by the whole cell microorganisms is economically and ecologically a competitive tool for the biotechnological professionals in search of new techniques to manufacture valuable chemicals, pharmaceutical and agrochemical compounds [1,2]. The production of steroid drugs and hormones is one of the best examples of the successful application of microbial technology in large scale industrial processes [3]. A large number of bacterial and fungal species are able to biotransform steroid compounds [4]. Among them, there are numerous fungi of the genus *Aspergillus* including *A. wentti, A. niger, A. nidulans, A. ochraceus, A. parasiticus, A. oryzae, A. flavus, A. tamari, A. parasiticus* and *A. fumigatus* which have been used for the biotransformation of many steroids and shown to mediate hydroxylation, oxidation, reduction, double bond formation and epoxidation of various steroid substances [5-7]. Insertion of a hydroxyl group to a steroid molecule is one of the most important steps in the production of steroidal derivatives which is carried out by many of filamentous fungi. Several positions in the steroid molecules can be hydroxylated by various microbial strains via their hydroxylase enzyme [8].

The filamentous fungi, *Aspergillus brasiliensis* is a biseriate black species, described and named within *Aspergillus* section *Nigri*, by Varga et al. in 2007. It is differentiable from the other black aspergilla because of its unique morphology, extrolite profiles and genotypic features [9]. Literature review shows that there is no report indicating the ability of this filamentous fungus to modify the structure of steroids. In the present work, the capability of *A. brasiliensis* was evaluated for the biotransformation of androsta-1,4-diene-3,17-dione (ADD) as an exogenous substrate. ADD is one of the most important steroids, which is used as a precursor for preparing some pharmaceutically-interesting steroids. It is commercially produced by the microbiological transformation of β-sitosterol and cholesterol [8]. It is presently used in the industrial synthesis of estradiol or estrone [4,10].

* Correspondence: farzadkf@yahoo.com
[2]Department of Medicinal Chemistry, School of Pharmacy, Shahid Beheshti University of Medical Sciences, Vali-e Asr Ave., Niayesh Junction, Tehran 1996835113, Iran
Full list of author information is available at the end of the article

Biotransformation of this substrate, has already been reported by some other fungi, such as *Mucor racemosus, Acremonium strictum, Cephalosporium aphidicola* and *Neurospora crassa* leading to the production of different compounds [11-14].

Experimental

Materials

ADD was purchased from Sigma- Aldrich. All other chemicals and reagents used, were of analytical grade and commercially available.

Microorganism

The fungal strain *A. brasilliensis* PTCC 5298 was purchased From Iranian Research Organization for Science and Technology (IROST).

Cultures of fungi were grown at 26°C for 5 days until good sporulation was obtained on Czapec medium, consisting of 30 g sucrose, 2.0 g $NaNO_3$, 1.0 g K_2HPO_4, 0.50 g $MgSO_4$, 0.50 g KCl, 0.01 g $FeSO_4$, 15 g Agar and 1000 ml DW, based on IROST catalogue for this fungus [15]. Stock cultures were maintained at 4°C on Czapec medium slopes and freshly subcultured before use in transformation experiments. The organism was transferred to fresh medium and refreshed every two weeks.

Inoculum preparation and biotransformation process

Spores freshly obtained from Czapec slopes were washed with distilled water (DW) containing Tween-80 and transferred aseptically into 500 ml flasks containing 100 ml sterile medium, in a biological safety cabinet (pH of the medium was adjusted to 7.4 before sterilization).

Volume of inoculums, containing 1×10^6 spores, was used in all experiments unless otherwise stated. After cultivation at 26°C for 2 days on a rotary shaker (125 rpm) and pellet formation, ADD (100 mg) was dissolved in 1 ml acetone and aseptically added to each flask. A parallel control without substrate and also a culture medium, containing substrate but no microorganism were run concurrently (as control cultures). Biotransformation was carried out under above condition for further 5 days.

Sampling was carried out every 24 h. The samples were extracted with three volumes of chloroform and the transformation was then checked using thin layer chromatography (TLC).

After detecting the transformation on TLC plate, the fermentation was conducted on the larger scale.

Ten 1000 ml-Erlenmeyer flasks were filled with 200 ml cultivation medium. The culture media were incubated under the same conditions and then 1000 mg of substrate, (dissolved in 10 ml acetone) was distributed evenly among the flasks and process continued for 5 days.

All the experiments were performed in duplicate.

Product isolation and analyses

At the end of incubation, the fungus mycelium was separated from the broth by filtration and the mycelium was rinsed with DW. Mycelia and the filtrate were separately extracted with chloroform (3 volumes), dried over anhydrous sodium sulfate and concentrated under vacuum. The residue was analyzed by TLC, then loaded on chromatography plates and fractionated with chloroform/acetone (6.5:3.5 v/v) as the eluent solvent. The metabolites were then separated from silica gel using a mixture of methanol/chloroform/acetone (three times). The transformation products were analyzed and identified using different spectroscopic data (^{13}C NMR, ^1H NMR, FTIR and MS).

Instruments

Melting points (mp) were determined on thermoscientific 9200 apparatus and were uncorrected.

^1H and ^{13}C nuclear magnetic resonances (NMR) spectra were recorded using a Bruker DRX (Avance 500) spectrometer (Rheinstetten, Germany) at 500 and 125 MHz, respectively, in $CDCl_3$ with tetramethylsilane (TMS) as the internal standard. Chemical shifts (δ) are given in parts per million (ppm) relative to TMS. The coupling constants (J) are given in hertz (Hz). Infrared (IR) spectra were recorded on a Perkin-Elmer 843 spectrometer with KBr as a diluent. Mass spectra (MS) were obtained using Agilent 6410 Triple Quadrupole mass spectrometer. TLC was conducted on 0.25 mm thick layers of silica gel G (Kieselgel 60 $HF_{254+366}$, Merck). Chromatography plates were developed with chloroform/acetone (3.5:6.5, v/v) and visualized by spraying the plates with a mixture of methanol/ sulfuric acid (6:1, v/v) and heating them in an oven at 100°C for 3 min until the colors developed. The compounds were also visualized under a UV lamp (Strstedt– Gruppe HP-UVIS) at 254 nm.

Results

Microbial transformation of ADD by *A. brasiliensis* in 5 days resulted in the formation of three hydroxysteroid-1,4-dien-3-one derivatives (II to IV), presented in Figure 1. No transformation occurred in the control media. Steroid products were characterized using different spectroscopic data (^{13}C NMR, ^1H NMR, FTIR and MS) and melting points.

The analytical data for compounds II–IV are mentioned in a respective order. ^{13}C NMR assignments for the substrates and metabolites are listed in Table 1.

17β-hydroxyandrost-1, 4-diene-3-one (Boldenone) (II)

Colorless crystalline compound; yield 24.5%; mp 169–172°C; R_f (acetone/chloroform 3.5:6.5, v/v): 0.71; IR ν_{max} 3489, 1666, 1619 cm^{-1}; MS (EI) m/z: 286 (M^+, $C_{19}H_{26}O_2$), 227, 159, 147, 121, 91, 77; ^1H NMR ($CDCl_3$, 500 MHz) δ 7.07 (1H, d, J = 10 Hz, H-1), 6.22 (1H, d, J = 10 Hz, H-2), 6.07

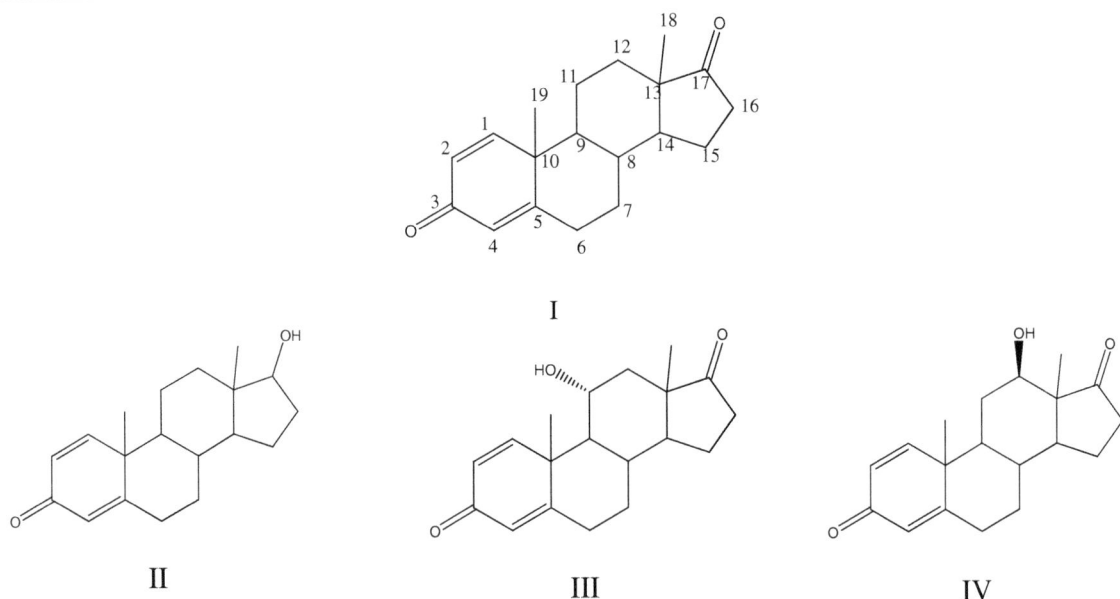

Figure 1 The structure of androstadienedione (I) and its metabolites; 17β-Hydroxyandrost-1,4-diene-3-one (II), 11α-Hydroxyandrost-1, 4-diene-3,17-dione (III) and 12β-Hydroxyandrost-1,4-diene -3,17-dione (IV).

Table 1 ^{13}C NMR data determined in CDCl$_3$ at 500 MHz for compounds I-IV

Carbon atom	I	II	III	IV
1	155.20	156.00	158.81	155.35
2	127.60	127.46	128.80	127.66
3	186.00	186.45	186.77	186.28
4	124.08	123.83	124.71	124.10
5	168.19	169.30	167.66	168.33
6	32.29	32.78	32.85	32.48
7	31.21	33.14	29.70	33.32
8	35.08	35.56	33.96	34.35
9	52.31	52.44	60.48	52.13
10	43.39	43.6	43.0	43.48
11	22.07	22.50	67.69	36.03
12	32.51	36.30	42.29	85.97
13	47.62	43.1	47.85	42.64
14	50.41	50.09	49.59	44.13
15	21.88	23.53	21.85	22.16
16	35.58	30.32	35.79	35.53
17	219.66	81.41	218.25	216.31
18	13.80	11.17	14.59	11.50
19	18.70	18.72	18.65	18.72

(1H, s, H-4), 3.64 (1H, t, J$_{17\alpha,16\alpha\beta}$ = 8.5 Hz, H-17α), 2.06 (1H, m, H-16α), 1.55 (1H, m, H-16β), 1.24 (3H, s, H-19), 0.82 (3H, s, H-18); ^{13}C NMR (CDCl$_3$) δ 186.4 (C-3), 169.3 (C-5), 156.0 (C-1), 127.5 (C-2), 123.8 (C-4), 81.4 (C-17), 18.7 (C-19), 11.1(C-18).

11α-hydroxyandrost-1,4-diene-3,17-dione (III)

Colorless crystalline compound; yield 9.6%; mp 210–214°C; R$_f$ (acetone/chloroform 3.5:6.5, v/v): 0.29; IR ν_{max} 3456, 1737, 1663, 1622 cm^{-1}; MS (EI) m/z: 300 (M$^+$, C$_{19}$H$_{24}$O$_3$), 282 , 231, 161, 124, 109, 84, 55; ^{1}HNMR (CDCl$_3$, 500 MHz): δ 7.27 (1H, d, J = 10 Hz, H-1), 6.15 (1H, d, J = 10 Hz, H-2), 6.08 (1H, s, H-4), 4.12 (1H, m, H-11$_\beta$), 2.31(1H, m, H-12$_\beta$), 1.54 (1H, m, H-12$_\alpha$), 1.24 (3H, s, H-19), 0.96 (3H, s, H-18); ^{13}CNMR (CDCl$_3$) δ 218.2 (C-17), 186.7 (C-3), 167.6 (C-5), 158.8 (C-1), 128.8 (C-2), 124.7 (C-4), 67.69 (C-11), 18.6 (C-19), 14.5 (C-18).

12β-hydroxyandrost-1,4-dien-3,17-dione (IV)

Colorless crystalline compound; yield 10.3%; mp 164–167°C; R$_f$ (acetone/chloroform, 3.5:6.5 v/v): 0.60; IR ν_{max} 3408, 1741, 1661, 1618 cm^{-1}; MS (EI) m/z 300 (M$^+$, C$_{19}$H$_{24}$O$_3$), 161, 147, 134, 122, 91, 55; ^{1}H NMR (CDCl$_3$, 500 MHz) δ 7.06 (1H, d, J = 10 Hz, H-1), 6.24 (1H, d, J = 10 Hz, H-2), 6.07 (1H, s, H-4), 3.74 (1H, s, H-12), 2.03, 1.45 (1H, m, H-11), 1.25 (3H, s, H-19), 0.79 (3H, s, H-18); ^{13}C NMR (CDCl$_3$) δ 216.3 (C-17), 186.3 (C-3), 168.3 (C-5), 155.3 (C-1), 127.6 (C-2), 124.1 (C-4), 85.97 (C-12), 18.7 (C-19), 11.50 (C-18).

Spectra interpretation

The EI-MS spectrum of compound II showed the M^+ at m/z 286 which corresponds to the molecular formula $C_{19}H_{26}O_2$, 2 a.m.u. higher than the molecular weight of parent compound and thus indicated a possible hydrogenation of compound I. The IR spectrum showed an absorbance at 3489 cm^{-1}, characteristic of a hydroxyl group. The lack of absorption band at 1736 cm^{-1} (17-ketone) and the existence of a peak at 3489 cm^{-1}, verify the reduction of the carbonyl group to a hydroxyl group at C-17 position. The ^{1}H-NMR spectrum of II showed an additional methine proton signal at δ 3.64 that is assigned to 17-H. This modification is confirmed by the appearance of a new methine carbon signal at δ 81.41 in ^{13}C-NMR spectra. The stereochemistry of the newly formed hydroxyl group was deduced to be β, based on the chemical shift of 17-H (δ 3.64), its coupling constant (J = 8.5 Hz) and splitting pattern (triplet) which is in agreement with the published data for a C-17α proton in 17β-hydroxysteroids [13,16]. This pattern is often seen when the 17β position is substituted with a hydroxyl group (e.g. pregnan-20-ones7 or androstan-17β-ols) [17]. In the case of 17α-hydroxy steroids, the splitting of H-17 β is generally a doublet [18].

The EI-MS spectrum of the transformed product III, showed the M^+ at m/z 300 (calcd for $C_{19}H_{24}O_3$ 300.1749), which was 16 a.m.u. higher than the molecular weight of compound I, thus suggesting the possible hydroxylation of it. The IR spectrum displayed hydroxyl signal at 3456 cm^{-1}. ^{1}H- and ^{13}C-NMR spectra were very similar to those of the substrate, except for a new downfield methine proton signal at δ 4.12 (ddd, $J_{11β,12β}$ = 12.2 Hz, $J_{11β,9α}$ = 10.3 Hz, $J_{11β,12α}$ = 5.4 Hz) which was assigned to the methine H-11 geminal to OH and with a downfield methine carbon signal at δ 67.69. This finding is also confirmed by the data reported in literature for this compound [13].

The mass spectrum for compound IV, showed the molecular ion peak at m/z 300 ($C_{19}H_{24}O_3$), which suggested the possible insertion of one oxygen atom in the structure of the substrate (I). The IR spectrum, showed two carbonyl absorption bands at 1741 and 1661 cm^{-1} for C-17 and C-3 respectively. The absorbance at 3408 cm^{-1}, confirmed the existance of a hydroxyl group. Melting point, ^{13}C-NMR and ^{1}H-NMR spectral data, assignments and chemical shifts for this compound were in agreement with those which have been reported by Zafar et al. in 2013 for 12β-hydroxyandrost-1,4-dien-3,17-dione [19].

Discussion

In light of the results obtained in this study, it appears that the A. brasiliensis transformation of ADD led to the formation of three major bioproducts. The bioconversion characteristics observed were 17-ketone reduction, 11α and 12β-hydroxylation.

ADD is one of the important intermediates for producing some valuable pharmaceutical steroid compounds and has been used in many studies as a substrate of the biotransformation experiments [20]. Compound II, Boldenone, also called 1-dehydrotestosterone or androsta-1, 4-dien-17β-ol-3-one, is a steroid which only differs from testosterone by one double bond at position 1. Reduction of 17-keto group of ADD results in formation of boldenone. Boldenone with its low androgenic characteristics but strong anabolic characteristics allows improving anabolic processes like growth and development of muscle mass without any undesired side-effects [21].

Reduction of 17-carbonyl group of ADD has been reported previously by Mucor racemosus and Acremonium strictum and Cephalosporium aphidicola fermention [11,12]. 11α-hydroxyandrost-1,4-diene-3,17-dione (III) which is used in the preparation of anti-osteoporosis active compounds, has been previously obtained by ADD biotransformation in Cephalosporium aphidicola, Rhizopus arrhizus and Aspergillus ochraceus culture media [13,20,22]. It has also been reported by fermentation of dihydrotestosterone (DHT) with Gibberella fujikuroi. This compound which is significant and specific inhibitor of butyrylcholinesterase (BChE), in comparison to standard drug, galanthamine. 12β-hydroxyandrost-1,4-diene-3,17-dione (IV) was also another hydroxylated steroid which has been obtained from DHT biotransformation by G. fujikuroi [19]. Although hydroxylation of steroidal substrates is common by filamentous fungi, hydroxylation at C-12 position is relatively rare [6]. The 12β-hydroxylation is proprietary reaction for filamentous fungi and is unknown in humans [23]. Introduction of a C-12 substituent and especially a β C-12 substituent into glucocorticoids improves their usefulness as topical anti-inflammatories by increasing their topical activity relative to their systemic activity [24]. Therefore from an industrial viewpoint, the ability of A. brasiliensis to carry out 12β-hydroxylation on ADD substrate may be interesting as a process for production of glucocorticoids.

Conclusion

The present research shows that the transformation of androstendienedione using A. brasiliensis whole cells yielded interesting transformation products. The observed modifications included hydroxylation at C-11α, C-12β and 17-carbonyl reduction into the related C-17β hydroxyl forms. These products were separated and characterized on the basis of their spectral data. To the best of our knowledge, there are only few reports for ADD biotransformation by microorganisms and also no report for A. brasiliensis. Therefore A. brasiliensis could be considered as efficient biocatalyst for preparation of new steroids with commercial significance.

Abbreviations

ADD: Androsta-1,4-diene-3,17-dione; DHT: Dihydrotestosterone; TLC: Thin layer chromatography; NMR: Nuclear magnetic resonances.

Competing interests

The authors declare that they have no competing interests.

Authors' contributions

All authors contributed to developing the study protocol. In addition, TH participated in project proposal and design, literature search, carried out whole analytic experiments, involved in analysis some part of data and interpretation of spectral data and drafted the manuscript. HV contributed to fermentation technique and supported the culture of microorganism. FK contributed to interpretation of the spectral data, structure elucidation and revising the manuscript. BN participated in project proposal and design, separation techniques and analysis of some part of data. All authors approved the final manuscript.

Acknowledgements

The authors would like to thank Research Deputy of Shahid Beheshti University of Medical Sciences in Iran for the financial support for this research. This study was a part of PhD thesis of Tahereh Hosseinabadi, proposed and approved in Faculty of Pharmacy, Shahid Beheshti University of Medical Sciences, Tehran, Iran.

Author details

[1]Department of Pharmacognosy and Biotechnology, School of Pharmacy, Shahid Beheshti University of Medical Sciences, Vali-e Asr Ave., Niayesh Junction, Tehran 1996835113, Iran. [2]Department of Medicinal Chemistry, School of Pharmacy, Shahid Beheshti University of Medical Sciences, Vali-e Asr Ave., Niayesh Junction, Tehran 1996835113, Iran.

References

1. Carballeira J, Quezada M, Hoyos P, Simeó Y, Hernaiz M, Alcantara A, Sinisterra J: Microbial cells as catalysts for stereoselective red–ox reactions. Biotechnol Adv 2009, 27:686–714.
2. Luo J, Liang Q, Shen Y, Chen X, Yin Z, Wang M: Biotransformation of bavachinin by three fungal cell cultures. J Biosci Bioeng 2014, 117:191–196.
3. Mohamed SS, El-Refai AMH, El-Raoof Sallam LA, Abo-Zied KM, Hashem AGM, Ali HA: Biotransformation of progesterone to hydroxysteroid derivatives by whole cells of Mucor racemosus. Malay J Microbiol 2013, 9:237–244.
4. Bhatti HN, Khera RA: Biological transformations of steroidal compounds: a review. Steroids 2012, 77:1267–1290.
5. Fernandes P, Cruz A, Angelova B, Pinheiro HM, Cabral JMS: Microbial conversion of steroid compounds: recent developments. Enzyme Microb Tech 2003, 32:688–705.
6. Mahato SB, Garai S: Advances in microbial steroid biotransformation. Steroids 1997, 62:332–345.
7. Hunter AC, Coyle E, Morse F, Dedi C, Dodd HT, Koussoroplis SJ: Transformation of 5-ene steroids by the fungus Aspergillus tamarii KITA: mixed molecular fate in lactonization and hydroxylation pathways with identification of a putative 3β-hydroxy-steroid dehydrogenase/Δ5-Δ4 isomerase pathway. BBA - Mol Cell Biol L 2009, 1791:110–117.
8. Donova MV, Egorova OV: Microbial steroid transformations: current state and prospects. Appl Microbiol Biot 2012, 94:1423–1447.
9. Varga J, Kocsubé S, Tóth B, Frisvad JC, Perrone G, Susca A, Meijer M, Samson RA: Aspergillus brasiliensis sp. nov., a biseriate black Aspergillus species with world-wide distribution. Int J Syst Evol Micr 2007, 57:1925–1932.
10. Sripalakit P, Wichai U, Saraphanchotiwitthaya A: Biotransformation of various natural sterols to androstenones by Mycobacterium sp. and some steroid-converting microbial strains. J Mol Catal B Enzym 2006, 41:49–54.
11. Faramarzi MA, Zolfaghary N, Yazdi MT, Adrangi S, Rastegar H, Amini M, Badiee M: Microbial conversion of androst-1,4-dien-3,17-dione by Mucor racemosus to hydroxysteroid-1,4-dien-3-one derivatives. J Chem Technol Biot 2009, 84:1021–1025.
12. Faramarzi MA, Yazdi MT, Jahandar H, Amini M, Monsef-Esfahani HR: Studies on the microbial transformation of androst-1,4-dien-3,17-dione with Acremonium strictum. J Ind Microbiol Biot 2006, 33:725–733.
13. ChoudHary MI, Musharraf SG, Shaheen F, Atta-Ur-Rahman: Microbial transformation of (+)-androsta-1, 4-diene-3, 17-dione by Cephalosporium aphidicola. Nat Prod Lett 2002, 16:377–382.
14. Faramarzi MA, Hajarolasvadi N, Yazdi MT, Amini M, Aghelnejad M: Microbiological hydroxylation of androst-1,4-dien-3,17-dione by Neurospora crassa. Biocatal Biotransform 2007, 25:72–78.
15. Atlas RM: Handbook of Microbiological Media. 3rd edition. Florida: CRC press; 2004.
16. Bridgeman J, Cherry P, Clegg A, Evans J, Jones ER, Kasal A, Kumar V, Meakins G, Morisawa Y, Richards E: Microbiological hydroxylation of steroids. Part I. Proton magnetic resonance spectra of ketones, alcohols, and acetates in the androstane, pregnane, and oestrane series. J Chem Soc C: Organic 1970, 2:250–257.
17. Kirk DN, Harold C, Robert W: A survey of the high-field 1H NMR spectra of the steroid hormones, their hydroxylated derivatives, and related compounds. J Chem Soc, Perkin Transactions 1990, 2:1567–1594.
18. Choudhary MI, Sultan S, Hassan Khan MT, Yasin A, Shaheen F, Atta-Ur-Rahman: Biotransformation of (+)-androst-4-ene-3, 17-dione. Nat Prod Res 2004, 18:529–535.
19. Zafar S, Choudhary MI, Dalvandi K, Mahmood U, Ul-Haq Z: Molecular docking simulation studies on potent butyrylcholinesterase inhibitors obtained from microbial transformation of dihydrotestosterone. Chem Cent J 2013, 7:164.
20. Holland HL, Chenchaiah PC: Microbial hydroxylation of steroids. 11. Hydroxylation of A-nor-, B-homo-Δ1-, and Δ1-testosterone acetates by Rhizopus arrhizus. Can J Chem 1985, 63:1127–1131.
21. Verheyden K, Noppe H, Zorn H, Van Immerseel F, Bussche JV, Wille K, Bekaert K, Janssen C, De Brabander H, Vanhaecke L: Endogenous boldenone-formation in cattle: alternative invertebrate organisms to elucidate the enzymatic pathway and the potential role of edible fungi on cattle's feed. J Steroid Biochem Mol Biol 2010, 119:161–170.
22. Bird TGC, Fredericks PM, Jones ER, Meakins GD: Microbiological hydroxylation. Part 23. Hydroxylations of fluoro-5α-androstanones by the fungi Calonectria decora, Rhizopus nigricans, and Aspergillus ochraceus. J Chem Soc, Perkin Transactions 1980, 1:750–755.
23. Ye M, Qu G, Guo H, Guo D: Specific 12β-hydroxylation of cinobufagin by filamentous fungi. Appl Environ Microbiol 2004, 70:3521–3527.
24. Avery MA, Detre G, Tanabe M, Yasuda D: Topically active steroidal anti-inflammatory agents. U.S. Patent 4,910,192, issued March 20, 1990.

9

Hydroxylation index of omeprazole in relation to CYP2C19 polymorphism and sex in a healthy Iranian population

Maryam Payan[1], Mohammad Reza Rouini[1*], Nader Tajik[2], Mohammad Hossein Ghahremani[3] and Reza Tahvilian[4]

Abstract

Background: Polymorphism of *CYP2C19* gene is one of the important factors in pharmacokinetics of CYP2C19 substrates. Omeprazole is a proton pump inhibitor which is mainly metabolized by cytochrome P450 2C19 (*CYP2C19*). The aim of present study was to assess omeprazole hydroxylation index as a measure of CYP2C19 activity considering new variant allele (*CYP2C19*17*) in Iranian population and also to see if this activity is sex dependent.

Methods: One hundred and eighty healthy unrelated Iranian individuals attended in this study. Blood samples for genotyping and phenotyping were collected 3 hours after administration of 20 mg omeprazole orally. Genotyping of *2C19* variant alleles *2, *3 and *17 was performed by using polymerase chain reaction-restriction fragment length polymorphism (PCR-RFLP) and semi-nested PCR methods. Plasma concentrations of omeprazole and hydroxyomeprazole were determined by high performance liquid chromatography (HPLC) technique and hydxroxylation index (HI) (omeprazole/ hydroxyomeprazole) was calculated.

Results: The *CYP2C19*17* was the most common variant allele in the studied population (21.6%). Genotype frequencies of *CYP2C19*17*17*, *1*17*, and *2*17* were 5.5%, 28.8% and 3.3% respectively. The lowest and the highest median omeprazole HI was observed in *17*17* and *2*2* genotypes respectively (0.36 vs. 13.09). The median HI of omeprazole in subjects homozygous for *CYP2C19*1* was 2.16-fold higher than individuals homozygous for *CYP2C19*17* (P < 0.001) and the median HI of *CYP2C19*1*17* genotype was 1.98-fold higher than *CYP2C19 *17*17* subjects (P < 0.001). However, subjects with *CYP2C19*2*17* (median HI: 1.74) and *CYP2C19*1*2* (median HI: 1.98) genotypes and also *CYP2C19*1*17* (median HI: 0.71) and *CYP2C19*1*1* (mean HI: 0.78) did not show any significantly different enzyme activity. In addition, no statistically significant difference was found between women and men in distribution of *CYP2C19* genotypes. Furthermore, the hydroxylation index of Omeprazole was not different between women and men in the studied population.

Conclusion: Our data point out the importance of *CYP2C19*2* and *CYP2C19*17* variant alleles in metabolism of omeprazole and therefore CYP2C19 activity. Regarding the high frequency of *CYP2C19*17* in Iranian population, the importance of this new variant allele in metabolism of CYP2C19 substrates shall be considered.

Keywords: CYP2C19, Enzyme activity, Genotype, Omeprazole, Phenotype

* Correspondence: rouini@tums.ac.ir
[1]Biopharmaceutics and Pharmacokinetics Division, Department of Pharmaceutics, School of Pharmacy, Tehran University of Medical sciences, Tehran, Iran
Full list of author information is available at the end of the article

Introduction

Cytochrome P450 includes a wide variety of phase I metabolizing enzymes which are involved in metabolism of drugs and endogenic substances [1,2]. CYP2C19 is one of the members of cytochrome iso enzyme superfamily which contributes in metabolism of important drugs such as proton pump inhibitors (PPI) [3] psychotic drugs like venlafaxine [4] and citalopram [5,6], voriconazol [7], and clopidogrel [8,9].

CYP2C19 is represented by a gene located on chromosome 10 [10]. Genetic polymorphism of CYP2C19 is one of the major reasons of inter-individual variability in response to CYP2C19 substrate [11-13]. The main CYP2C19 polymorphisms that are associated with difference in therapeutic response are attributed to CYP2C19*2, CYP2C19*3 and CYP2C19*17 [14,15].

A point mutation in exon 5 (681 G > A, designated *2) causes a cryptic splice defect (CYP2C19*2) and a single nucleotide polymorphism (SNP) in exon 4 (636 G > A designated *3) creates a stop codon. Both mutations predominantly result in decreased CYP2C19 activity [9,16]. A recently discovered SNP in 5′ –flanking region (−806 C > T and −3402 C > T) leads to increased CYP2C19 activity and therefore produces ultra rapid metabolizer phenotype [17,18].

The CYP2C19*2*2 and *3*3 genotypes are more prevalent in oriental and Asian populations than in Caucasian (12-23% vs 3-5%). In contrast the CYP2C19*17*17 is more frequent in Caucasian than in Asian populations (18-26% vs 0.4-1.4%) [19,20].

Omeprazole is a proton pump inhibitor that is administered in treatment of gastric acid related disease [21]. Polymorphism of CYP2C19 can affect pharmacokinetic and therefore efficacy of proton pump inhibitors [21,22]. Additionally non genetic factors like age, liver disease and combination therapy can result in resistance to Helicobacter Pylori eradication treatment [23,24].

Several studies have used hydroxylation index of omeprazole as an indicator of CYP2C19 activity however this enzyme activity, was mainly measured in relation to *2 and *3 variant alleles and not the new variant allele (*17) [16,25-28]. Although Sim et al. studied the effect of CYP2C19*17 variant allele on enzyme activity, they only reported this activity in extensive metabolizers (*17*17, *1*17 and *1*1) and they did not determine CYP2C19 activity in CYP2C19*2*17 carriers [17]. CYP2C19*2 leads to decreased enzyme activity and CYP2C19*17 causes increased enzyme activity [16,17] but the impact of combined alleles (CYP2C19*2*17) on CYP2C19 activity has not been reported comprehensively and it is unknown that the effect of which allele is more predominant in CYP2C19*2*17 carriers.

Furthermore there are some controversies in publications about impact of sex on CYP2C19 activity [29,30].

To our best knowledge, currently there is no published data regarding CYP2C19 activity in relation to new variant allele in Iranian population. Thus, the objects of this study were to assess effect of CYP2C19*17 on enzyme activity and also to see if there is any sex-dependent difference in CYP2C19 activity and finally to investigate genotype-phenotype relationship of CYP2C19 considering new variant allele (CYP2C19*17) in Iranian population.

Material and methods

Study subjects

The study protocol was approved by ethics committee of Tehran University of Medical Sciences (ethical no. 11208). Generally one hundred and eighty (60 women and 120 men) unrelated healthy Iranian volunteers with the mean age of between 20–55 years and average body weight of 45–89 kg took part in this study. All participants signed written informed consent of this project. The study was completed by contribution of faculties of pharmacy of Tehran, Yazd, Kermanshah and Kerman University of Medical Sciences. The participants were students or stuffs of pharmacy schools, with no history of any illness or medicine consumption. No smoking and consumption of medicine that would affect CYP2C19 activity was permitted for one week before and during the study.

CYP2C19 phenotyping

After an overnight fast for at least 8 hours, volunteers took 20 mg omeprazole capsule (Abidi pharmaceuticals) with 250 milliliter tap water. Ten ml venous blood sample was collected from each subject 3 hours after administration of omeprazole and transferred into tubes containing 10 µl of 10% EDTA. Five ml of blood samples were centrifuged for 5 min at 4000 rpm and the plasma was separated and transferred to Eppendorf tube and stored at –80°C up to the day of analysis. The other 5 ml blood samples were stored directly in –80°C for genotyping analysis.

Analytical procedure

Omeprazole powder was purchased from TMAD (Iran). 5-hydroxyomeprazole was a kind donation by AstraZeneca (Sweden). The concentration of omeprazole and 5-hydroxyomeprazole was analyzed by HPLC method as described by Rezk et al. with a few modifications [31]. Briefly 500 µl plasma was extracted by liquid-liquid extraction using 1500 µl ethyl acetate. After orbital mixing for 10 min and centrifuging at 4000 × g for 10 min, the upper organic layer was separated and transferred to glass tube and then evaporated to dryness under gentle stream of air. Finally the residue was dissolved in 250 µl mobile phase and 100 µl of this sample was injected to HPLC system. The mobile phase was a combination of dibasic sodium phosphate buffer (0.025 mol/lit, pH 6): acetonitrile: methanol (73: 18: 8 V/V/V). The HPLC apparatus consisted of a low pressure HPLC pump, UV detector (λ = 302 nm) all from Knauer (Berlin, Germany). The chromatographic separation was performed by using Chromolit™ Performance RP-18e 100 mm × 4.6 mm, 5 μm particle size. Flow rate was adjusted to 1 ml/min. The limits of quantification were about 15 μg/ml for both compounds. Intraday and between day precisions were < 5% for both omerpazole and 5-hydroxyomeprazole.

CYP2C19 genotyping
The DNA was extracted from blood leucocytes by standard salting out method as explained by Miller et al. [32]. The extracted DNA was dissolved in sterile distilled water and stored at 4 °C until the day of analysis. Amplification of CYP2C19*2 and *3 allele was implemented using polymerase chain reaction-restriction fragment length polymorphism (PCR-RFLP) as described by De Morias [33]. The PCR product of each reaction was digested by specific endonuclease (all from New England Biolabs GmbH, Frankfurt, Germany); the 169 bp CYP2C19*2 product was digested by SmaI to 40 and 129 bp fragments. The 329 bp PCR product of CYP2C19*3 was digested by BamHI to 233 and 96 bp pieces. Genotyping of CYP2C19*17 -3402 C > T and −806 C > T polymorphisms was done by PCR-RFLP and nested-PCR assays as defined by Sim et al. [17]. For CYP2C19*17 -3402 C > T the PCR product (504 bp) was digested by MnlI and resulted in 224 and 280 bp fragments. But the PCR product of CYP2C19*17 -806 C > T (200 bp) was separated directly on 2.5% agarose gel without any digestion. In all PCR-RFLP assays mutation caused abolishment of restriction site and thus PCR product was not digested.

Statistical analysis
The allele frequencies differences between population were estimated using two-tailed Fisher's exact test. The 95% confidence intervals (CI) were calculated using Confidence Interval Analysis software. The relation of sex and genotype was assessed by two tailed Fisher's exact test. The observed and expected frequencies were calculated by using Hardy-Weinberg equation. The two-tailed Fisher's exact test was used to evaluate deviation of genotype frequencies in the studied population from Hardy-Weinberg equilibrium. The enzyme activity was compared by using omeprazole hydroxylation index. The hydroxylation index (HI) of omeprazole 3 hours after administration of omeprazole was calculated by dividing omeprazole to 5-hydroxyomeprazol plasma concentration. The mean HI in different genotypes were compared by Mann–Whitney two tailed test. The impact of sex on HI of omeprazole was also evaluated using Mann–Whitney two tailed test. The inter-individual variability in metabolism of

omeprazole was represented by probit plot. For drawing probit plot, the log of HI was calculated, the antimode value was determined using Microsoft office excel 2010. The normality of HI distribution was analyzed by frequency distribution histogram and also by Kolmogorov-Smirnov test. All statistical analyses were performed by Sigma Plot version 12.0 and Graph Pad Prism version 5 softwares and $P < 0.05$ was considered as statistically significant difference.

Results
The genotype and allele frequencies of CYP2C19 are reported in Table 1. According to the data presented in Table 1, CYP2C19 *17*17, *1*17 and *1*1 were detected in 10 (5.5%), 52 (28.9%) and 75 (41.7%) subjects respectively. The CYP2C19 *2*17 and *1*2 were identified in 6 (3.3%) and 33 (18.3%) individuals and finally the CYP2C19*2*2 was recognized in 4 (2.2%) of volunteers. CYP2C19*17 was the most common variant allele in Iranian population.

The hydroxylation index of omeprazole as mean ± SD, median and 95% confidence interval is reported in Table 2. Subjects with CYP2C19 *17*17 genotype had a very high metabolic capacity with median hydroxylation index of 0.36 and were classified as Ultra-Rapid Metabolizers (URM). The median hydroxylation index of omeprazole in subjects homozygous for CYP2C19*1 was 2.17 fold higher than individual homozygous for CYP2C19*17 ($P < 0.001$) and the median hydroxylation index of CYP2C19*1*17 genotype was 1.97 fold higher than CYP2C19*17*17 subjects ($P < 0.001$). There was not a significant difference between HI of omeprazole in CYP2C19*1*17 and *1*1 carriers ($P > 0.05$) and these two groups were stratified as extensive metabolizers (EM).

The median HI of omeprazole was 1.74 in CYP2C19*2*17 and 1.98 in CYP2C19*1*2 carriers respectively. The difference in HI of omeprazole in CYP2C19*1*2 carriers were statistically significant with other CYP2C19 genotypes ($P < 0.05$) except for CYP2C19*2*17 genotype ($p > 0.05$). Individuals in these two groups had intermediate metabolic capacity and were designated as Intermediate-Metabolizers (IM). Homozygous carrier of CYP2C19*2 had a very low metabolic capacity with the median hydroxylation index of 13.03 and they were classified as poor metabolizers (PM). There was a significant difference between HI index of homozygous carriers of CYP2C19*2 with the other five genotypes ($p < 0.001$).

The plasma concentration of omeprazole and hydroxyomeprazole is illustrated in Figure 1. According to this figure there is a significant difference between omeprazole plasma concentration in individuals with CYP2C19*17*17 genotype with all other groups ($P < 0.01$), but the omeprazole plasma concentration was neither different between 1*17 and 1*1(EM) ($P > 0.5$) nor between 2*17 and 1*2 (IM)

Table 1 Genotype and allele frequencies of CYP2C19 in 180 healthy Iranian volunteers

CYP2C19 Genotype	Number of subjects		Frequency (%)	95% CI
	Men (120)	Women (60)		
*17*17	5	5	5.5	2.7 - 10.0
*1*17	37	15	28.8	22.4 - 36.1
*1*1	53	22	41.7	34.4 - 49.2
*1*2	20	13	18.3	13.0 - 24.7
*2*17	4	2	3.3	1.23 - 7.1
*2*2	1	3	2.2	0.6 - 5.5
CYP2C19 Alleles	**No. of alleles**		**Frequency (%)**	**95% CI**
CYP2C19*17	78		21.6	17.5 - 26.3
CYP2C19*1	235		65.3	60.1 - 70.2
CYP2C19*2	47		13.1	9.7 - 16.9
CYP2C19*3	0		0	0

*CI: Confidence Interval. (The 95% confidence intervals (CI) were calculated using Confidence Interval Analysis software).

genotypes. However, omeprazole plasma concentration was significantly different between EM (*1*17* and *1*1*) and IM (*2*17* and *1*2*). The plasma concentration of hydroxyomeprazole was significantly different between *2*2 and all other 5 genotypes while the plasma concentration of hydroxyomeprazole was not significantly different between other 5 genotypes (*17*17, 1*17, *1*1, 2*17, 1*2*).

Figure 2 indicates the hydroxylation index of omeprazole in 6 genotypes and also in predicted phenotype groups. As it is observed there is no significant difference between hydroxylation index of omeprazole in *1*17* and *1*1* groups or between *2*17* and *1*2* groups. While the difference between *17*17* or *2*2* with all other genotype groups were statistically significant.

The summary of omeprazole, hydroxyomeprazole plasma concentration and omeprazole HI in the total population, women and men is reported in Table 3. Omeprazole plasma concentration was significantly higher in *2*2* genotype than other genotype groups. Additionally there was a significant difference in omeprazole plasma concentration between different groups (P < 0.001) except for *CYP2C19*1*17* and *1*1* (P > 0.05), *CYP2C19*1*2* and *CYP2C19*2*17* (P > 0.05). Mean omeprazole plasma concentration was 19.0 fold higher in *CYP2C19*2*2* than *CYP2C19*17*17* and 11 fold higher than *CYP2C19*1*1* (P < 0.001), however hydroxyomeprazole concentration

was not statistically different among genotype groups (P > 0.05) except for *CYP2C19*2*2*. Moreover, omeprazole and hydroxyomeprazole plasma concentrations as well as omeprazole HI were not statistically different among women and men in the studied population (P > 0.05).

The effect of sex on hydroxylation index of omeprazole is illustrated in Figure 3. According to this figure there is not any significant difference between median hydroxylation index in women (0.84) and men (0.86) (p > 0.05).

The frequency distribution histogram of omeprazole hydroxylation index in 180 healthy Iranian volunteers is indicated in Figure 4. The graph shows a bimodal distribution with the antimode of around 0.8. Kolmogorov-Smirnov test showed that the omeprazole hydroxylation index was not normally distributed in the studied population (K-S Dist. = 0.296 p < 0.001). The bimodal distribution was also confirmed by probit plot.

The correlation of CYP2C19 genotype and phenotype was tested using Spearman rank correlation, and the results showed a well correlation between CYP2C19 genotype and phenotype (r_s = 0.64, P < 0.0001).

Discussion

Inter-individual variability in drug response always has been one of the main concerns in drug discovery and development. The important factors resulting in such

Table 2 Hydroxylation index of omeprazole (omeprazole/hydroxyomeprazole) in relation to CYP2C19 genotype in 180 healthy Iranian subjects

	*17*17	*1*17	*1*1	*2*17	*1*2	*2*2
Mean (SD)	0.35(0.06)	0.75(0.28)	0.85(0.30)	2.02(0.84)	2.27(1.04)	13.59(3.13)
Median	0.36[a]	0.71	0.78	1.74[b]	1.98[b]	13.03[a]
95% CI	0.31 - 0.39	0.68 -0.83	0.79 – 0.92	1.33 – 2.72	1.92 – 2.63	10.51– 16.67

[a]Represent statistically significant difference with other 5 genotypes.
[b]Represent statistically significant difference with *17*17, *1*17, *1*1 and *2*2.
CI: Confidence Interval.

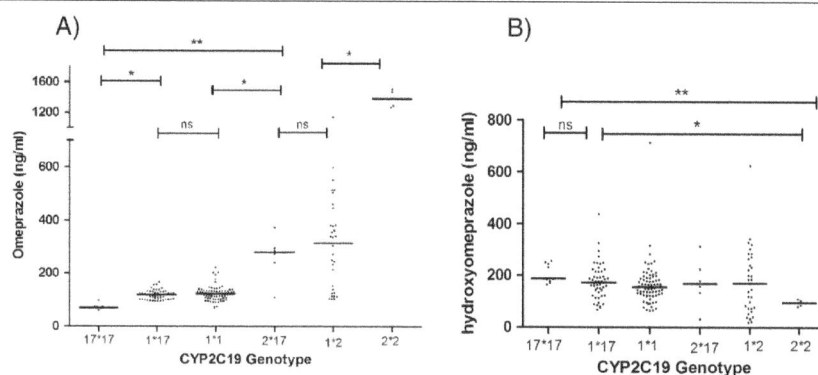

Figure 1 Plasma concentrations of Omeprazole (A) and hydroxyomerpazole (B) in different genotypes 3 hours after administration of Omeprazole orally. ns: not significant, * p < 0.05, ** p < 0.001.

variation include genetic, nongenetic and physiologic agents like change in protein structure, combination therapy, alcohol, smoking, sex, age and disease condition [34].

CYP2C19*17 is a new variant allele which is associated with increased gene transcription and therefore higher enzyme activity [17]; which may lead to several clinical consequences including the lower susceptibility to breast cancer risk [35], higher risk of peptic ulcer disease [36], greater response to clopidogrel treatment and more risk of bleeding [37] in addition to a better treatment with tamoxifen [38].

In this study, omeprazole HI after 3 hours administration of omeprazole was used as indicator of CYP2C19 activity. The HI in CYP2C19*17*17 was significantly different with CYP2C19*1*17 and CYP2C19*1*1 genotypes and people in this group had very high metabolic activity, which is in agreement with what was reported by Sim et al. They found that median HI of omeprazole in homozygous carriers of CYP2C19*1 is 2 fold higher than homozygous carriers of CYP2C19*17 and 1.2 fold higher

than CYP2C19*1*17 [17]. Ramsjö et al. has also reported that mean HI of omeprazole in CYP2C19*1*1 was 3.2 fold higher than CYP2C19*17*17 and 1.1 fold higher than CYP2C19*1*17 [27].

CYP2C19*2 allele is associated with decreased enzyme activity and CYP2C19*17 variant allele is connected with increased enzyme activity. In Most of the genotype phenotype studies of CYP2C19*17 variant allele, only HI of omeprazole in CYP2C19*17*17, CYP2C19*1*17 and CYP2C19*1*1 genotypes has been reported [17,27]. However, the capacity of CYP2C19 enzyme activity in people carrying both defective mutant alleles of *2 and *17 (CYP2C19*2*17) was still unclear. Although Ragia et al. in the study for evaluation of distribution of CYP2C19*17 genetic polymorphism in Greece people defined CYP2C19*2*17 carriers as EM and people with CYP2C19*1*2 as IM, they only predicted phenotype based on genotype and CYP2C19 activity was not determined by using a probe drug [39]. Sugimito et al. did not see any difference between metabolic capacities of CYP2C19*1*1, *1*17, 2*17 and 1*2 for metabolism of

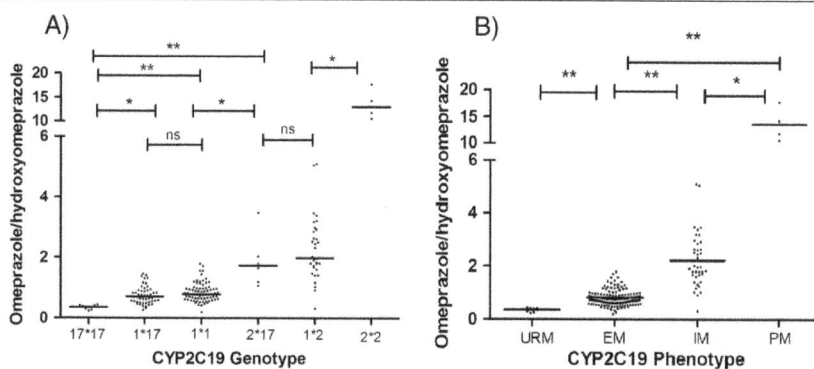

Figure 2 The hydroxylation index of Omeprazole in different genotypes (A) and in predicted phenotype groups (B) 3 hours after administration of Omeprazole orally. ns: not significant, * p < 0.05, ** p < 0.001.

Table 3 Plasma concentration of omeprazole (OMP) and hydroxyomeprazole (OH-OMP) and hydroxylation index (HI) of omeprazole in relation to genotype in 60 women and 120 men 3 hour after administration of single oral dose of 20 mg omeprazole

Genotype	No of subjects	Mean OMP concentration (ng/ml) ± SD	Mean OH-OMP concentration (ng/ml) ± SD	Mean HI ± SD
17*17	Total (10)	71.01 ± 10.28	203.31 ± 34.93	0.35 ± 0.06
	Women (5)	68.32 ± 5.73	204.92 ± 41.35	0.34 ± 0.08
	Men (5)	73.71 ± 13.67	201.69 ± 32.08	0.36 ± 0.04
1*17	Total (52)	118.28 ± 10.19	177.05 ± 37.53	0.75 ± 0.28
	Women (15)	120.22 ± 20.12	174.51 ± 28.01	0.72 ± 0.18
	Men (37)	117.49 ± 16.10	178.07 ± 44.57	0.77 ± 0.32
1*1	Total (75)	124.75 ± 27.18	163.74 ± 32.25	0.85 ± 0.30
	Women (22)	128.06 ± 39.90	194.40 ± 60.84	0.78 ± 0.27
	Men (53)	123.38 ± 20.83	151.01 ± 26.38	0.89 ± 0.30
2*17	Total (6)	289.01 ± 97.45	172.79 ± 63.58	2.02 ± 0.54
	Women (4)	324.25 ± 39.90	178.72 ± 33.59	1.97 ± 0.62
	Men (2)	271.39 ± 118.56	169.82 ± 84.95	2.05 ± 0.67
1*2	Total (33)	319.45 ± 150.34	177.79 ± 38.39	2.27 ± 1.04
	Women (13)	364.92 ± 265.16	194.66 ± 52.56	2.24 ± 0.79
	Men (20)	289.89 ± 167.55	165.53 ± 23.55	2.29 ± 1.19
2*2	Total (4)	1388.99 ± 123.41	104.67 ± 10.55	13.59 ± 3.13
	Women (3)	1359.84 ± 133.23	105.03 ± 13.80	13.37 ± 3.80
	Men (1)	1476.4	103.58	14.25

HI = (omerpazole concentration/hydroxyomeprazole concentration).

omeprazole and stratified these individuals as EM [20]. The omeprazole HI in subjects with *CYP2C19*2*17* genotype in this study was not significantly different from *CYP2C19*1*2* genotype (P = 0.33) so we designated them as IM. It seems that in heterozygous carriers of *CYP2C19*2* and *17* allele, the effect of *2* allele is more predominant than *17* allele and it can suppress induced enzyme activity by *17* allele. This observation is in agreement with classification of *CYP2C19*2*17* as IM by Gurbel *et al.* based on the study for genotype phenotype analysis of 2C19 in stented patient [40]. In contrast to these findings, in a study for evaluation of CYP2C19 enzyme activity in Turkish children using lansoprazole as a probe drug, individuals with *CYP2C19*2*17* had similar enzyme activity to *CYP2C19*1*17* and *CYP2C19*1*1*; and this activity was significantly different from *CYP2C19*1*2* [41]. Involvement of individual with different age groups could possibly explain such different observations. Our study was conducted in adult individuals with the average age of 32 years but Gumus implemented the study in children with mean age of 10.2 years. The lower frequency of *CYP2C19*2*17* in our studied subjects in comparison to Turkish individuals (6 vs 16) can be considered as another justification.

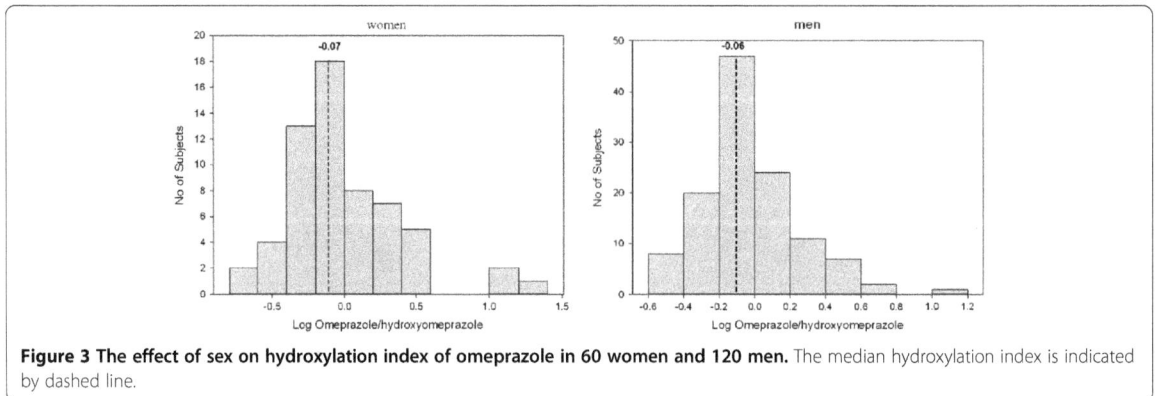

Figure 3 The effect of sex on hydroxylation index of omeprazole in 60 women and 120 men. The median hydroxylation index is indicated by dashed line.

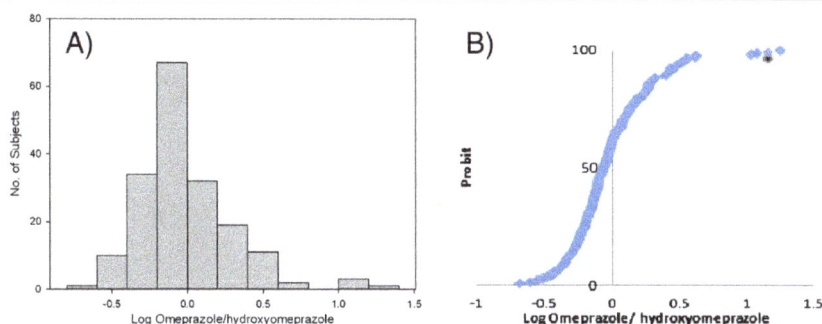

Figure 4 A) **Frequency histogram distribution and** B) **Probit plot of log omeprazole hydroxylation index in 180 healthy Iranian volunteers.** Subjects with log HI > 1.0 were phenotyped as poor metabolizers.

In the present study effect of CYP2C19 genetic polymorphism and sex on metabolic activity of CYP2C19 was also assessed. Sex is an important factor in activity of some cytochrome P450 enzymes. CYP3A4 is an example of cytochrome enzymes which has higher activity in women than men [2]. There were some controversies in the previous published reports for impact of sex on CYP2C19 activity. Ramsjö et al. indicated a sex difference in CYP2C19 activity between Korean subjects and not in Swedish volunteers using Omeprazole as a probe drug [27]. Tamminga et al. observed a sex related decreased CYP2C19 activity in women when used mephenytoin as a probe for evaluation of CYP2C19 activity, however the author declared this reduction was more obvious in those who used oral contraceptive [42]. In contrast, Hägg et al. did not see any sex differences in CYP2C19 activity after administration of mephenytoin in Norwegian population [43]. By considering these reports one may conclude that sex dependency of CYP2C19 activity is influenced by environmental and epigenetic factors like diet and ethnic differences. The other possibility can be attributed to some new genetic mutation in some populations which has not been studied well. The result of this study represents no effect of sex on CYP2C19 activity which is in line with what is reported in Swedish and Norwegian population.

The frequency of PM and URM in Iranian population in this study was about 2.2% and 5.5% which is close to the study by Zand et al. [44] and other Caucasian population. In previous report by Akhlaghi et al. in Iranian patients with coronary artery disease the genotype frequency of CYP2C19*2*2 was reported 4.7% which is quite different from our results [45]. This can be due to difference in studied population (healthy volunteer's vs specific patients). The genotype frequency of CYP2C19*17*17 (URM) was 4% in Swedish and 3% in Ethiopian [17], 5.1% in Danish [19], 3.18% in Greece [39], 7% in Saudi Arabian [46] 1.2% in Indian [16] and 0% in Japanese, Korean and Thai population [20,27,47]. Accordingly the genotype frequency of

CYP2C19*2*2 (PM) is 2.2% in Danish [19], 2.1% in Greece [39], 0.4% in Saudi Arabian [46], 18.4% in Indian [16] and 18% in Japanese people [20].

To the best of authors' knowledge, this is the first study evaluating CYP2C19 genotype and phenotype in Iranian population in relation to new variant allele (CYP2C19*17). In the previous report, Zendehdel et al. investigated impact of CYP2C19 on therapeutic efficacy of omeprazole in Iranian patients with erosive reflux esophagitis; patients were genotyped only for CYP2C19*2 and CYP2C19*3, Individuals with HetEM genotype had better response to treatment with omeprazole than EM (95% vs 43% successful treatment response respectively) [48]. The high frequency of CYP2C19*17 allele (21.6%) detected in this study maybe one justification for 50% resistance rate in the EM group in Iranian patients in previous report. However impact of this variant allele (CYP2C19*17) on the efficacy of PPIs like omeprazole shall be evaluated in controlled clinical trials.

In this study the antimode of 0.8 was calculated for Iranian population. Different antimodes for HI of omeprazole have been reported in different ethnics groups: 14.4 in Indian [16], 7.0 in Koreans [25] and Thai population [47], 0.63 in Colombians [26], and 3.98 in West Mexicans [49]. The calculated antimode for Iranian population is similar to Colombian population, indicating comparable CYP2C19 activity in Iranians and Colombians and faster enzyme activity than Asian people.

A complete genotype phenotype correlation was observed in this study. However it should be noted that enzyme activity and therefore metabolic ratio may vary during some disease condition which may result in discrepancy in genotype-phenotype relationship of specific enzyme. Kimura et al. [50] indicated discordance of genotype-phenotype relationship of omeprazole in 14.5% of EM patients who had peptic ulcer disease. However this discrepancy was not observed in healthy individuals. Reduced hepatic enzyme activity as a result of old age or liver disease was reported as an explanation for such finding. Long term treatment with omeprazole which has auto inhibition effect was the other possibility. Williams *et al.* [51] also did not see genotype-phenotype relationship of 2C19 using omeprazole in patients with advanced cancer. The authors concluded that increased level of some signaling molecules like interleukin (IL) and tumor necrosis factors (TNFα) may result in down-regulation of metabolizing enzymes [51,52]. So it should be considered that factors like age, disease state, and concomitant medication may have pronounced effect on enzyme activity. Although omeprazole hydroxylation index has been used as an indicator of CYP2C19 activity, it should be considered that hydroxyomeprazole which is formed by CYP2C19 is further metabolized by CYP3A4 to hydroxyomeprazole sulfone [53] which in turn may indirectly affect the hydroxylation index of omeprazole. Therefore the high concentration of CYP3A4 in liver microsomes of some human can explain the deviation from CYP2C19 genotype and also the sex dependent enzyme activity observed in some ethnic groups [54].

The prevalence of *CYP2C19*2*17* in this study was only 6% which is a limitation of this study. Future studies to investigate impact of *CYP2C19*2*17* genotype on CYP2C19 enzyme activity in larger groups specially by using drugs with narrow therapeutic window is suggested.

In conclusion, the result of this study shows that *CYP2C19*2*17* has an intermediate metabolic activity which maybe important for drug dose adjustment regimens for treatment, specially in those having narrow therapeutic indices like clopidogrel. Additionally no effect of sex on CYP2C19 activity was observed in this study. Regarding the high frequency of *CYP2C19*17* in Iranian population, the importance of this new variant allele in metabolism of CYP2C19 substrates shall be considered.

Abbreviations
CYP2C19: Cytochrome P450 2C19; PCR-RFLP: Polymerase chain reaction-restriction fragment length polymorphism; HPLC: High performance liquid chromatography; HI: Hydroxylation index; SNP: Single nucleotide polymorphism; URM: Ultra-rapid metabolizers; EM: Extensive metabolizers; IM: Intermediate metabolizers; PM: Poor metabolizers; OMP: Omeprazole; OH-OMP: Hydroxyomepazole.

Competing interests
The authors declare that they have no competing interests.

Authors' contributions
M-RR, MP, NT, M-H GH and RT conceived the study. MP performed the experimental work. All authors were involved in data analysis and interpretation. MP prepared the manuscript. All authors read and approved the final version.

Acknowledgement
This project was supported by a grant from Tehran University of Medical Sciences. We thank Dr. Kjell Andersson, AstraZeneca, Sweden, for kind donation of pure powder of 5 -hydroxyomeprazole. We are grateful to Dr. Mehdi Ansari Dogaheh, Department of Pharmaceutics, Faculty of Pharmacy, Kerman Medical Sciences and Dr. Mohsen Nabimeybodi, Department of pharmaceutics, Faculty of Pharmacy, Yazd University of Medical Sciences, for kind assistance in collection of blood samples.

Author details
[1]Biopharmaceutics and Pharmacokinetics Division, Department of Pharmaceutics, School of Pharmacy, Tehran University of Medical sciences, Tehran, Iran. [2]Cellular and Molecular Research Center (CMRC), Iran University of Medical Sciences, Tehran, Iran. [3]Department of Pharmacology and Toxicology, School of Pharmacy, Tehran University of Medical sciences, Tehran, Iran. [4]Department of pharmaceutics, School of Pharmacy, Kermanshah University of Medical Sciences, Kermanshah, Iran.

References
1. Sim SC, Nordin L, Andersson TM-L, Virding S, Olsson M, Pedersen NL, Ingelman- Sundberg M: Association Between CYP2C19 Polymorphism and Depressive Symptoms. *Am J Med Genet* 2010, 153(B):1160–1166.
2. Zanger UM, Schwab M: Cytochrome P450 enzymes in drug metabolism: Regulation of gene expression, enzyme activities, and impact of genetic variation. *J Pharmacol Ther* 2013, 138:103–141.
3. Qiao H-L, Hu Y-R, Tian X, Jia L-J, Gao N, Zhang L-R, Guo Y-z: Pharmacokinetics of three proton pump inhibitors in Chinese subjects in relation to the CYP2C19 genotype. *Eur J Clin Pharmacol* 2006, 62:107–112.
4. Weide JVD, Baalen-Benedek EHV, Kootstra-Ros JE: Metabolic ratios of psychotropics as indication of cytochrome P450 2D6/2C19 genotype. *Ther Drug Monit* 2005, 27:478–483.
5. Yu B-N, Chen G-L, He N, Ouyang D-S, Chen X-P, Liu Z-Q, Zhou HH: Pharmacokinetic of citalopram in relation to genetic polymorphism of CYP2C19. *Drug Metabol Dispos* 2003, 31(10):1255–1259.
6. Mrazek DA, Biernacka JM, O'Kane DJ, Black JL, Cunningham JM, Drews MS, Snyder KA, Stevens SR, Rush AJ, Weinshilboum RM: CYP2C19 variation and citalopram response. *Pharmacogenet Genomics* 2011, 21:1–9.
7. Wang G, Lei HP, Li Z, Tan Z-R, Guo D, Fan L, Chen Y, Hu D-L, Wang D, Zhou H-H: The CYP2C19 ultra rapid metabolizer genotype influences the pharmacokinetics of voriconazol in healthy male volunteers. *Eur J Clin Pharmacol* 2009, 65:281–285.
8. Sibbing S, Koch W, Gebhard D, Schuster T, Braun S, Stegherr J, Morath T, Scho˙mig A, Beckerath NV, Kastrati A: Cytochrome 2C19*17 allelic variant, platelet aggregation, bleeding events, and stent thrombosis in clopidogrel-treated patients with coronary stent placement. *Circulation* 2010, 121:512–518.
9. Hulot JS, Collet JP, Silvain J, Pena A, Bellemain-Appaix A, Barthélémy O, Cayla G, Beygui F, Montalescot G: Cardiovascular risk in clopidogrel-treated patients according to cytochrome P450 2C19*2 loss-of-function allele or proton pump inhibitor coadministration: a systematic meta-analysis. *J Am Coll Cardiol* 2010, 56(2):134–143.
10. Mathijssen RHJ, Schaik RHN: Genotyping and phenotyping cytochrome P450: Perspectives for cancer treatment. *Eur J Cancer* 2006, 42:141–148.
11. Gabriella Scordo M, Caputi AP, D'Arrigo C, Fava G, Spina E: Allele and genotype frequencies of CYP2C9, CYP2C19 and CYP2D6 in an Italian population. *Pharmacol Res* 2004, 50:195–200.
12. Ingelman-Sundberg M, Sim SC, Ingelman-Sundberg A, Rodriguez-Antona C: Influence of cytochrome P450 polymorphism on drug therapies: Pharmacogenetic and clinical aspects. *Pharmacol Ther* 2007, 116:496–526.
13. Chaudhry AS, Kochhar R, Kohli KK: Genetic polymorphism of CYP2C19 & therapeutic response to proton pump inhibitors. *Indian J Med Res* 2008, 127(6):521–530.
14. Lee S-J, Kim W-Y, Kim H, Shon J-H, Lee SS, Shin J-G: Identification of new CYP2C19 variants exhibiting decreased enzyme activity in the metabolism of S-Mephenytoin and Omeprazole. *Drug Metab Dispos* 2009, 37(11):2262–2269.
15. Li-Wan-Po A, Girard T, Farndon P, Cooley C, Lithgow J: Pharmacogenetics of CYP2C19: functional and clinical implications of a new variant CYP2C19*17. *Br J Clin Pharmacol* 2010, 69(3):222–230.
16. Rosemary J, Adithan C, Padmaja N, Shashindran CH, Gerard N, Krishnamoorthy R: The effect of the CYP2C19 genotype on the hydroxylation index of Omeprazole in south Indians. *Eur J Clin Pharmacol* 2005, 61:19–23.
17. Sim SC, Risinger C, Dahl ML, Aklillu E, Christensen M, Bertilsson L, Ingelman-Sundberg M: A common novel CYP2C19 gene variant causes ultrarapid drug metabolism relevant for the drug response to proton pump inhibitors and antidepressants. *Clin Pharmacol Ther* 2006, 79:103–113.

18. Anichavezhi D, Roa C, Shewade DG, Krishnamoorthy R, Adithan C: Distribution of *CYP2C19*17* allele and genotype in an Indian population. *J Clin Pharmacy Ther* 2012, 37:313–318.

19. Pedersen RS, Brasch-Andersen C, Sim SC, Bergmann TK, Halling J, Petersen MS, Weihe P, Edvardsen H, Kristensen VN, Brøsen K, Ingelman-Sundberg M: Linkage disequilibrium between the *CYP2C19*17* allele and wide type CYP2C8 and CYP2C9 alleles: identification of CYP2C haplotypes in healthy Nordic population. *Eur J Clin Pharmacol* 2010, 66:1199–1205.

20. Sugimito K, Uno T, Yamazaki H, Tateishi T: Limited frequency of the *CYP2C19*17* allele and its minor role in a Japanese population. *Br J Clin Pharmacol* 2008, 65(3):437–439.

21. Sakai T, Aoyama N, Kita T, Sakaeda T, Nishiguchi K, Nishitora Y, Hohda T, Sirasaka D, Tamura T, Tanigawara Y, Kasuga M, Okumura K: CYP2C19 genotype and pharmacokinetics of three proton pump inhibitors in healthy subjects. *Pharm Res* 2001, 18(6):72–77.

22. Cho H, Choi MK, Cho DY, Yeo CW, Jeong HE, Shon JH, Lee JY: Effect of CYP2C19 genetic polymorphism on pharmacokinetics and pharmacodynamics of a new proton pump inhibitor, ilaprazole. *J Clin Pharmacol* 2012, 52(7):976–984.

23. Ammon S, Treiber G, Kees F, Klotz U: Influence of age on the steady state disposition of drugs commonly used for the eradication of *Helicobacter pylori*. *Aliment Pharmacol Ther* 2000, 14(6):759–766.

24. Ishizawa Y, Yasui-Furukori N, Takahata T, Sasaki M, Tateishi T: The effect of aging on the relationship between the cytochrome P450 2C19 genotype and Omeprazole pharmacokinetics. *Clin pharmacokinetics* 2005, 44:1179–1189.

25. Chong E, Ensom M: Pharmacogenetics of the Proton Pump Inhibitors: A Systematic Review. *Pharmacotherapy* 2003, 23(4):460–471.

26. Isaza C, Henao J: Isaza Martínez J H, Sepúlveda Arias J, Beltrán L: Phenotype-genotype analysis of CYP2C19 in Colombian mestizo individuals. *BMC Clin Pharmacol* 2007, 7(6):1–5.

27. Ramsjö M, Aklillu E, Bohman L, Ingelman-Sundberg M, Roh HK: CYP2C19 activity comparison between Swedish and Koreans: effect of genotype, sex, oral contraceptive use and smoking. *Eur J Clin Pharmacol* 2010, 66:871–877.

28. Niioka T, Uno T, Sugimoto K, Sugawara K, Hayakari M, Tateishi T: Estimation of CYP2C19 activity by the Omeprazole hydroxylation index at a single point in time after intravenous and oral administration. *Eur J Clin Pharmacol* 2007, 63(11):1031–1038.

29. Xie HG, Huang SL, Xu ZH, Xiao ZS, He N, Zhou HH: Evidence for the effect of gender on activity of (S)-mephenytoin 4′-hydroxylase (CYP2C19) in a Chinese population. *Pharmacogenetics* 1997, 7(2):115–119.

30. Laine K, Tybring G, Bertilsson L: No sex-related differences but significant inhibition by oral contraceptives of CYP2C19 activity as measured by the probe drugs mephenytoin and Omeprazole in healthy Swedish white subjects. *Clin Pharmacol Ther* 2000, 68(2):151–159.

31. Rezk NL, Brown KC, Kashuba ADM: A simple and sensitive bioanalytical assay for simultaneous determination of Omeprazole and its three major metabolites in human blood plasma using RP-HPLC after a simple liquid–liquid extraction procedure. *J Chromatogr B* 2006, 844:314–321.

32. Miller SA, Dykes DD, Polesky HF: A simple salting out procedure for extracting DNA from human nucleated cells. *Nucleic Acids Res* 1988, 16:1215.

33. De Morais SM, Wilkinson GR, Blaisdell J, Nakamura K, Meyer UA, Goldstein JA: The major genetic defect responsible for the polymorphism of S-mephenytoin metabolism in humans. *J Bio Chem* 1994, 269(22):15419–15422.

34. Qiang M, Anthony YHL: Pharmacogenetics, Pharmacogenomics, and Individualized Medicine. *Pharmacol Rev* 2011, 63:2437–2459.

35. Justenhoven C, Hamann U, Pierl CB, Baisch C, Harth V, Rabstein S, Spickenheuer A, Pesch B, Brüning T, Winter S, Ko YD, Brauch H: CYP2C19*17 is associated with decreased breast cancer risk. *Breast Cancer Res Treat* 2009, 115(2):391–396.

36. Musumba CO, Jorgensen A, Sutton L, Eker DV, Zhang E, Hara NO, Carr DF, Pritchard DM, Pirmohamed M, Eker DV, Zhang E, Hara NO, Carr DF, Pritchard DM, Pirmohamed M: CYP2C19*17 Gain-of-function polymorphism is associated with peptic ulcer disease. *Clin Pharmacol Ther* 2013, 93(2):195–203.

37. Li Y, Tang HL, Hu YF, Xie HG: The gain-of-function variant CYP2C19*17: a double-edged sword between thrombosis and bleeding in clopidogrel-treated patients. *J Thromb Haemost* 2012, 10(2):199–206.

38. Schroth W, Antoniadou L, Fritz P, Schwab M, Muerdter T, Zanger UM, Simon W, Eichelbaum M, Brauch H: Breast cancer treatment outcome with adjuvant tamoxifen relative to patient CYP2D6 and CYP2C19 genotypes. *J Clin Oncol* 2007, 25(33):5187–5193.

39. Ragia G, Arvanitidis KI, Tavridou A, Manolopoulos VG: Need for reassessment of reported CYP2C19 allele frequencies in various populations in view of *CYP2C19*17* discovery: the case of Greece. *Pharmacogenomics* 2009, 10(1):43–49.

40. Gurbel PA, Shuldiner AR, Bliden KP, Ryan K, Pakyz RE, Tantry US: The relation between CYP2C19 genotype and phenotype in stented patients on maintenance dual antiplatelet therapy. *Am Heart J* 2011, 161:598–604.

41. Gumus E, Karaca O, Babaoglu MO, Baysoy G, Balamtekin N, Demir H, Uslu N, Bozkurt A, Yuce A, Yasar U: Evaluation of lansoprazole as a probe for assessing cytochrome P450 2C19 activity and genotype-phenotype correlation in childhood. *Eur J Clin Pharmacol* 2012, 68(5):629–636.

42. Tamminga WJ, Wemer J, Oosterhuis B, Weiling J, Wilffert B, de Leij LF, de Zeeuw RA, Jonkman JH: CYP2D6 and CYP2C19 activity in a large population of Dutch healthy volunteers: indications for oral contraceptive-related gender differences. *Eur J Clin Pharmacol* 1999, 55(3):177–184.

43. Hägg S, Spigset O, Dahlqvist R: Influence of gender and oral contraceptives on CYP2D6 and CYP2C19 activity in healthy volunteers. *Br J Clin Pharmacol* 2001, 51(2):169–173.

44. Zand N, Tajik N, Moghaddam AS, Milanian I: Genetic polymorphisms of cytochrome P450 enzymes 2C9 and 2C19 in a healthy Iranian population. *Clin Exp Pharmacol Physiol* 2007, 34(1–2):102–105.

45. Akhlaghi A, Shirani S, Ziaie N, Pirhaji O, Yaran M, Shahverdi G, Sarrafzadegan N, Khosravi A, Khosravi E: Cytochrome P450 2C19 Polymorphism in Iranian Patients with Coronary Artery Disease. *ARYA Atheroscler* 2011, 7(3):106–110.

46. Saeed LH, Mayet AY: Genotype-Phenotype analysis of CYP2C19 in healthy Saudi individuals and its potential clinical implication in drug therapy. *Int J Med Sci* 2013, 10:1497–1502.

47. Tassaneeyakul W, Tawalee A, Tassaneeyakul W, Kukongaviriyapan V, Blaisdell J, Goldstein JA, Gaysornsiri D: Analysis of the CYP2C19 polymorphism in a North-eastern Thai population. *Pharmacogenetics* 2002, 12:221–225.

48. Zendedel N, Biramijamal F, Hossein-Nezad A, Zendedel N, Sarie H, Doughaiemoghaddam M, Pourshams A: Role of Cytochrome P450 2C19 genetic polymorphism in the therapeutic efficacy of omeprazole in Iranian patients with erosive reflux esophagitis. *Arch Iran Med* 2010, 13(5):406–412.

49. Gonzalez HM, Romero EM, Peregrina AA, de J Chavez T T, Escobar-Islas E, Lozano F, Hoyo-Vadillo C: CYP2C19- and CYP3A4-dependent Omeprazole metabolism in West Mexicans. *J Clin Pharmacol* 2003, 43:1211–1215.

50. Kimura M, Ieiri I, Wada Y, Mamiya K, Urae A, Iimori E, Sakai T, Otsubo K, Higuchi S: Reliability of the omeprazole hydroxylation index for CYP2C19 phenotyping: possible effect of age, liver disease and length of therapy. *Br J Clin Pharmacol* 1999, 47(1):115–119.

51. Williams ML, Bhargava P, Cherrouk I, Marshall JL, Flockhart DA, Wainer IW: A discordance of the cytochrome P450 2C19 genotype and phenotype in patients with advanced cancer. *Br J Clin Pharmacol* 2000, 49(5):485–488.

52. Helsby NA, Lo WY, Sharples K, Riley G, Murray M, Spells K, Dzhelai M, Simpson A, Findlay M: CYP2C19 pharmacogenetics in advanced cancer: compromised function independent of genotype. *Br J Cancer* 2008, 99(8):1251–1255.

53. Hagymási K, Müllner K, Herszényi L, Tulassay Z: Update on the pharmacogenomics of proton pump inhibitors. *Pharmacogenomics* 2011, 12(6):873–888.

54. Yamazaki H, Inoue K, Shaw PM, Checovich WJ, Guengerich FP, Shimada T: Different contributions of cytochrome P450 2C19 and 3A4 in the oxidation of omeprazole by human liver microsomes: effects of contents of these two forms in individual human samples. *J Pharmacol Exp Ther* 1997, 283(2):434–442.

10

Enhanced oxygen transfer rate and bioprocess yield by using magnetite nanoparticles in fermentation media of erythromycin

Ghazal Labbeiki[1], Hossein Attar[1*], Amir Heydarinasab[1], Sayed Sorkhabadi[2,3] and Alimorad Rashidi[4]

Abstract

Background: Magnetite nanoparticles have widespread biomedical applications. In the aerobic bioprocesses, oxygen is a limiting factor for the microbial metabolic rate; hence a high availability of oxygen in the medium is crucial for high fermentation productivity. This study aimed to examine the effect of using magnetite nanoparticles on oxygen transfer rate in erythromycin fermentation culture.

Methods: Magnetite nanoparticles were synthetized through co-precipitation method. After observing the enhanced oxygen transfer rate in deionized water enriched with magnetite nanoparticles, these nanoparticles were used in the media of by *Saccharopolyspora erythraea* growth to explore their impact on erythromycin fermentation titer. Treatments comprised different concentrations of magnetite nanoparticles, (0, 0.005, 0.02 v/v).

Results: In the medium containing 0.02 v/v magnetite nanoparticles, KLa was determined to be 1.89 time higher than that in magnetite nanoparticle-free broth. An improved 2.25 time higher erythromycin titer was obtained in presence of 0.02 v/v nanoparticles.

Conclusions: Our results, demonstrate the potential of magnetite nanoparticles for enhancing the productivity of aerobic pharmaceutical bioprocesses.

Keywords: Bioprocess, Oxygen transfer rate, Mass transfer coefficient (KLa), Magnetite nanoparticles, Pharmaceutical biotechnology, Fermentation, *Saccharopolyspora erythraea*

Background

Oxygen is one of the most important substrate influencing productivity of aerobic bioprocesses [1]. While oxygen has a low solubility in most fermentation media, the uptake of the major amount of oxygen by microorganisms during the fermentation decreases the dissolved oxygen level in liquid to less than the critical concentration, rendering oxygen the limiting factor for productivity. A significantly low rate of oxygen transfer from gas into liquid, will lead to a decreased microbial metabolic rate, thereby low fermentation performance. Therefore an adequate supply of O_2 is required for achieving a high fermentation productivity, particularly in high-cell

density bioprocesses [2] such as erythromycin fermentation by *Saccharopolyspora erythraea*.

The Oxygen Transfer Rate (OTR) is usually determined by volumetric mass transfer coefficient (KLa). This variable is affected by several factors, including composition of medium, and geometrical and operating characteristic of the bioreactor [3]. Several methods have been proposed for improving KLa, including use of more effective agitation and aeration systems, enriching air with pure oxygen, reducing gas bubbles' size and enhancing gas hold up [2], and modifying physical properties of the medium by adding dispersed phases containing particles in size of μm [4] capable of solubilizing O_2 more than water.

Recent studies have shown that nanomaterials have potential to positively influence the variables affecting biochemical processes. For instance, Olle et al. [4] showed that O_2 mass transfer improves in the presence of colloidal nanoparticle dispersion. In addition, Nagi et al. [5]

* Correspondence: Attar.h@srbiau.ac.ir
[1]Department of Chemical Engineering, Science and Research Branch, Islamic Azad University(IAU), Tehran, Iran
Full list of author information is available at the end of the article

reported an enhanced oxygen mass transfer rate in the presence of nano-size particles.

Following this growing line of research, in the present study, first aqueous solution of magnetite nanoparticles (MNPs) was prepared. The solution was then added to the fermentation media of *S. erythraea* to examine the possible effects of magnetite nanoparticles on O_2 transfer rate and final titer of fermentation product.

Methods

Materials
The erythromycin-producing strain *Saccharopolyspora erythraea* PTCC 1685 was obtained from Persian Type Culture Collection I-124, Iran. Soybean flour was supplied from Maxsoy Co., Iran. Chemical reagents and media were purchased from Merck or Sigma.

Synthesis of nanoparticles
Several procedures have been developed for synthesis of iron oxide nanoparticles [6,7]. In this study, co-precipitation technique was used for synthesis of magnetite nanofluid, which is based on the simultaneous precipitation of Fe_{3+}, Fe_{2+} ions in basic aqueous media [6]. Some advantages of this method include being straightforward, cheap, and environment-friendly, and producing a uniform size distribution of nanoparticles.

To prepare solution of MNPs, 23.5 g $FeCl_3.6H_2O$ and 8.6 g $FeCl_2.4H_2O$ were dissolved in 25 ml deionized water in an Erlenmeyer flask under Nitrogen sparging, 80°C and vigorous mechanical stirring. After 30 min, 45 ml of an aqueous solution of NH_4OH was added to the mixture dropwise, after which the color of solution changes from light-brown to black, an indication of MNPs formation. The reaction was continued at 80°C under stirring and Nitrogen sparging conditions for 30 min to allow the substance completely crystalize. Afterwards the solution was cooled at room temperature [4,8-10]. The process reaction follows the following formula:

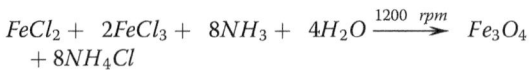

$$FeCl_2 + 2FeCl_3 + 8NH_3 + 4H_2O \xrightarrow{1200\ rpm} Fe_3O_4 + 8NH_4Cl$$

Due to their strong magnetic properties, the synthetic MNPs were aggregated near the magnet. MNPs were then washed with deionized water three time sat the end of process. Next, NPs were dried in oven at 80°C overnight to be characterized by XRD and TEM analysis [4].

Experimental determination of the volumetric mass transfer coefficient (KLa) by dynamic method
According to the Dynamic method [11] for determining mass transfer coefficient, first the concentration of the dissolved oxygen in the liquid phase in reduced by means of Nitrogen bubbling until the oxygen concentration falls to zero. Afterwards, by bubbling the air into the reaction container the concentration of dissolved oxygen is increased [11-13]. The KLa can then be calculated using the two-film theory. According to this theory, the rate of oxygen transfer from gas phase into liquid phase (at cell-free systems) is represented by:

$$\frac{dc}{dt} = K_La(C^* - C_L) \tag{1}$$

where dc/dt is the accumulation rate of the oxygen in the liquid phase, KLa represents the lumped volumetric mass transfer coefficient, C^* denotes the saturate concentration of the dissolved oxygen in the broth, and C_L represents the dissolved oxygen concentration in the aqueous phase [14]. Integrating Equation 1 will result in Equation 2:

$$\int_{C_{L1}}^{C_{L2}} \frac{dC_L}{C^* - C_L} = \int_{t1}^{t2} K_La \cdot dt \tag{2}$$

With CL1 = 0 at t1 = 0, the integrated form of Equation (2) can be represented as the Equation 3:

$$ln\frac{C^* - C_{L2}}{C^*} = -K_La \cdot t_2 \tag{3}$$

A plot of $ln\frac{C^* - C_L}{C^*}$ vs. t will result in a straight line with slope of -KLa [12,14].

Media and cultural method
Spores of *S. erythraea* were produced on slants of CSL agar medium after 14 days in incubator at 30°C [15]. Ingredients of the sporulation medium used in this study was (per liter): 10 g CSL, 10 g starch, 2.5 g $CaCO_3$, 3 g $(NH_4)2SO_4$, 3 g NaCl, 20 g agar, 2 ml trace element ($MgSO_4.7H_2O$, $FeSO_4.7H_2O$, $ZnSO_4.7H_2O$, $CuSO_4.5H_2O$, $CoCl_2.6H_2O$, HCL 37%), pH 7 ± 0.1 [15]. A volume of 1 ml of spore suspension of strain was inoculated in a 1000 ml Erlenmeyer flask containing 100 ml of seeding medium and incubated at 30°C and 220 rpm for 48 hours on a shaker-incubator. The composition of seeding medium used in this study was (per liter): 30 g soybean meal, 10 g glucose, 10 g glycerol, 3.5 g $(NH_4)2SO_4$, 1 g $(NH_4)2HPO_4$, 5 g $CaCO_3$, pH 7 ± 0 [15]. Based on strain's morphology (Figure 1), culture's pH and biomass, the best inoculum was selected to be inoculated (5% v/v) into fermentation flasks. Fermentations were carried out in 9 Erlenmeyer flasks of 1000 ml, containing 150 ml of fermentation media. The composition of fermentation media was (per liter): 30 g soybean meal, 40 g dextrin, 30 g starch, 2 g$(NH_4)2SO_4$, 0.15 g $(NH_4)2HPO_4$, 10 g $CaCO_3$, 50 g rapeseed oil, pH 6.8. Two concentrations of MNPs (0.005, 0.02 v/v) were added to each fermentation flask. Flasks were then put in shaker-incubator at 33°C

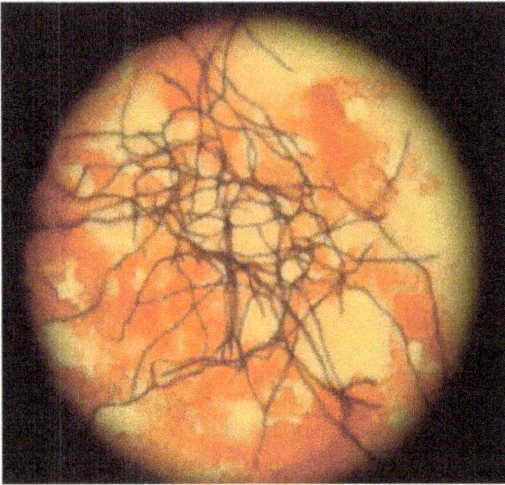

Figure 1 The mycelia of strain used as inoculum.

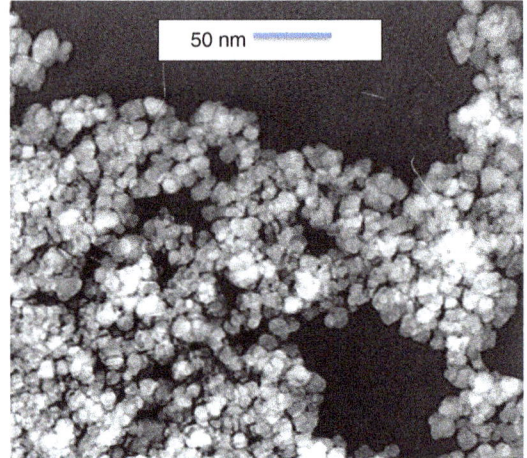

Figure 3 TEM image of magnetite nanoparticles.

and 220 rpm for 11 days [15-17]. All experiments were performed in triplicate in six batches. Samples of 7 ml were taken on days 6, 8, and 10 for further analysis. Investigation of S. erythraea morphology indicated that the hyphae of the strain were lysed on day 12, hence, no further erythromycin production was occurred.

Erythromycin assay

Purification of erythromycin was carried out by centrifugation of the samples (4000 rpm, 20 min) followed by using magnet to separate the possibly remaining magnetite nanoparticles from the supernatant. The supernatant was then diluted with 0.2 M carbonate-bicarbonate buffer of pH9.6 and the total erythromycin was extracted with chloroform. The extracted erythromycin was then mixed with the bromophenol blue reagent. The absorbance of

organic phase was measured at 415 nm by spectrophotometry [15-17].

Statistical analysis

T-test was used to examine the significance of the mean differences. KLa was calculated from regression analysis. $P < 0.05$ was considered as the statistical significance.

Results and discussion

Nanoparticles characterization

NPs' crystal structure

The crystal structure of the synthetized MNPs is characterized by X-ray powder diffraction (XRD) [9]. Figure 2 displays the structural properties of the MNPs as determined by XRD (Bruker axs D4, cu, step size 0.02). The XRD pattern shows the diffraction peaks at $2\theta = 18.270°$, 30.035°, 35.423° (strongest line), 43.053°, 53.392°, 56.944°,

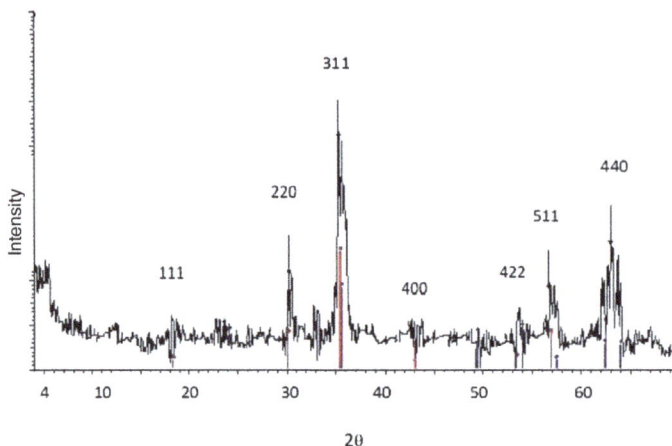

Figure 2 XRD pattern of synthetic nanoparticles.

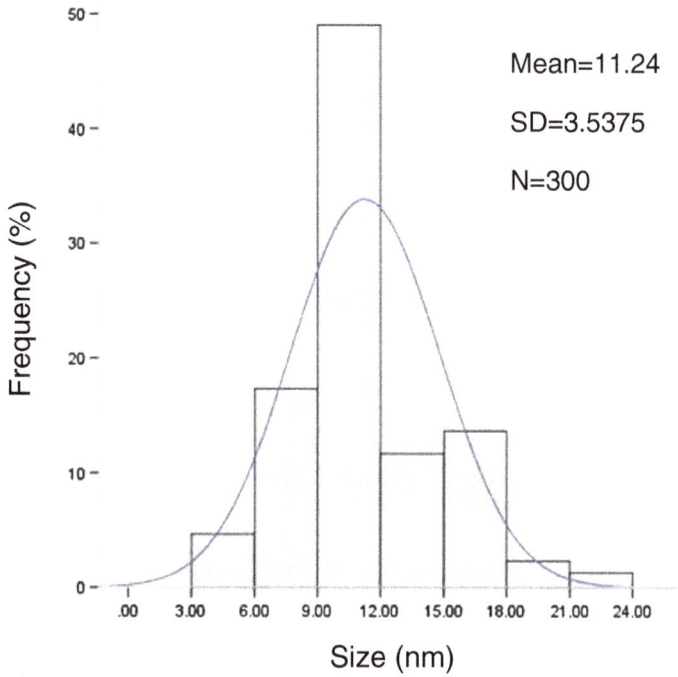

Figure 4 The size distribution of magnetite nanoparticles.

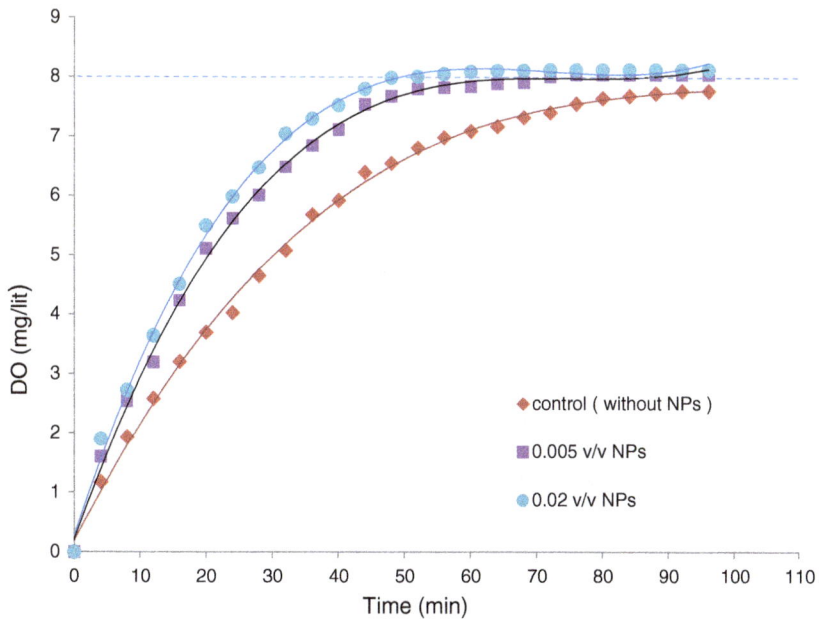

Figure 5 The dissolved oxygen at different concentrations of MNPs (each value in the figure is the mean of corresponding values from 3 repeated experiments).

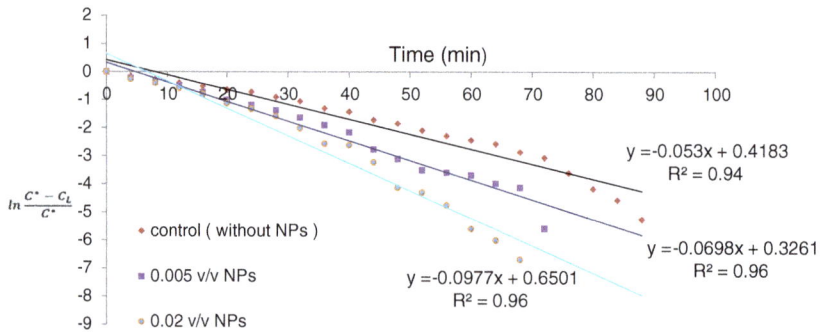

Figure 6 The linearized curve of dissolved oxygen at different concentrations of MNPs (the slope of the curve represents-KLa).

62.516°, which correspond to the (111), (220), (311), (400), (422), (511), (440) reflections, respectively [9,18-20].The XRD results show that the synthetized MNPs are well crystallized and the relative intensity of the diffraction peaks matches well with the reported XRD data for magnetite nanoparticles in the literature.

NPs' size
Morphology and size of the prepared MNPs was determined by Transmission Electron Microscopy (TEM) (Figure 3) [10,21-23]. A small amount of dried MNPs were dissolved in ethanol. The solution was then sonicated for better dispersion. A drop of the solution was then placed on a 200 mesh Copper grid and dried in the air. The sample was analyzed by TEM at 100 KV.

Diameter of the MNPs was determined directly from the TEM image [24]. Figure 4 displays the histogram of NPs' size distribution (n = 300). A mean (SD) size of particles is 11.24 (3.5) nm was calculated.

Effect of nanoparticles on mass transfer coefficient
The changes in concentration of dissolved oxygen in deionized water at different concentrations of MNPs were measured during the absorption process, based on Dynamic method [11,12], and compared with nanoparticle-free water, as the control. As shown in Figure 5, at all concentrations of MNPs, the amount of DO has increased and the time for achieving saturate concentration has decreased, when compared with the control. KLa was determined using the linearized curve of DO *vs.* time (see Methods). As shown in Figure 6, MNPs positively

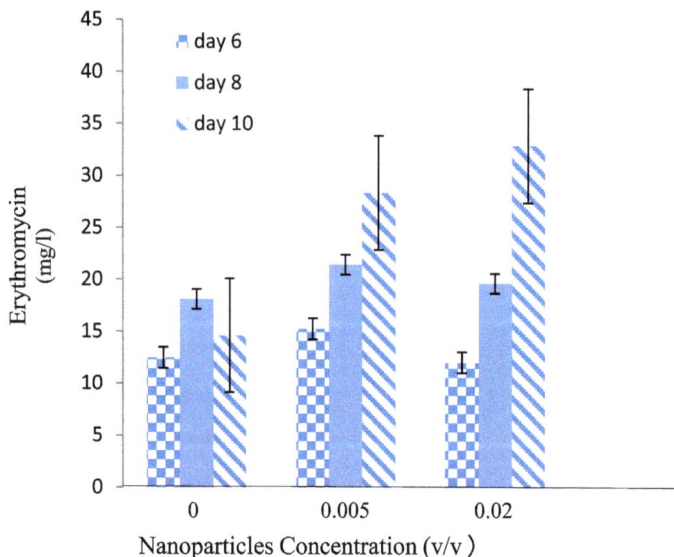

Figure 7 Effect of different concentrations of nanoparticles on the production of erythromycin by S. *erythraea* (each value on the figure is the mean of corresponding values from 12 repeated experiments).

affects the mass transfer coefficient; KLa in water containing 0.02 v/v MNPs is 1.85 times higher than that in the control.

Effect of MNPs on erythromycin titer

Magnetite MNPs with initial concentrations of zero (control medium), 0.005, 0.02 v/v were used in fermentation media of *S. erythraea* and their effect on erythromycin titer was examined. As shown in Figure 7, while the maximum concentration of erythromycin is 18.1 mg/lit in the control medium, in the medium with 0.02 v/v MNPs, a maximum titer of 32.86 mg/lit has obtained which is 2.25 times higher. Erythromycin final titer (day 10) in both 0.005 and 0.02 (v/v) media shows significant difference as compared with the control ($P < 0.05$). Figure 6 shows that this higher titer is due to the more prolonged production of erythromycin in MNP-containing medium compared to the control medium. It could be aurged that this higher titer is due to an extended viability of the microorganism as a result of higher OTR in the presence of MNPs.

The chief objective of the present study was to explore the impact of MNPs on OTR and thereby titer of bioprocess product. MNPs are strong oxygen absorbent due to their increased surface area at nano scale. These nanoparticles have proven useful when used as recyclable oxygen carriers in aerobic fermentation [25]. A number of mechanisms proposed for the positive impact of MNPs on OTR include enhancing oxygen solubility in the fermentation medium, inducing microconvection in the surrounding fluid by Brownian motion [4], and enlarging the gas-liquid interfacial surface through being adsorbed on the air bubbles, preventing them from coalescence [26].

Results obtained in this study, which are in close agreement with the findings from previous researches [4,25-27], add weight to the notion of MNPs being candidate members of O_2-vectors that promote the oxygen transfer in stirred aerobic bioprocesses.

Composition of fermentation medium plays an important role in the titer of secondary metabolites and the cost of fermentation product [15]. Because the erythromycin producing bacterium, *S. erythraea* is an aerobic actinomycete, proper oxygenation is crucial to achieve a high yield of this substance. Our results clearly indicate that presence of MNPs remarkably enhance the erythromycin production by *S. erythraea*.

Possible toxicity of nanoparticles is a major concern, particularly when used in pharmaceutical bioprocesses [28,29]. The fact that MNPs can be efficiently separated from fermentation medium, virtually eliminate the risk of possible toxic effects. On the other hand, the wide use of MNPs in environmental applications, including pollutant removal, toxicity mitigation, and water and waste treatment [30] indicates the safety of its use at limited doses. These advantages together with their positive impact on fermentation productivity as supported in this study, introduce use of them as a viable strategy for an improved pharmaceutical bioprocessing.

Conclusions

The metabolic rate and growth of microbial biocatalysts are controlled by oxygen; hence, for an improved yield of aerobic bioprocesses, there is a need for strategies enabling a high rate oxygen transfer, while maintain affordable energy consumption. Our results indicate that MNPs can improve the efficiency of oxygen transfer in the fermentation medium. Use of MNPs in the erythromycin fermentation culture enhanced erythromycin titer, presumably via promotion of microbial growth and viability. The straightforward and inexpensive synthetize of these biocompatible, non-toxic and non-volatile nanoparticles, together with their positive impact on oxygen transfer rate, introduce them as promising agents for achieving an enhanced productivity of the industrial bioprocesses.

Competing interests

The authors declare that they have no competing interests.

Authors' contributions

HA and AH jointly conceived and designed the study and contributed to the revision of the manuscript. GL made the major contribution to performing the experiments, summarizing and interpretation of the results, and drafting the manuscript. AR was involved in statistical analyses and drafting the manuscript. SMRS coordinated the study procedure and contributed to revision of the manuscript. All authors read and approved the final manuscript.

Acknowledgements

The authors wish to thank Dr. Meysam Mobasheri for participating in statistical analysis and revision of the manuscript.

Author details

[1]Department of Chemical Engineering, Science and Research Branch, Islamic Azad University(IAU), Tehran, Iran. [2]Department of Pharmacology, School of Advanced Sciences and Technologies in Medicine, Tehran University of Medical Sciences, Tehran, Iran. [3]Department of Toxicology and Pharmacology, Islamic Azad University of Pharmaceutical Sciences Branch, Tehran, Iran. [4]Catalyst and Nanotechnology Division, Research Institute of Petroleum Industry, Tehran, Iran.

References

1. Garcia-Ochoa F, Gomez E, Santos VE, Merchuk JC: **Oxygen uptake rate in microbial processes.** *Biochem Eng J* 2010, 49:289–307.
2. Fadavi A, Chisti Y: **Gas-Liquid mass transfer in a novel forced circulation loop reactor.** *Chem Eng J* 2005, 112:73–80.
3. Moutafchieva D, Popova D, Dimitrova M, Tchaoushev S: **Experimental determination of the volumetric mass transfer coefficient.** *J Chem Technol Metallurgy* 2013, 48(4):351–356.
4. Olle B, Bucak S, Holmes TC, Bromberg L, Hatton TA, Wang DIC: **Enhancement of oxygen mass transfer using functionalized magnetic nanoparticles.** *Ind Eng Chem Res* 2006, 45:4355–4363.
5. Nagy E, Feczko T, Koroknai B: **Enhancement of oxygen mass transfer rate in the presence of nanosized particles.** *Chem Eng Sci* 2007, 62:7391–7398.
6. Figuerola A, Di Corato R, Manna L, Pellegrino T: **From iron oxide NPs towards advanced iron-based inorganic materials designed for biomedical applications.** *J Pharmacol Res* 2010, 62:126–143.

7. Lu AH, Salabas EL, Schuth F: **Magnetic NPs: synthesis, protection, functionalization, and application.** *Angew Chem Int Ed Engl* 2007, **46**:1222–1244.

8. Sun J, Zhou SH, Hou P, Yang Y, Weng J, Li X, Li M: **Synthesis and characterization of biocompatible Fe3o4 Nanoparticles.** *J Biomed Mater Res* 2006, **A**:333–341.

9. Awwad AM, Salem NM: **A green and facile approach for synthesis of magnetite NPs.** *Nanosci Nanotechnol* 2012, **2**(6):208–213.

10. Kafayati ME, Raheb J, TorabiAngazi M, Alizadeh SH, Bardania H: **The Effect of magnetic Fe3O4 NPs on the growth of genetically manipulated bacterium,** *Pseudomonas aeruginosa.* *Iran J Biotechnol* 2013, **11**(1):41–46.

11. Garcia-Ochoa F, Gomez E: **Bioreactor scale-up and oxygen transfer rate in microbial processes: an overview.** *Biotechnol Adv* 2009, **27**:153–176.

12. Juarez P, Orejas J: **Oxygen transfer in a stirred reactor in laboratory scale.** *Lat Am Appl Res* 2001, **31**:433–439.

13. Haribabu K, Sivasubramanian V: **Determination of mass transfer coefficient in an inverse fluidized bed reactor using statistical and dynamic method for a non-Newtonian fluid.** *J Sci Ind Res* 2013, **72**:485–490.

14. Nielsen DR, Daugulis AJ, McLellan PJ: **A novel method of simulating oxygen mass transfer in two-phase partitioning bioreactors.** *J Biotech Bioeng* 2003, **83**(6):735–742.

15. Hamedi J, Malekzadeh F, Saghafi-nia AE: **Enhancing of erythromycin production by** *Saccharopolysporaeryhtraea* **with common and uncommon oils.** *J Microb Biotechnol* 2004, **31**:447–456.

16. Rostamza M, Noohi A, Hamedi J: **Enhancement in production of erythromycin by** *Saccharopolyspora erythraea* **by the Use of suitable industrial seeding-media.** *Daru J Pharm Sci* 2008, **1**:13–17.

17. Hamedi J, Khodagholi F, Hassani-Nasab A: **Increased erythromycin production by alginate as a medium ingredient or immobilization support in cultures of** *Saccharopolyspora erythraea.* *Biotechnol Lett* 2005, **27**:661–664.

18. Wang B, Wei Q, Qu SH: **Synthesis and characterization of uniform and crystalline magnetite nanoparticles via oxidation-precipitation and modified co-precipitation method.** *Int J Electrochem Sci* 2013, **8**:3786–3793.

19. Shaker S, Zafarian SH, Chakra SH, Rao KV: **Preparation and characterization of magnetite nanoparticles by Sol-Gel method for water treatment.** *Int J Inn Res Sci Eng Technol* 2013, **2**(7):2969–2973.

20. Bahrampour F, Raheb J, Rabiei Z: **Alteration in protein profile of** *Pseudomonas aeruginosa* **(PTSOX4) coated with magnetic nanoparticles.** *J Nanostructure Chem* 2013, **3**(58):1–8.

21. Wang R, Zuo SH, Zhu W, Zhang J, Fang J: **Rapid synthesis of Aqueous-Phase magnetite nanoparticles by atmospheric pressure Non-Thermal microplasma and their application in magnetic resonance imaging.** *Plasma Process Polym* 2014, **11**(5):448–454.

22. Giraldo L, Moreno-Pirajan JC: **Synthesis of magnetite nanoparticles and exploring their application in the removal of Pt2+ andAu3 + ions from aqueous solutions.** *Eur Chem Bull* 2013, **7**:445–452.

23. Mahmed N, Eczko OH, Soderberg O, Hannula SP: **Room temperature synthesis of magnetite nanoparticles by a simple reverse Co-Precipitation method.** *Mater Sci Eng* 2011, **18**:1–4.

24. Ghalamboran MR, Ramsden J, Ansari F: **Growth rate enhancement of** *Bradyrhizobium japanicum* **due to magnetite nanoparticles.** *J Bionanosci* 2009, **3**:1–6.

25. Bromberg LE, Hatton TA, Wang IC, Yin J, Olle B: **Bioprocesses enhanced by magnetic nanoparticles, United States patent.** 2006, **US0040388A1**:1–23.

26. Dobre T, Ohreac BS, Parvulescu OC, Danciu TD: **Effect of solid carriers on oxygen mass transfer in a stirred tank bioreactor.** *REVCHIM (Bucharest)* 2014, **65**(4):489–496.

27. Saeednia L, Hashemi Pour H, Afzali D: **Effect of nanoparticles on gas-liquid mass transfer coefficient.** *Iran Chem Eng J* 2013, **12**(66):50–57.

28. Mostafalou S, Mohammadi H, Ramazani A, Abdollahi M: **Different biokinetics of nanomedicines linking to their toxicity; an overview.** *Daru J Pharm Sci* 2013, **21**:14.

29. Mogharabi M, Abdollahi M, Faramarzi M: **Toxicity of nanomaterials; an undermined issue.** *Daru J Pharm Sci* 2014, **22**:59.

30. Tang SCN, Lo IMC: **Magnetic nanoparticles: essential factors for sustainable environmental applications.** *J Water Res* 2013, **47**:2613–2632.

Trend analysis of the pharmaceutical market in Iran; 1997–2010; policy implications for developing countries

Abbas Kebriaeezadeh[1,2*], Nasser Nassiri Koopaei[1], Akbar Abdollahiasl[1*], Shekoufeh Nikfar[1] and Nafiseh Mohamadi[3]

Abstract

Background: So far, no detailed study of the Iranian pharmaceutical market has been conducted, and only a few studies have analyzed medicine consumption and expenditure in Iran. Pharmaceutical market trend analysis remains one of the most useful instruments to evaluate the pharmaceutical systems efficiency. An increase in imports of medicines, and a simultaneous decrease in domestic production prompted us to investigate the pharmaceutical expenditure structure. On the other hand, analyzing statistics provides a suitable method to assess the outcomes of national pharmaceutical policies and regulations.

Methods: This is a descriptive and cross-sectional study which investigates the Iranian pharmaceutical market over a 13-year period (1997–2010). This study used the Iranian pharmaceutical statistical datasheet published by the Iranian Ministry of Health. Systematic searches of the relevant Persian and English research literature were made. In addition, official government documents were analyzed as sources of both data and detailed statements of policy.

Results: Analysis of the Iranian pharmaceutical market in the 13-year period shows that medicine consumption sales value growth has been 28.38% annually. Determination of domestic production and import reveals that 9.3% and 42.3% annual growth, respectively, have been experienced.

Conclusions: The Iranian pharmaceutical market has undergone great growth in comparison with developing countries and the pharmerging group, and the market is expanding quickly while a major share goes to biotechnology drugs, which implies the need to commercialization activities in novel fields like pharmaceutical biotechnology. This market expansion has been in favor of imported medicine in sales terms, caused by the reinforcement of suspicious policies of policy makers that necessitates fundamental rearrangements.

Keywords: Pharmaceutical market trends, Therapeutic categories, Pharmaceutical biotechnology, Commercialization

Background

Total expenditure on health in Iran is increasing, while the public sector's share is decreasing. Private sector expenditure as out-of-pocket payment is remarkably high as it accounts for more than 50% of the whole expenditure [1]. The modern Iranian pharmaceutical system commenced 100 years ago with the opening of the first modern-style pharmacy by German, French, and Austrian pharmacists in Tehran. Pharmacy training was initiated by European instructors at Darolfonoon, which was remodeled with the inauguration of the Tehran Faculty of Pharmacy in 1934 which undertook a very important role in the Iranian pharmaceutical industry. Established in 1946, Abidi was the first Iranian pharmaceutical company, followed by Tolid Darou and Darou Pakhsh in 1958 and 1963, respectively [2]. After the Islamic revolution, two major motions caused fundamental changes: nationalization of the pharmaceutical industries, and generic scheme. Governmental industry privatization and transition to the semi-governmental sector was one of the major actions taken by the government in the 1988 to 1993 period. This study examines the present situation of the pharmaceutical system

* Correspondence: kebriaee@tums.ac.ir; abdollahiasl@gmail.com
[1]Department of Pharmacoeconomics and Pharmaceutical Administration, Faculty of Pharmacy, Tehran University of Medical Sciences, P.O. Box 14155–6451, Tehran 14174, Iran
[2]Department of Toxicology and Pharmacology, Faculty of Pharmacy, Tehran University of Medical Sciences, P.O. Box 14155–6451, Tehran 14174, Iran
Full list of author information is available at the end of the article

in Iran, including the domestic production companies, importing companies, distribution, regulations, human resources in the pharmaceutical system, and market trend analysis [3].

Present situation of the Iranian pharmaceutical industry

Pharmaceutical production consisted mainly of 89 companies in 2010. The market concentration ratio is low. In 2010, the Herfindahl–Hirschman Index (HHI) was 295.11 for the domestic production companies, indicating little market power. Raw and packaged materials are provided by the domestic and import suppliers. Regarding sales, ten top pharmaceutical companies in 2009–2010 are shown in Table 1. Tamin Pharmaceutical Investment Company (Social Security Organization), Sobhan Pharma Group, and Shafadarou corporation (Melli Bank Investment Corporation) are the most important public owners of the pharmaceutical industry. Based on these structures, pharmaceutical holdings (Groups) sales are shown in Table 2. Data reveals an increasing rate of privatization in pharmaceutical sector.

Import companies

There are 93 private companies engaged in importing medicine, and 30 designated emergency medicine centers besides national medicine and medical equipment corporations. There is Red Crescent (Ministry of Health), Darou pakhsh trade development (Tamin Investment Corporation), and KBC (Sobhan Pharmaceutical Group), which are all public. In 2010, the HHI was 781, which is higher in comparison with that of the domestic production companies. Ten top importer companies in 2009–2010 are shown in Table 3.

Distribution

There were 35 nationwide drug distribution companies, among which the first four distribute approximately 70% of the entire market's drugs. All major holdings have their own nationwide drug distribution companies that are ranked in the top four. HHI was 1387, which was significantly higher than that of the domestic production.

Regulations

Passed in 1955, the medicine, drug, food, and drink affairs law act is the cornerstone for the current pharmaceutical procedures in Iran. Most of the bylaws and ordinances are designed and approved in the drug affairs department [2].

Licensing

Production, importation, and distribution of medicinal products are performed under strict control by the authorities, and involve registration and licensure by the food and drug organization (formerly, Undersecretary of Food and Drug).

Pricing

Medicine price is controlled by the food and drug organization through pricing commission regulations in a cost plus basis through comparison with selected companies according to published regulations.

Reimbursement

Medicine cost reimbursement is mainly undertaken by three major organizations: Social Security Organization (public), Medical Services Insurance Organization (governmental), and Medical Insurance Services Organization of Armed Forces (governmental), all of which reimburse the cheapest medicine registered. The emerging supplementary insurance companies are putting constraints on pharmaceutical expenditure. There is a positive list of medicines fully covered by the government that contains specialty drugs.

Human resources

Pharmacists are considered a major source for the pharmaceutical system. Most of the 13000 pharmacist society members are involved in pharmacies. About 6%

Table 1 Ten top domestic production pharmaceutical companies in Iran; 2009-2010

Rank	Company name	Market share	Cumulative market share
1	Darou Pakhsh Pharma	6.6%	6.6%
2	Exir Pharma	6.1%	12.7%
3	Jaber Ebne Hayyan	5.8%	18.5%
4	Farabi	5.3%	23.8%
5	Tehran Chemie	5.2%	29.0%
6	Alborz Darou	3.8%	32.8%
7	Sobhan Darou	3.7%	36.5%
8	Osvah	3.6%	40.1%
9	Dana	2.9%	42.9%
10	Aboureihan	2.8%	45.7%

Table 2 Major holdings in domestic pharmaceutical production in Iran; 2009-2010

Rank	Pharmaceutical holdings	Market share	Cumulative market share
1	Tamin Investment Corporation	29%	29%
2	Sobhan Pharmaceutical Group	16%	45%
3	Shafadarou Corporation	10%	55%
4	Tehran Chimi Corporation (Private)	10%	65%

Table 3 Ten top importer companies in Iran; 2009-2010

Rank	Company name	Market share	Cumulative market share
1	Cobel	17.2%	17.2%
2	Akbarieh	12.3%	29.6%
3	Behestan Darou	11.6%	41.2%
4	Shafayab Gostar	8.4%	49.6%
5	Jahan Behbood	5.7%	55.3%
6	Ahran Tejarat	5.0%	60.3%
7	Gostaresh Bazargani Daroupakhsh	4.8%	65.1%
8	Actover	3.4%	68.4%
9	KBC	2.6%	71.0%
10	Kavosh Gostar Darou	2.2%	73.2%

of the pharmacists work in the industry. In the industry itself, less than 2% of the trained and scientific workforce is engaged in research and development.

Active pharmaceutical ingredients

A growing number of companies are engaged in the production of Active Pharmaceutical Ingredient (API). Each holding has its own API-producing branch, and there are more than 30 companies engaged in production of APIs. Formal policies of the Ministry of Health actively promote motions towards independence in the API industry. Companies active in the field of API production are mainly possessed by the private sector, contrary to the finished products and distribution companies [4].

Methods

This is a descriptive and cross-sectional study which investigates the Iranian pharmaceutical market over a 13-year period (1997–2010). This study used the Iranian pharmaceutical statistical datasheet published by the Iranian Ministry of Health. Drug consumption statistics are collected by the Food and Drug Organization (FDO) through the data received from the drug distribution companies. All distribution companies deliver their data on drug sales to the pharmacies as a unified format to the food and drug organization on a monthly basis. That data, after revision, is published as the Iranian pharmaceutical statistical datasheet yearly as sales volume (by unit) for any medicine delivered, and cost per medicine unit. Although that data does not represent real drug consumption and the subsidy paid by the government and only reveals the sales of drug to the pharmacies, it is the most unique and convenient method to monitor the pharmaceutical market. Systematic searches of the relevant Persian and English research literature were made, using electronic databases in addition to written reports. Official government documents were also analyzed as sources of data and detailed statements of policy.

Different sources, such as statistics published by the Iranian Ministry of Health, pharmaceutical production companies syndicate, and the national medicine assemblies were also researched for statistics and data on medicine consumption in a domestic production and importation separation basis, production and importation statistics, pharmaceutical expenditure, medicine consumption per capita, and drug utilization by sales value in different therapeutic categories.

Results

The trend analysis shows that Iranian pharmaceutical medicine market has been drastically grown in the recent decade. In the period, the population of the country has grown from 61 to 74 million, namely a total and annual growth of 21.3% and 1.53%, respectively. Total medicine market sales value reached $2.467 billion in 2010 from $0.139 billion in 1997, representing a 1669% increase (Figure 1). The annual growth rate was 28.38%. Domestic pharmaceutical production sales value reached $1.639 billion in 2010 in comparison with $0.125 billion in 1997, a 1213% growth. The average annual sales value growth is 9.3%. The correlation coefficient (R^2) of 0.9293 shows a fairly consistent growth, though the 2011 estimate shows a decrease in market sales value. The imported medicine market sales value rose to $0.828 billion in 2010 from $0.015 in 1997, showing a dramatic total growth of 5499%, and an annual growth of 42.3%. In the period under investigation, sales value percentile proportion of imports to total drug consumption has reached 39% from 10.59% in the base year, showing a huge growth of 28.41%. The average sales value percentile proportion of imports to total medicine consumption has been 2.1% (R^2: 0.9612) (Figure 2). The sales value percentile proportion of domestic production to total medicine consumption has reduced from 89.41% to 61% in 2010, revealing a significant decrease of 28%.

Per capita drug consumption sales value

Over the 13-year period, the data indicates that the index has reached $34.43 from $2.28 in 1997, which shows an overwhelming growth of 1405%, and an annual average growth of 10.8% (R^2: 0.9235) (Figure 3). These figures show marked growth in comparison to population growth (20%).

Per capita value of domestic pharmaceutical medicine consumption

This index has reached $22.86 from $2.05 in 1997, with a total and an annual growth of 1018% and 10.8%, respectively (R^2: 0.9397).

Per capita value of the imported medicine consumption

This index has reached $11.57 from $0.24 in 1997, with a total growth of 4373% (R^2: 0.8907).

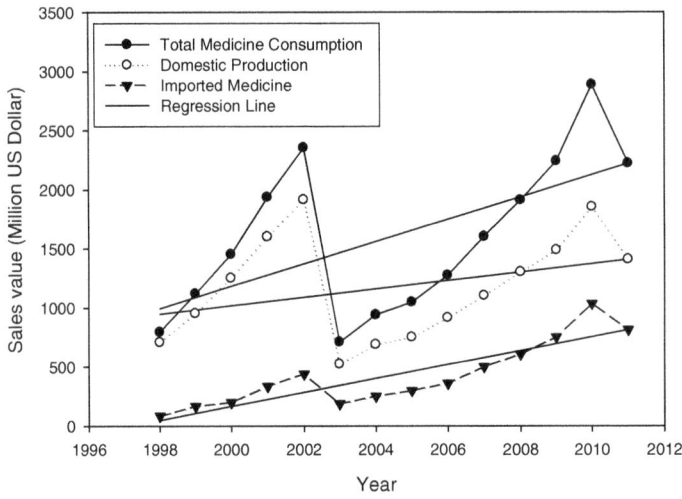

Figure 1 Total, domestic production and imported medicine consumption by value; 1998–2011.

Average sales value of the medicines by unit

The index reached an estimated $0.084 in 2011 from $0.009 in 1997, with a growth rate of 847% (R^2: 0.9407) (Figure 4). The average sales value of domestic and imported medicines by unit also shows a total growth rate of 631% (R^2: 0.9506) and 1930% (R^2: 0.8345), respectively.

Drug consumption by therapeutic categorization (by ATC codes)

As the graph depicts, the market shows a point drop in the year 2000 that was due to the nationwide currency exchange rate variation (Figure 5). The data shows that antiinfectives preparations for systemic use and then

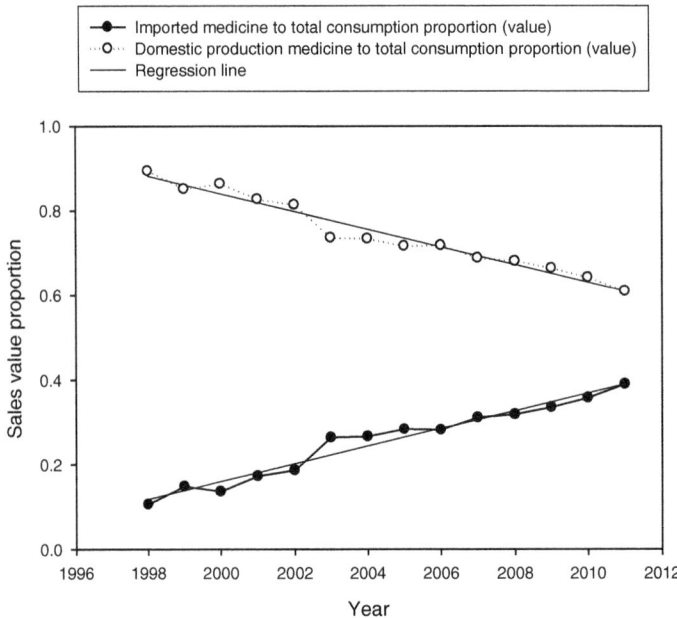

Figure 2 Sales value percentile proportion of imports and domestic production to the total medicine consumption; 1998–2011.

antineoplastics and immunomudulating agents seize the most shares in the market and have had the steepest slope among the categories. Alimentary tract and metabolism and nervous system products also show high growth rates. The two recently mentioned categories contain the most prevalent utilization among all in terms of volume (data not shown).

Discussion

This study presents the market environment of the pharmaceutical sector in Iran, and highlights its challenges and future prospects. In order to study a country's medicine market systematically, various indicators can be applied, e.g. market behavior about specific dosage forms or quantity or quality trends [3]. Most owners of the pharmaceutical industry were either dependent on the former regime or foreigners who left Iran after the revolution, so young domestic pharmacists began to manage the pharmaceutical system of the country. Iran-Iraq War (1980–1988) also prompted the need for strict monitoring of the market. The revolutionary government exerted fundamental changes in the food and drug organization in order to assess the need for pharmaceuticals in both general society and for the military forces. With the establishment of the planning office in the food and drug organization, some experts were ascribed to closely monitor the needs and prepare the production and the import scheme. In 1986, the government in office assumed private ownership and liberalization in the economic system, which resulted in magnificent growth in the market. In 1999, the government allowed domestic production companies usage of their free capacity to cross the borders of planning by the food and drug organization. In 2001, further liberalization in the

pharmaceutical system and the lack of subsidized currency caused an increase in prices. This liberalization in the pharmaceutical system also augmented imports. Throughout the period, domestic production constituted a major share in the market [3]. The major reasons for the growing demand are as follows [4,5]:

- Iran's demographic structure and population growth;
- increased insurance coverage of the population;
- increased level of income and gross domestic product (GDP) per capita;
- incidence of new diseases and epidemiologic transition, e.g. types of cancer and multiple sclerosis;
- intentionally lowered medicine price; and
- medical sciences advances.

In the period under investigation, accessibility to health services and insurance coverage has grown remarkably, possibly as a result of GDP growth. The government has approached the medicine accessibility positively, and a number of medicines have been included in the medicine list. However, insurance coverage has not expanded simultaneously and proportionately. Health sector budget share in the GDP did not develop acceptably, causing a drastic increase in the public's out-of-pocket payment. Insurance coverage expansion was through three major organizations: the Social Security Organization, Medical Services Insurance Organization, and Medical Insurance Services Organization of Armed Forces. The universal insurance coverage act obliges the population to register for an insurance service which contributes to the goal. Iranian pharmaceutical industries mostly manufacture traditional medicines, and deficiency in the investments needed for monoclonal antibodies and other biotechnology-derived

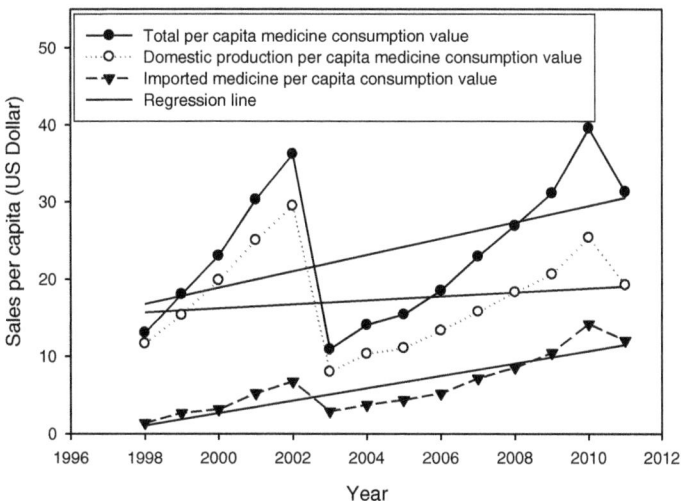

Figure 3 Total, domestic production and import value per capita medicine consumption; 1998–2011.

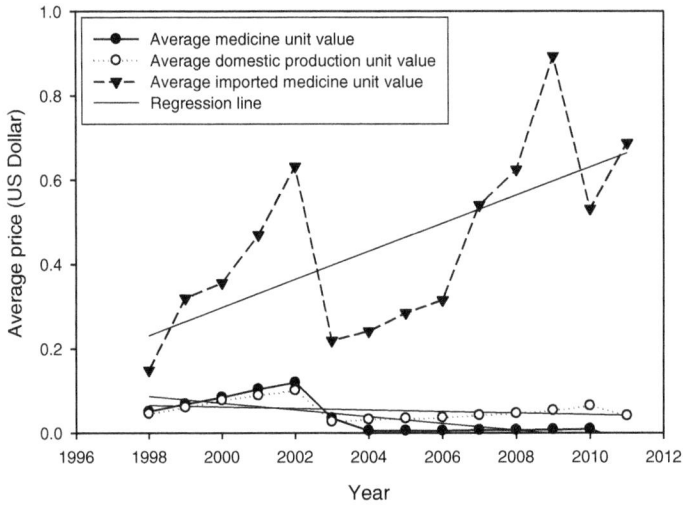

Figure 4 Average sales value of the total, domestic production and imported medicines by unit; 1998–2011.

products, as a consequence, helped the higher share of imported medicine. The Iranian pharmaceutical industry's private sector has not yet developed as much as required. More than 70% of the domestic industries are owned by the government and its related bodies or the public organizations. As evidenced by the two existing biotechnology companies, both of which are privately-owned, privatization can lead to greater sustainable development in domestic industries [6,7]. Currently, total pharmaceutical market value is about $3.2 billion, or as much as $4-4.5 billion according to some estimates on the real market size [8]. The present difference between real and estimated value is attributed to the price suppression policies of the authorities [9]. It should also be noted that national currency has experienced a drastic devaluation against USD. Iran experiences

an average growth rate of 28.38%, which is significantly more than developing countries such as China and India which have around 11 to 15% growth [10,11]. The results show that the domestic production sales value has grown, but not in concordance with that of the imported medicine sales value. The results also imply that the current pharmaceutical policies are in favor of imports, as the slope of the import and domestic production lines illustrate. The rise in Iranian pharmaceutical expenditure is expected to continue at a significant, even higher rate than expected from developing countries, based on factors mentioned above and the deliberate deficiencies of pharmaceutical policy [12,13]. Medicines are regarded as both public and industry goods. Iranian patients are entitled to have access to high-quality, timely, and cost-effective medicine [14,15]. The Iranian

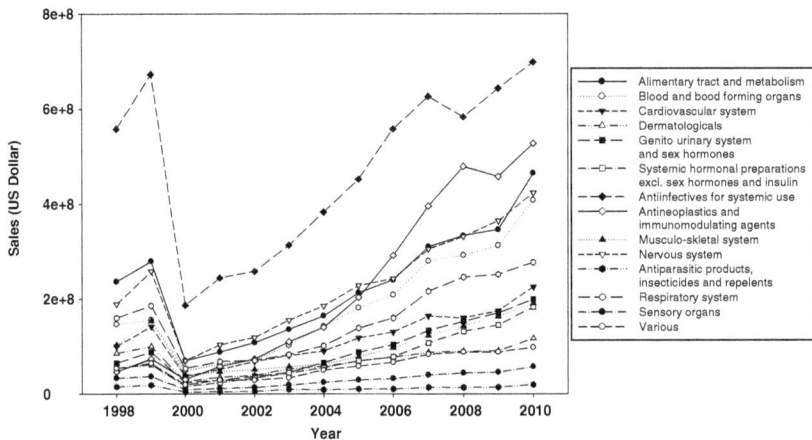

Figure 5 Medicine consumption by value in therapeutic categories; 1998–2010.

pharmaceutical market is predicted to maintain its growth for years to come. Currently, 20% of Iran's total health expenditure, on average, goes on medicine (reimbursed by the insurance organizations, based on their reports to the supreme insurance council for last year). Antibiotics, antineoplastics and immunomudulating agents (medicines mostly used for organ transplantation rejection prohibition), antidiabetics, and alimentary tract medications gain the most value in the market (Figure 5). Regarding sales volume, analgesics, antibiotics, and second generation antidiabetics are the best sellers. Investigating the mostly used products among the two top categories it is obvious that pharmaceutical biotechnology derived medicines such as proteins and monoclonal antibodies take major positions (results not presented). Considering the items mentioned, it is concluded that new and high tech medicines are seizing a large share of the market; which should incite policy makers to change for the better. If the market continues its growth, a great financial load will be imposed on the health system. Iran contains nearly 1% of the world's population, but only about 0.3% of the world market, so if the two are in an agreement, Iran should assume $7-8 billion in 2010, and $10-12 billion in 2020. Generic medicine use is an important component of the government's health plan that was obligatory through the generic scheme shortly after the revolution. The policy assisted the country pass the constraints of the 1980s, but vitally restricted research and development in the domestic industry, while exerting severe price containment policies [16]. Current issues of interest for the Iranian pharmaceutical market include a rise in imports and simultaneous fall in domestic production. Low rates of investment, capital asset substitution, scarce attention to modern technologies like pharmaceutical biotechnology, and a branded medicine market are possible reasons for this domestic medicine market shrinkage [17,18]. The investment activity of pharmaceutical companies is dependant mainly on product demand, profits, technological developments, and capital availability. It is vital to notice the steady decrease in investment rate for capital equipment replacement. This is associated with the market shift towards imported medicines and the lack of well-designed, long-term policies to support the domestic pharmaceutical industry that would potentiate reasonable conditions to encourage domestic production [19]. Meanwhile vast research projects have been conducted in the universities and research centers but few of them have been commercialized into medicines. Performing studies aligned with the needs of the biopharmaceutical industry could be seen as a choice. Policy makers and authorities could contribute the national production capabilities by establishing the basements to commercialize the researches, revising the policies, forming close relationships and cooperative committees with the biopharmaceutical industries and applying evidence based decision making procedures.

Conclusions

The absence of significant basic and applied biopharmaceutical research that can result in industrial breakthroughs and attain competitive advantage in Iran has induced a state of regression in the domestic industry that has accelerated a drain on the capital and energy of the industry. Such conditions, along with price suppression, increase imports [20,21]. It is advised that policy makers take all necessary measures towards establishing an appropriate pharmaceutical business environment that favors domestic production, as well as controlling rising expenditure in the pharmaceutical sector [22]. We can conclude that the average value of imported medicine per unit is growing, which suggests technological content is in continuous improvement in comparison with domestic ones [23-25]. Medicine consumption per capita shows that this index is high in Iran. Therefore, it is proposed that conducting applied research projects ordered by the biopharmaceutical industries along with preparing the requirements for commercialization of novel fields like pharmaceutical biotechnology which assigns a great share in the national pharmaceutical expenditure be in the top agenda.

Abbreviations

HHI: Herfindahl–Hirschman Index; API: Active Pharmaceutical Ingredient; FDO: Food and Drug organization; GDP: Gross Domestic Product; ATC: Anatomical Therapeutic Chemical Classification System.

Competing interests

The authors declare that they have no competing interests.

Authors' contributions

AK conceived the strategy of study and supervised the project, NNK conceived and implemented the strategy, performed the data analysis and statistical interpretation and drafted the paper, AA gave consultation on designing the study, complemented the data and statistical analysis, SN gave consultation on the study methodology and edited the draft, NM performed the data analysis. All authors read and approved the final manuscript.

Acknowledgements

The authors are thankful to the Food and Drug Organization (FDO) and Department of Planning and Statistics for providing the data for the project.

Author details

[1]Department of Pharmacoeconomics and Pharmaceutical Administration, Faculty of Pharmacy, Tehran University of Medical Sciences, P.O. Box 14155–6451, Tehran 14174, Iran. [2]Department of Toxicology and Pharmacology, Faculty of Pharmacy, Tehran University of Medical Sciences, P.O. Box 14155–6451, Tehran 14174, Iran. [3]Management Information System Division, Osvah Pharmaceutical Company, Tehran, Iran.

References

1. Ensor T, Weinzierl S: Regulating health care in low- and middle-income countries: Broadening the policy response in resource constrained environments. Soc Sci Med 2007, 65:355–366.
2. Kebrieezadeh A, Eslamitabar S, Khatibi M: Iranian pharmaceutical law and regulations. 2nd edition. Tehran: Razico; 2009.
3. Reinhardt UE: An information infrastructure for the pharmaceutical market. Health Aff 2004, 23(1):107–112.

4. Davari M, Walley T, Haycox A: Pharmaceutical policy and market in Iran:
    past experiences and future challenges. *J Pharm Health Serv Res* 2011,
    2:47–52.
5. Cheraghali AM: Pharmacoeconomics: An Effective Tool for Prioritization
    in Iran Healthcare System. *Iranian J Pharm Res* 2008, 7(2):89–91.
6. Kebriee-zadeh A: Overview of National Drug Policy of Iran. *IJPR* 2003:1–2.
7. Faden L, Vialle-Valentin C, Ross-Degnan D, Wagner A: Active
    pharmaceutical management strategies of health insurance systems to
    improve cost-effective use of medicines in low- and middle-income
    countries: A systematic review of current evidence. *Health Policy* 2011,
    100:134–143.
8. Cheraghali AM: Pharmaceutical Market. *IJPR* 2006, 1:1–7.
9. Rusu A, Kuokkanen K, Heier A: Current trends in the pharmaceutical
    industry - A case study approach. *Eur J Pharm Sci* 2011, 44:437–440.
10. Drews J: Strategic trends in the drug industry. *Drug Discov Today* 2003,
    8(9):411–420.
11. Nikfar S, Kebriaeezadeh A, Majdzadeh R, Abdollahi M: Monitoring of
    National Drug Policy (NDP) and its standardized indicators; conformity
    to decisions of the National Drug Selecting Committee in Iran. *BMC Int
    Health Hum Rights* 2005, 5:5.
12. Kontozamanis V, Mantzouneas E, Stoforos C: An overview of the Greek
    pharmaceutical market. *Eur J Health Econ* 2003, 4:327–333.
13. Eisenberg DM, Davis RB, Ettner SL, Appel S, Wilkey S, Rompay MV, *et al*:
    Trends in alternative medicine use in the United States, 1990–1997,
    results of a follow-up national survey. *JAMA* 1998, 280(18):1569–1575.
14. Tokgöz T: The Turkish pharmaceutical market. *JGM* 2010, 7:270–274.
15. Tetteh EK: Providing affordable essential medicines to African
    households: The missing policies and institutions for price containment.
    Soc Sci Med 2008, 66:569–581.
16. Cameron A, Ewen M, Ross-Degnan D, Ball D, Laing R: Medicine prices,
    availability, and affordability in 36 developing and middle-income
    countries: a secondary analysis. *Lancet* 2009, 373:240–249.
17. Oortwijn W, Mathijssen J, Banta D: The role of health technology
    assessment on pharmaceutical reimbursement in selected middle-
    income countries. *Health Policy* 2010, 95:174–184.
18. Kutaini D: Pharmaceutical industry in Syria. *J Med Life* 2010, 3(3):348–350.
19. Ghislandi S, Krulichova I, Garattini L: Pharmaceutical policy in Italy: towards
    a structural change? *Health Policy* 2005, 72:53–63.
20. Merkur S, Mossialos E: A pricing policy towards the sourcing of cheaper
    drugs in Cyprus. *Health Policy* 2007, 81:368–375.
21. Aaserud M, Dahlgren AT, Kosters JP, Oxman AD, Ramsay C, Sturm H:
    Pharmaceutical policies: effects of reference pricing, other pricing, and
    purchasing policies. *Cochrane Database Syst Rev* 2006, 2: .
22. Lockhart M, Babar ZUD, Garg S: Evaluation of policies to support drug
    development in New Zealand. *Health Policy* 2010, 96:108–117.
23. Kisa A: Analysis of the pharmaceuticals market and its technological
    development in Turkey. *Int J Technol Assess Health Care* 2006,
    22(4):537–542.
24. Abdollahiasl A, Kebriaeezadeh A, Nikfar S, Farshchi A, Ghiasi G, Abdollahi M:
    Patterns of antibiotic consumption in Iran during 2000–2009. *Int J
    Antimicrob Agents* 2011, 37:489–490.
25. Abdollahiasl A, Nikfar S, Kebriaeezadeh A, Dinarvand R, Abdollahi M: A
    model for developing a decision support system to simulate national
    drug policy indicators. *Arch Med Sci* 2011, 5:744–746.

12

Design, synthesis, docking study and cytotoxic activity evaluation of some novel letrozole analogs

Mohsen Vosooghi[1], Loghman Firoozpour[2], Abolfazl Rodaki[2], Mahboobeh Pordeli[3], Maliheh Safavi[4], Sussan K Ardestani[3], Armin Dadgar[1], Ali Asadipour[5], Mohammad Hassan Moshafi[5] and Alireza Foroumadi[5,6*]

Background: Breast cancer is the most common type of female cancer. One class of hormonal therapy for breast cancer drugs -non steroidal aromatase inhibitors- are triazole analogues. In this work, some derivatives of these drugs was designed and synthesized. All synthesized compounds were evaluated for their cytotoxic activities on breast cancer cell lines (MDA-MB-231, T47D and MCF-7).

Methods: Our synthetic route for designed compounds started from 4-bromotolunitrile which was reacted with 1*H*-1,2,4-triazole to afford 4-(4-cyanobenzyl)-1,2,4-triazole. The reaction of later compound with aromatic aldehydes led to formation of the designed compounds. Eleven novel derivatives 1a-k were tested for their cytotoxic activities on three human breast cancer cell lines.

Results: Among the synthesized compound, 4-[2-(3-chlorophenyl)-1-(1*H*-1,2,4-triazol-1-yl)ethenyl]benzonitrile (**1c**) showed the highest activity against MCF-7 and MDA-MB-231 cell lines and 4-[2-(4-methoxyphenyl)-1-(1*H*-1,2,4-triazol-1-yl)ethenyl]benzonitrile (**1 h**) exhibited highest activity against T47D cell line. According to cytotoxic activities results, compound 4-[2-(4-dimethylamino)-1-(1*H*-1,2,4-triazol-1-yl)ethenyl]benzonitrile (**1 k**) showed comparative activity against T47D and MDA-MB-231 cell lines with compound (**1 h**) and our reference drug Etoposide.

Conclusion: In the process of anti-cancer drug discovery, to find new potential anti-breast cancer agents, we designed and synthesized a novel series of letrozole analogs. Cytotoxicity evaluation revealed that compounds (**1c**) and (**1 k**) were the most potent compounds with comparative activity with Etoposide. The results revealed that π-π interactions are responsible for the enzyme inhibitions of compounds (**1 c**) and (**1 k**).

Keyword: Breast cancer, Non-steroidal aromatase inhibitor, Cytotoxic activity

Background

Breast cancer is the most common female cancer. According to the American cancer society's report about 12% of women in the U.S. will develop some invasive breast cancer during their lifetime. However breast cancer treatment has a complicated process and problems, chemotherapy resistance, surgery and available anti-tumor drugs side effects make it more difficult to gain the appropriate treatment regimen; consequently, there is great demand to introduce new active compounds with more anticancer activity and less unwanted reaction [1,2].

There is some different type of systemic therapy for breast cancer, one kind is hormonal therapy. Hormonal therapy can be given to women whose breast cancers test positive for estrogen to lower estrogen levels. Letrozole is a third generation of non-steroidal aromatase inhibitor – one class of hormonal therapy drugs- that was first introduces by Novartis to the market as Femara® for the treatment of local or metastatic breast cancer [3-5].

Non-steroidal aromatase inhibitors (as shown in Figure 1) are triazole or imidazole analogues that bind to the active site of enzyme by coordinating the heme iron atom of active site through a heterocyclic nitrogen lone pair [5,6].

As it shown in Figure 1, 1-benzyl-1*H*-1,2,4-triazole scaffold is a conservative section of aromatase inhibitors which contains various moieties attached to the aliphatic carbon part of this scaffold. In continuation of our research program to find a novel anticancer agent [7-11], and considering the above mentioned data, in the current study, we

* Correspondence: aforoumadi@yahoo.com
[5]Neuroscience Research Center, Institute of Neuropharmacology, Kerman University of Medicinal Sciences, Kerman, Iran
[6]Pharmaceutical Sciences Research Center, Tehran University of Medical Sciences, Tehran, Iran
Full list of author information is available at the end of the article

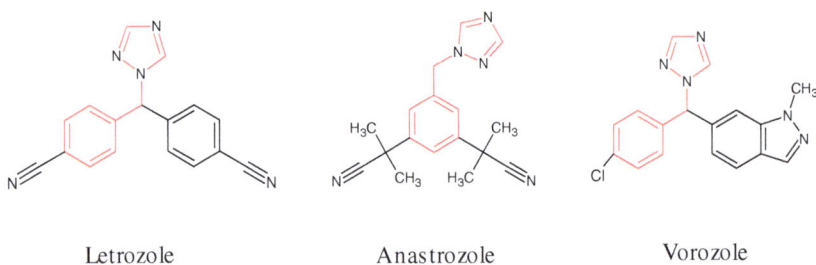

Figure 1 Structure of non-steroidal aromatase inhibitors.

report the synthesis of a novel series of substituted ethe-nylbenzene derivatives which linked to1-benzyl-1H-1,2,4-triazole (**1a-k**) and evaluated against three human breast cancer cell lines (Scheme 1).

Methods
Chemistry
All raw-materials, solvents and reagents were provided from Aldrich Chemicals and Merck AG. A Kofler hot stage apparatus was used for determination of melting points. The IR and ^{1}HNMR Spectra were determined on a Shimadzu 470 (potassium bromide disks) and a Bruker 500 spectrophotometer respectively. Tetramethylsilane (TMS) was used as internal standard and chemical shifts are re-ported in ppm relative to it. The elemental analysis for C, H and N were taken by a Perkin-Elmer 843 spectrometer with using KBr as diluent. Electrospray ionization mass spectra (ESI-MS) were recorded by using Agilent 6410 Triple Quad. LC/MS.

Key intermediate 4-(4-cyanobenzyl)-1,2,4-triazole was prepared according to Doiron J. and his collogues report [12].

General procedure for preparing of 4[2-aryl-1-(1H-1, 2, 4-triazol-1-yl)ethenyl]benzonitrile (1a-k)
4-(4-Cyanobenzyl)-1,2,4-triazole (1Gr) and 1,4-Dioxane (10 mL) were added to the reaction vessel and stirred. Sodium hydride (0.27 Gr 60%) was added to the reaction mixture in 0–5°C and stirred for 30 minutes. Corre-sponding aldehyde (0.5 mmol) was added to the mixture and stirred at room temperature for 30 minutes. Ethanol (3 mL) was added to the reaction mixture at 60°C and

stirred for an hour. Reaction mixture cooled to room temperature and mixture of ice-water (25 Gr) was added. Precipitate was filtered and recrystallized in etha-nol to yield corresponding compound (**1a-k**).

4-[2-Phenyl-1-(1H-1, 2, 4-triazol-1-yl)ethenyl]benzonitrile (1a)
Yield: 73%, mp 141–146°C. IR (KBr, cm^{-1}) ν_{max}: 2245 (nitrile), 1630 (C = C). ^{1}H NMR (500 MHz, CDCl$_3$): δ 8.25(s, 1H, triazole), 8.05 (s, 1H, triazole), 7.70-7.68 (d, J = 8.55 Hz,2H, benzonitrile), 7.35-7.33 (d, J = 8.55 Hz, 2H, benzonitrile), 7.30-7.26 (m, phenyl and ethenyl), 6.88-6.87 (d, J = 7.3 Hz, 1H, phenyl), ESI-Mass m/z: 272 [M]$^+$.

4-[2-(2-Chlorophenyl)-1-(1H-1,2,4-triazol-1-yl)ethenyl] benzonitrile (1b)
Yield: 70%, mp 141–144°C. IR (KBr, cm^{-1}) ν_{max}: 2240 (nitrile), 1622 (C = C). ^{1}H NMR (500 MHz, CDCl$_3$): δ 8.16(s, 1H, triazole), 7.96 (s, 1H, triazole), 7.72-7.71 (d , J = 8.45 Hz, 2H, benzonitrile), 7.43 (s, 1H, ethenyl), 7.45 (d, J = 7.75 Hz, 1H, phenyl), 7.40-7.39 (d, J = 8.45 Hz, 2H, benzonitrile), 7.27-7.23 (t, J = 7.9 Hz, 1H, phenyl), 7.08-7.05 (t, J = J = 7.15 Hz, 1H, phenyl), 6.61-6.59 (d, J = 7.75 Hz, 1H, phenyl), ESI-Mass m/z: 306 [M]$^+$.

4-[2-(3-Chlorophenyl)-1-(1H-1,2,4-triazol-1-yl)ethenyl] benzonitrile (1c)
Yield: 74%, mp 137–140°C. IR (KBr, cm^{-1}) ν_{max}: 2242 (nitrile), 1631 (C = C).^{1}H NMR (500 MHz, CDCl$_3$): δ 8.25(s, 1H, triazole), 8.04 (s, 1H, triazole), 7.70-7.69 (d, J = 8.5 Hz, 2H, benzonitrile), 7.35-7.33 (d, J = 8.5 Hz, 2H, benzoni-trile), 7.29-7.26 (m, 1H, phenyl), 7.22 (s, 1H, phenyl), 7.20-7.18 (d, J = 7.95 Hz, 1H, phenyl), 6.93 (s, 1H,

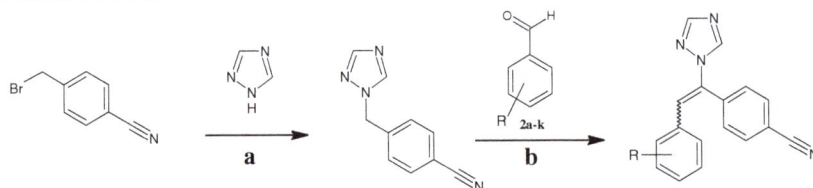

Scheme 1 The Synthesis rout of 4-[2-aryl-1-(1H-1,2,4-triazol-1-yl)ethenyl] benzonitriles 1a-k. (a) MeOH, KOH, DMF, (b) 1,4-Dioxane, recrystallized in EtOH.

ethenyl), 6.69-6.68 (d, $J = 8.2$ Hz, 1H, phenyl), ESI-Mass m/z: 306 [M]$^+$.

4-[2-(4-Chlorophenyl)-1-(1H-1,2,4-triazol-1-yl)ethenyl] benzonitrile (1d)

Yield: 71%, mp 139–146°C. IR (KBr, cm^{-1}) v_{max}: 2237 (nitrile), 1630 (C = C).^{1}H NMR (500 MHz, CDCl$_3$) δ 8.25(s, 1H, triazole), 8.04 (s, 1H, triazole), 7.70-7.69 (d, $J =$ 8.86 Hz,2H, benzonitrile), 7.34-7.33 (d, $J = 8.6$ Hz, 2H, benzonitrile), 7.27-7.25 (d, $J = 8.5$ Hz, 2H, phenyl),7.24 (s, 1H, ethenyl), 6.80-6.79(d, $J = 8.5$ Hz, 2H, phenyl), ESI-Mass m/z: 306 [M]$^+$.

4-[2-(2,4-Dichlorophenyl)-1-(1H-1,2,4-triazol-1-yl)ethenyl] benzonitrile (1e)

Yield: 74%, mp 150–153°C. IR (KBr, cm^{-1}) v_{max}: 2248 (nitrile), 1629 (C = C).^{1}H NMR (500 MHz, CDCl$_3$): δ 8.16 (s, 1H, triazole), 7.96 (s, 1H, triazole), 7.74-7.72 (d, $J =$ 8.35 Hz, 2H, benzonitrile) , 7.42-7.40 (m, 4H, benzonitrile and ethenyl), 7.04-7.01 (m, 1H, phenyl), 6.56-6.55 (m, 1H, phenyl), ESI-Mass m/z: 340 [M]$^+$.

4-[2-(3-Fluorophenyl)-1-(1H-1,2,4-triazol-1-yl)ethenyl] benzonitrile (1f)

Yield: 74%, mp 145–150°C. IR (KBr, cm^{-1}) v_{max}: 2244 (nitrile), 1634 (C = C).^{1}H NMR (500 MHz, CDCl$_3$): δ 8.25 (s, 1H, triazole), 8.05 (s, 1H, triazole), 7.71-7.69 (d, $J =$ 8.5 Hz,2H, benzonitrile), 7.35-7.33 (d, $J = 8.5$ Hz, 2H, benzonitrile), 7.30-7.26 (m, 1H, phenyl), 7.25 (s, 1H, ethenyl), 7.03-6.99 (m, 1H, phenyl), 6.68-6.66 (d, $J = 7.75$ Hz, 1H, phenyl), 6.58-6.56 (d, $J = 7.8$ Hz, 1H, phenyl), ESI-Mass m/z: 290 [M]$^+$.

4-[2-(3-Methoxyphenyl)-1-(1H-1,2,4-triazol-1-yl)ethenyl] benzonitrile (1 g)

Yield: 74%, mp 128–132°C. IR (KBr, cm^{-1}) v_{max}: 2242 (nitrile), 1631 (C = C).^{1}H NMR (500 MHz, CDCl$_3$): δ 8.24 (s, 1H, triazole), 8.05 (s,1H, triazole), 7.69-7.67 (d, $J =$ 8.1 Hz, 2H, benzonitrile), 7.34-7.33 (d, $J = 8.1$ Hz, 2H, benzonitrile), 7.27 (s, 1H, ethenyl), 7.21-7.18 (t, $J = 7.9$ Hz, 1H, phenyl), 6.86-6.84 (d, $J = 7.6$ Hz, phenyl), 6.54-6.53 (d, $J = 7.43$ Hz, phenyl), 6.31 (s, 1H, phenyl), 3.66 (s,3H,OMe), ESI-Mass m/z: 302 [M]$^+$.

4-[2-(4-Methoxyphenyl)-1-(1H-1,2,4-triazol-1-yl)ethenyl] benzonitrile (1 h)

Yield: 74%, mp 140–143°C. IR (KBr, cm^{-1}) v_{max}: 2244 (nitrile), 1632 (C = C).^{1}H NMR (500 MHz, CDCl$_3$) δ 8.27 (s, 1H, triazole), 8.08 (s,1H, triazole), 7.67-7.65 (d, $J =$ 8.7 Hz,2H, benzonitrile) , 7.30-7.29 (d , $J = 8.7$ Hz, 2H, benzonitrile), 7.25 (s, 1H, ethenyl), 6.80-6.78 (d, $J = 9.2$ Hz, 2H, phenyl), 6.77-6.76 (d, $J = 9.2$ Hz, 2H, phenyl), 3.80 (s,3H, OMe), ESI-Mass m/z: 302 [M]$^+$.

4-[2-(2,4-Dimethoxyphenyl)-1-(1H-1,2,4-triazol-1-yl)ethenyl] benzonitrile (1i)

Yield: 74%, mp 158–161°C. IR (KBr, cm^{-1}) v_{max}: 2239 (nitrile), 1632 (C = C). ^{1}H NMR (500 MHz, CDCl$_3$): δ 8.22 (s, 1H, triazole), 8.06 (s,1H, triazole), 7.66-7.65 (d, $J =$ 8.3 Hz,2H, benzonitrile), 7.50 (s, 1H, ethenyl), 7.31-7.30 (d, $J = 8.3$ Hz, 2H, benzonitrile), 6.44-6.27 (m, 3H, phenyl), 3.84 (s,3H, OMe), 3.79 (s,3H, OMe), ESI-Mass m/z: 332 [M]$^+$.

4-[2-(2,3,4-Trimethoxy)-1-(1H-1,2,4-triazol-1-yl)ethenyl] benzonitrile (1j)

Yield: 75%, mp 188–191°C. IR (KBr, cm^{-1}) v_{max}: 2246 (nitrile), 1634 (C = C).^{1}H NMR (500 MHz, CDCl$_3$): δ 8.20 (s, 1H, triazole), 8.09 (s,1H, triazole), 7.67-7.65 (d, $J =$ 8.3 Hz,2H, benzonitrile), 7.51 (s, 1H, ethenyl), 7.33-7.30 (d, $J = 8.3$ Hz, 2H, benzonitrile), 6.46-6.25 (m, 2H, phenyl), 3.86 (s,3H, OMe), 3.81 (s,3H, OMe), 3.76 (s,3H, OMe), ESI-Mass m/z: 3362 [M]$^+$.

4-[2-(4-Dimethylamino)-1-(1H-1,2,4-triazol-1-yl)ethenyl] benzonitrile (1 k)

Yield: 72%, mp 158–161°C. IR (KBr, cm^{-1}) v_{max}: 2241 (nitrile), 1633 (C = C).^{1}H NMR (500 MHz, CDCl$_3$) δ 8.26 (s, 1H, triazole), 8.05 (s,1H, triazole), 7.66-7.65 (d, $J =$ 8.5 Hz,2H, benzonitrile), 7.32-7.27 (d, $J = 8.5$ Hz, 2H, benzonitrile), 7.25 (s, 1H, ethenyl), 6.79-6.75 (d, $J = 9.1$ Hz, 2H, phenyl), 6.74-6.72 (d, $J = 9.1$ Hz, 2H, phenyl), 3.79-3.75 (m,6H, Me), ESI-Mass m/z: 315 [M]$^+$.

Physicochemical prediction

Marvin was used for chemical drawing, displaying and characterizing chemical structures, calculator plugins were used for structure property prediction and calculation, (version: Marvin 6.0.3, 2013, ChemAxon scientific package, http://www.chemaxon.com).

Molecular modeling study

Docking studies for selected compounds were performed using Autodock Vina (ver. 1.1.1) [13]. The crystal structure of human placental aromatase cytochrome P450 in complex with androstenedione (code ID: 3EQM, resolution [Å]: 2.90) was retrieved from protein data bank [14-17]. Crystal structure was cleaned from Co-crystallized ligand and water molecules and the protein was converted to pdbqt format using Autodock Tools (1.5.4) [18]. 2Dstructures of ligands converted to 3D in pdbqt format by Openbabel (ver. 2.3.1) [18]. The docking parameters were set on vina docking parameter as follow: center_x = 85.027; center_y = 54.737; center_z = 46.428; size_x =50; size_y =50; size_z =50;. The other parameters were left as default for the program. Finally, the conformation for the best free energy of binding was selected for analyzing the interactions between the macromolecule and selected inhibitors. 3D

Table 1 Target structures and physicochemical properties

No.	Comp. Code	Ar	MW	Formula	Vander Waals Surface	Polar Surface	Log P
1.	1a	(phenyl)	272	$C_{17}H_{12}N_4$	363.21	54.50	3.12
2.	1b	(2-Cl-phenyl)	306.75	$C_{17}H_{11}ClN_4$	376.65	54.50	3.72
3.	1c	(Cl-phenyl)	306.75	$C_{17}H_{11}ClN_4$	378.12	54.50	3.72
4.	1d	(Cl-phenyl)	306.75	$C_{17}H_{11}ClN_4$	378.12	54.50	3.72
5.	1e	(diCl-phenyl)	341.19	$C_{17}H_{10}Cl_2N_4$	393.15	54.50	4.33
6.	1f	(F-phenyl)	290.29	$C_{17}H_{11}FN_4$	369.04	54.50	3.22
7.	1g	(OMe-phenyl)	302.33	$C_{18}H_{14}ON_4$	410.22	63.73	2.96
8.	1h	(OMe-phenyl)	302.33	$C_{18}H_{14}ON_4$	409.36	63.73	2.96
9.	1i	(diOMe-phenyl)	332.36	$C_{19}H_{16}O_2N_4$	457.69	72.96	2.80
10.	1j	(triOMe-phenyl)	362.38	$C_{20}H_{18}O_3N_4$	504.76	82.19	2.65
11.	1k	(N,N-dimethylamino-phenyl)	315.37	$C_{19}H_{17}N_5$	448.10	57.74	3.23

models of ligand-receptor interactions are generated by using the Autodock Tools (1.5.4) [19].

Biological assay
Cell lines and cell culture
Three human breast cancer cell lines including MDA-MB-231, MCF-7 and T-47D were obtained from National Cell Bank of Iran (NCBI, Iran). The cells were grown in RPMI-1640 medium supplemented with 10% heat-inactivated fetal calf serum (GibcoeBRL, UK), 100 mg/ml strepto-mycin and 100 U/ml penicillin at 37°C/95% rh/5% CO_2.

In vitro cytotoxicity assay
The in-vitro cytotoxic activity of all synthesized compounds **1a-k** was achieved against three human breast cancer cell lines using MTT colorimetric assay according

Table 2 *In vitro* **cytotoxic activity (IC$_{50}$, µg/ml) of compounds 1a-k against breast cancer cell lines[a]**

No.	Comp. Code	Cell lines		
		MCF-7	MDA-MB-231	T-47D
1.	1a	57.1 ± 2.1	87.5 ± 2.5	64.3 ± 1.9
2.	1b	63.2 ± 2.6	97.3 ± 3.1	77.1 ± 2.8
3.	1c	27.1 ± 1.2	14.5 ± 2.1	76.25 ± 7.0
4.	1d	52.3 ± 2.2	43.3 ± 3.4	83.3 ± 5.2
5.	1e	78.3 ± 5.7	83.3 ± 7.2	92.3 ± 6.2
6.	1f	72.3 ± 5.5	85.3 ± 7.4	87.3 ± 7.5
7.	1 g	40.3 ± 2.8	77.4 ± 6.5	69.4 ± 5.7
8.	1 h	74.6 ± 6.5	82.3 ± 7.4	14.3 ± 1.1
9.	1i	75.3 ± 4.4	89.4 ± 6.1	79.1 ± 7.7
10.	1j	69.3 ± 5.3	45.05 ± 6.2	63.3 ± 6.6
11.	1 k	55.3 ± 5.1	19.7 ± 1.8	16.8 ± 2.1
12.	Etoposide	7.9 ± 0.5	11.1 ± 1.1	8 ± 0.8

[a]The IC$_{50}$ values represent an average of three independent experiments (mean $\pm$ SD).

to the method of Mosman [20]. Cells were seeded in 96-well plates (Nunc, Denmark) and incubated overnight in a humidified air atmosphere at 37°C with 5% CO$_2$ to allow cell attachment. The cells were then incubated for another 48 h with various concentrations of compounds **1a-k**. The final concentration of DMSO in the highest concentration of the applied compounds was 1%. In each plate, there were three control wells (cells without test compounds) and three blank wells (the medium with 1% DMSO) for cell viability. Etoposide were used as positive controls for cytotoxicity. After 48 h, the culture medium was removed and 200 µl phenol red-free medium containing MTT (final concentration 0.5 mg/mL) was added to wells, followed by 4 h incubation.

After incubation, the culture medium was then replaced with 100 µl of DMSO and the absorbance of each well was measured by using a microplate reader at 492 nm. For each compound, the concentration causing 50% cell growth inhibition (IC$_{50}$) compared with the control containing 1% DMSO was calculated from concentration response curves by regression analysis.

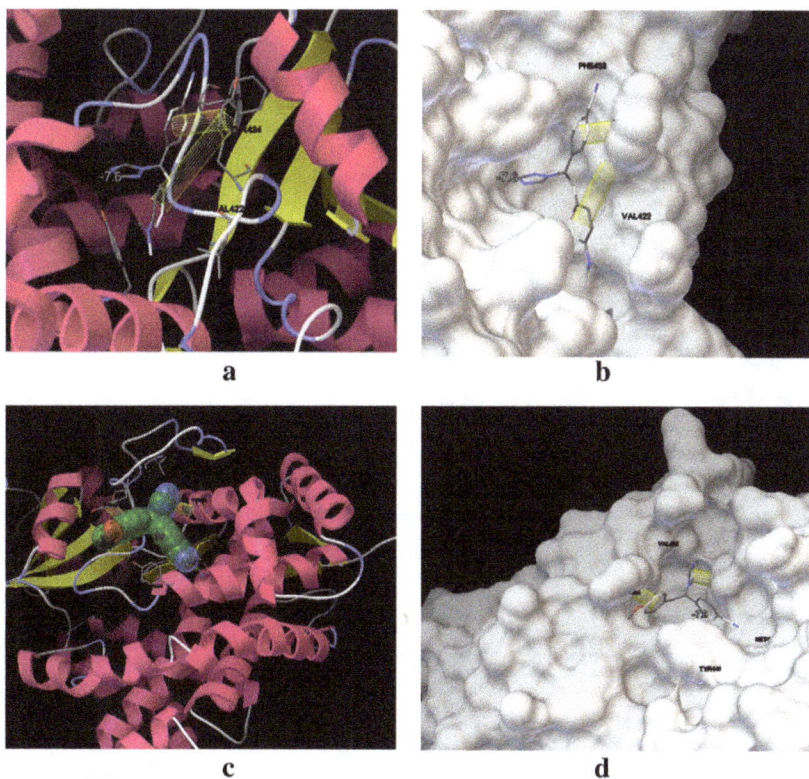

Figure 2 Presentation of compounds (1c) and (1 k) with aromatase enzyme, π-π interactions showed in yellow cylindrical shape. (a, b) visualization of compound **(1c)** in enzyme with ribbon and molecular surface views; **(c, d)** binding mode of **(1 k)** in enzyme with ribbon and molecular surface views.

Results and discussions

Chemistry

4-Bromotolunitrile was converted to 4-(4-cyanobenzyl)-1,2,4-triazole and subsequently to corresponding product, 4-[2-aryl-1-(1H-1,2,4-triazol-1-yl)ethenyl]benzonitrile (1a-k) according to the procedure presented in Scheme 1. Chemical structures, molecular formula and molecular weight of compounds (1a-k) are illustrated in Table 1. Reaction yields are presented in chemistry section of methods in this report.

Physicochemical prediction

In order to investigate the physicochemical properties of products, Vander Waals surface, polar surface and partition-coefficient (Log P) of compounds (1a-k) were predicted by Marvin program and are reported in Table 1. As it shown primary physicochemical criteria were passed by all designed compounds (1a-k).

Cytotoxic activity

The in vitro cytotoxic activity of 4[2-aryl-1-(1H-1,2,4-triazol-1-yl)ethenyl]benzonitrile (1a-k), were tested against three human breast cancer lines including MDA-MB-231, T47D and MCF-7. The various concentrations of the synthetic compounds (final concentration 5, 10, 20, 40, 80 and 100 μg/ml) were applied to calculate IC_{50}. The 50% growth inhibitory concentration (IC_{50}) for products were calculated and depicted in Table 2.

According to MTT assay results in Table 2, 4-[2-(3-chlorophenyl)-1-(1H-1,2,4-triazol-1-yl)ethenyl]benzonitrile (1c) showed the highest activity against MCF-7 and MDA-MB-231 cell lines with IC_{50} values of 27.1 ± 1.2 and 14.5 ± 2.1 μg/ml, respectively and 4-[2-(4-methoxyphenyl)-1-(1H-1,2,4-triazol-1-yl)ethenyl]benzonitrile (1 h) exhibited highest activity against T47D cell line with IC_{50} value of 14.3 ± 1.1 μg/ml. As can be seen in Table 2, compound 4-[2-(4-dimethylamino)-1-(1H-1,2,4-triazol-1-yl)ethenyl]benzonitrile (1 k), showed comparative activity against T47D and MDA-MB-231 cell lines with compound 1 h and Etoposide withIC$_{50}$ values of 16.8 ± 2.1 and 19.7 ± 1.8 μg/ml, respectively. As it shown in MTT assay results all other synthesized compound did not show good activity against tested cell lines.

Docking study

In order to understand the binding mode of active compounds in the active site pocket of aromatase, docking study was performed using Autodock Vina. To attain this aim, the potent compounds, 1c and 1 k were docked into target enzyme. Docking strongly suggested that the π-π interaction between adjacent phenyl rings and hydrophobic moieties in enzyme residues –Tyrosine 424 and Tyrosine 361- are effective in activity of biologically active synthesized compounds. According to Figure 2, selected compounds fit in the pocket of aromatase enzyme completely, however missing the potentially hydrogen bond between ligands and macromolecule is responsible for moderate activities of compounds (1c) and (1 k).

Conclusion

In the process of anti-cancer drug discovery, to find new potential anti-breast cancer agents, we designed and synthesized a novel series of letrozole analogs. Cytotoxicity evaluation revealed that compounds (1c) and (1 k) were the most potent compounds with comparative activity with Etoposide. Physicochemical properties of products predicted and the binding mode of (1c) and (1 k) were predicted by docking simulation; the results revealed that π-π interactions are responsible for the enzyme inhibitions of compounds (1c) and (1 k).

Competing interests

The authors declare that they have no competing interests.

Authors' contributions

MV: design and synthesis of the title compound, manuscript preparations. LF: computational design for prediction of physicochemical properties. AR: collaboration in the synthesis of the target compounds. MP: collaboration in cytotoxic assay. MS: collaboration in cytotoxic assays and IC$_{50}$ calculations. SKA: supervision of the pharmacological part. AD: reporting the spectra and writing experimental section. AA: collaboration in the synthesis of intermediates. KD: collaboration in cytotoxic assays. AF: design of target compounds and the synthetic rout. All authors read and approved the final manuscript.

Acknowledgments

This work was supported by a grant from Iran National Science Foundation (INSF).

Author details

[1]Department of Medicinal Chemistry, Faculty of Pharmacy, Tehran University of Medical Sciences, Tehran, Iran. [2]Drug Design and Development Research Center, Tehran University of Medical Sciences, Tehran, Iran. [3]Institute of Biochemistry and Biophysics, University of Tehran, PO Box 13145–1384, Tehran, Iran. [4]Department of Biotechnology, Iranian Research Organization for Science and Technology, Tehran, Iran. [5]Neuroscience Research Center, Institute of Neuropharmacology, Kerman University of Medicinal Sciences, Kerman, Iran. [6]Pharmaceutical Sciences Research Center, Tehran University of Medical Sciences, Tehran, Iran.

References

1. Dutta U, Pant K: **Aromatase inhibitors: past, present and future in breast cancer therapy.** Med Oncol 2008, 25:113–124.
2. Vicini F, Beitsch P, Quiet C, Gittleman M, Zannis V, Fine R, Whitworth P, Kuerer H, Haffty B, Keisch M, Lyden M: **Five-year analysis of treatment efficacy and cosmesis by the American society of breast surgeons mammo site breast brachytherapy registry trial in patients treated with accelerated partial breast irradiation.** Int J Radiant Oncol Biol Phys 2011, 79:808–817.
3. Smith GL, Xu Y, Buchholz TA, Giordano SH, Jiang J, Shih YC, Smith BD: **Association between treatment with brachytherapy vs. whole-breast irradiation and subsequent mastectomy, complications , and survival among older women with invasive breast cancer.** JAMA 2012, 307:1827–1837.
4. Cox JA, Swanson TA: **Current modalities of accelerated partial breast irradiation.** Nat Rev Clin Oncol 2013, 10:344–356.
5. Caporuscio F, Rastelli G, Imbriano C, Delrio A: **Structure-based design of potent aromatase inhibitors by high-throughput docking.** J Med Chem 2011, 54:4006–4017.

6.   Dowsett M, Cuzick J, Ingle J, Coates A, Forbes J, Bliss J, Buyse M, Baum M, Buzdar A, Colleoni M, Coombes C, Snowdon C, Gnant M, Jakesz R, Kaufmann M, Boccardo F, Godwin J, Davies C, Peto R: **Meta-analysis of breast cancer outcomes in adjuvant trials of aromatase inhibitors versus tamoxifen.** *J Clin Oncol* 2010, **28:**509–518.

7.   Zonouzi A, Mirzazadeh R, Safavi M, Kabudanian Ardestani S, Emami S, Foroumadi A: **2-Amino-4-(nitroalkyl)-4H-chromene-3-carbonitriles as New Cytotoxic Agents.** *Iran J Pharm Res* 2013, **12:**679–685.

8.   Vosooghi M, Yahyavi H, Divsalar K, Shamsa H, Kheirollahi A, Safavi M, Ardestani SK, Sadeghi-Neshat S, Mohammadhosseini N, Edraki N, Khoshneviszadeh M, Shafiee A, Foroumadi A: **Synthesis and In vitro cytotoxic activity evaluation of (***E***)-16-(substituted benzylidene) derivatives of dehydroepiandrosterone.** *Daru J Pharm Sci* 2013, **21:**34.

9.   Ketabforoosh S H M E, Kheirollahi A, Safavi M, Esmati N, Ardestani S K, Emami S, Firoozpour L, Shafiee A, A Foroumadi A: **Synthesis and anti-cancer activity evaluation of new dimethoxylated chalcone and flavanone analogs.** *Arch. Pharm. (Weinheim)* 2014, in press: doi:10.1002/ardp.201400215.

10. Noushini S, Alipour E, Emami S, Safavi M, Ardestani SK, Gohari AR, Shafiee A, Foroumadi A: **Synthesis and cytotoxic properties of novel (***E***)-3-benzylidene-7-methoxychroman-4-one derivatives.** *Daru J Pharm Sci* 2013, **2:**31.

11. Alipour E, Mousavi Z, Safaei Z, Pordeli M, Safavi M, Firoozpour L, Mohammadhosseini N, Saeedi M, Ardestani SK, Shafiee A, Foroumadi A: **Synthesis and cytotoxic evaluation of some new[1,3]dioxolo[4,5-g] chromen-8-one derivatives.** *Daru J Pharm Sci* 2014, **22:**41.

12. Doiron J, Soultan AH, Richard R, Touré MM, Picot N, Richard R, Cuperlović-Culf M, Robichaud GA, Touaibia M: **Synthesis and structure-activity relationship of 1- and 2-substituted-1,2,3-triazole letrozole-based analogues as aromatase inhibitors.** *Eur J Med Chem* 2011, **46:**4010–4024.

13. Trott O, Olson AG: **Software news and update AutoDockVina: improving the speed and accuracy of docking with a new scoring function, efficient optimization, and multithreading.** *J Comput Chem* 2010, **31:**455–461.

14. Ghosh D, Griswold J, Erman M, Pangborn W: **Structural basis for androgen specificity and oestrogen synthesis in human aromatase.** *Nature* 2009, **457:**219–223.

15. Suvannang N, Nantasenamat C, Isarankura-Na-Ayudhya C, Prachayasittikul V: **Molecular docking of aromatase inhibitors.** *Molecules* 2011, **16:**3597–3617.

16. Thakur A, Timiri AK: **Designing of potential new aromatase inhibitor for estrogen dependent disease: a computational approach.** *World J Pharm Sci* 2014, **2:**13–24.

17. Mirzaie S, Chupani L, Barzegari Asadabadi E, Shahverdi AR, Jamalan M: **Novel inhibitor discovery against aromatase through virtual screening and molecular dynamic simulation: a computational approach in drug design.** *EXCLI J* 2013, **12:**168–183.

18. Sanner MF: **Python: a programming language for software integration and development.** *J Mol Graph Mod* 1999, **17:**57–61.

19. O'Boyle NM, Banck M, James CA, Morley C, Vandermeersch T, Hutchison GR: **Open babel: an open chemical toolbox.** *J Cheminform* 2011, **3:**33.

20. Mosmann T: **Rapid colorimetric assay for cellular growth and survival: application to proliferation and cytotoxicity assays.** *J Immunol Methods* 1983, **65:**55–63.

13

A randomized controlled trial of gonadotropin-releasing hormone agonist versus gonadotropin-releasing hormone antagonist in Iranian infertile couples: oocyte gene expression

Fatemeh Sadat Hoseini[1], Seyed Mohammad Hossein Noori Mugahi[2], Firoozeh Akbari-Asbagh[3], Poopak Eftekhari-Yazdi[4], Behrouz Aflatoonian[5], Seyed Hamid Aghaee-Bakhtiari[6], Reza Aflatoonian[7] and Nasser Salsabili[8*]

Abstract

Background: The main objective of the present work was to compare the effects of the gonadotropin-releasing hormone agonist (GnRH-a) and GnRH antagonist (GnRH-ant) on the gene expression profiles of oocytes obtained from Iranian infertile couples undergoing in vitro fertilization (IVF).

Methods: Fifty infertile couples who underwent IVF between June 2012 and November 2013 at the Infertility Center of Tehran Women General Hospital, Tehran University of Medical Sciences, were included in this study. We included women that had undergone IVF treatment because of male factor, tubal factor, or unexplained infertility. The women randomly underwent controlled ovarian stimulation (COS) with either the GnRH-a (n = 26) or the GnRH-ant (n = 24). We obtained 50 germinal vesicle (GV) oocytes donated by women in each group. After the sampling, pool of 50 GV oocytes for each group was separately analyzed by quantitative polymerase chain reaction (qPCR).

Result: The expression levels of Adenosine triphosphatase 6 (ATPase 6), Bone morphogenetic protein 15 (BMP15), and Neuronal apoptosis inhibitory protein (NAIP) genes were significantly upregulated in the GnRH-ant group compared to the GnRH-a group, with the fold change of 3.990 (SD ± 1.325), 6.274 (SD ± 1.542), and 2.156 (SD ± 1.443), respectively, (P < 0.001). Growth differentiation factor 9 (GDF9) mRNA did not have any expression in the GnRH-a group; however, GDF9 mRNA was expressed in the GnRH-ant group. Finally, it was found that the genes involved in the DNA repairing and cell cycle checkpoint did not have any expression in either group.

Conclusion: The present study showed, for the first time, the expression levels of genes involved in the cytoplasmic maturity (BMP15, GDF9), adenosine triphosphate production (ATPase 6), and antiapoptotic process (NAIP), in human GV oocytes were significantly higher in the GnRH-anta group than in the GnRH-a group in COS. Higher expression level of these genes when GnRH-ant protocol is applied, this protocol seems to be a more appropriate choice for women with poly cystic ovarian syndrome, because it can probably improve the expression of the aforementioned genes.

Trial registration: Current Controlled Trials: IRCT 2014031112307 N3.

Keywords: Gene expression, Controlled ovarian stimulation, GnRH antagonist, GnRH agonist

* Correspondence: nsalsabili56@yahoo.com
[8]Department of Physiotherapy, School of Rehabilitation of Tehran University of Medical Sciences, Tehran, Iran; Lab director Assisted Conception Unit, Tehran Women General Hospital, Tehran University of Medical Sciences, Tehran, Iran
Full list of author information is available at the end of the article

Background

Controlled ovarian stimulation (COS) is an important part of reproductive medicine; it also plays a vital role in inducing a pregnancy through assisted reproductive technology (ART). Higher pregnancy and implantation rates, compared to natural cycles, can be achieved using COS. Currently, three objectives are commonly followed when using COS for ART: ovulation induction, suppression of hypophyseal activity, and the growth stimulation of multiple follicles. For this purpose, two kinds of drugs are commonly used: gonadotropin releasing hormone agonists (GnRH-a) and gonadotropin releasing hormone antagonists (GnRH-ant). Multi-follicular recruitment causes a rapid increase in serum 17-beta estradiol (E2) levels during stimulated cycles, which in turn results in an untimely release of LH. The use of GnRH analogs can prevent the luteinizing hormone (LH) surge, which in turn improves the oocyte yield with more embryos and allows for better selection and therefore an increased pregnancy rate [1].

GnRH-a have been the most widely used drug for women undergoing COS, either for ICSI or for IVF [2]. GnRH-ant, on the other hand, has been introduced in clinical practice as a valid alternative in the last decade. In contrast to GnRH-a that decrease the number of receptors, GnRH-ant competitively inhibit endogenous GnRH from binding to its receptors. Consequently, they induce a direct, dose-dependent block of GnRH-receptors that are quickly reversible, which help avoid a flare effect [1].

Since 2001, several studies have compared the efficacy of the two GnRH analogs [2,3]. A recent Cochrane review indicated no evidence of a statistically significant difference in the rates of live births or ongoing pregnancies of the two GnRH analogs. In addition, the incidence of ovarian hyperstimulation syndrome (OHSS) in GnRH-ant treatment was lower than that of the GnRH-a treatment [3-5]. Furthermore, the following characteristics of the two protocols have also been compared: the number of oocytes retrieved and embryos transferred, the quality of oocyte morphology, implantation rate, the cycle cancellation rate, endometrial receptivity, follicular microenvironment, the percentage of granulosa cells with positive DNA fragmentation and apoptosis, genes expression in cumulus cells, and the distribution pattern and activity of human mature oocyte mitochondria [6-9].

It should be noted that the quality of oocytes obtained following controlled ovarian stimulation (COS) may vary significantly. Most oocytes are capable of being fertilized; however, nearly half of the fertilized ones can complete preimplantation development and even fewer ones can still implant. It has been shown that defects or variations in the ovulation or maturation processes have significant associations with gene expression alterations in oocytes and their supporting cells [10].

As mentioned earlier, although different clinical and molecular studies have been conducted to compare the efficacy of GnRH-a and GnRH-ant in assistant reproductive technique (ATR), results have been mostly inconsistent; Microarray studies conducted on human oocytes have indicated that some genes are expressed in both GV and MII stages, though with different levels. In fact, the more the oocytes move towards the maturity, the expression level of these genes increases [10-28]. These genes include those involved in the maturity of human oocytes (BMP15 and GDF9, both from the TGF beta category) [29,30], those involved in the cellular cycle and meiosis (BUB1, MAD2L1, CDC20, ATR, and ATM) [10-28,31], the energy-producing, mitochondrial gene (ATPase6) [27], and NAIP, which indicates oocytes viability [32-34]. Additionally, it is reported that COS can affect the gene expression level of oocytes [10]. During ovulation, mature and immature oocytes are obtained at the same time; however, the mature oocyte is used to treat patients. If differences are observed in the expression levels of the above mentioned genes in the cytoplasm of the GV oocytes due to different COS protocols (i.e. GnRH-ant or GnRH-a), the same conditions are expected to exist in the cytoplasm of mature oocytes. In other words, if increased levels of cytoplasmic maturity factors are observed following a COS protocol compared to the other, it highly likely to observe the same conditions in the cytoplasm of mature oocytes (MII) which co-exist with the GV oocytes in the same cycle. Therefore, for the first time, we decided to investigate the expression levels of nine genes involved in the cytoplasmic maturity, antiapoptotic process, cell cycle checkpoint, DNA repairing, and adenosine triphosphate production in germinal vesicle oocytes regarding the type of controlled ovarian stimulation in human. No studies have so far compared the genes expression in oocytes of women undergoing IVF/ICSI cycles between the GnRH-a and GnRH-ant protocols.

Materials

Subjects

Fifty infertile couples who underwent IVF/intracytoplasmic sperm injection (ICSI) between June 2012 and November 2013 at the Infertility Center of Tehran Women General Hospital, Tehran University of Medical Sciences, were included in this study. They were in good physical and mental conditions. We included the women that had undergone IVF treatment because of male factor, tubal factor, or unexplained infertility. These women did not have ovulatory dysfunction, were aged ≤40 years, and had a normal baseline follicle stimulating hormone (FSH) and luteinizing hormone (LH) (<10 mIU/mL).

Methods

Ovarian Stimulation and Oocyte Collection

The women underwent controlled ovarian stimulation with either the GnRH-a long protocol (n = 26) or the GnRH-ant fixed multi-dose protocol (n = 24), which was randomly assigned by the statistician [11,12].

The mean age (SD) of the participants was 31.7 (±5.7) years. In the GnRH-a long protocol group (n = 26), the treatment started by administering oral contraception pill (OCP) on the 2nd or the 3rd day of the pervious menstrual cycle. The daily administration of Buserelin acetate 500 μg (Suprefact, Aventis, Germany) was started preceding the IVF cycle from day 21 until pituitary down-regulation (serum E2 < 50 pg/ml in the absence of follicular structures larger than 10 mm). The Buserelin dose was reduced to 250 μg/d until the day of human chorionic gonadotropin (hCG) injection when pituitary down-regulation was achieved.

In the GnRH-ant fixed multi-dose protocol group (n = 24), Cetrorelix acetate 0.25 mg/day (Cetrotide, Serono, Switzerland) was initiated on the sixth day of the gonadotropin stimulation.

Ovarian stimulation was started on the 3rd day of the current menstrual cycle by injection of rFSH Follitropin alfa (Gonal F, Serono, Italy) at a daily dose of 150 to 225 IU in each group.

Administration of Buserelin and Cetrorelix was continued until hCG was injected. When at least 3 follicles with a mean diameter of 17 mm were developed (evaluated by transvaginal sonography), hCG 5000 IU/2/IM (Choriomon, IBSA Institut Biochimique S.A., Switzerland) was injected. About 34–36 h later, ultrasound-guided transvaginal oocyte retrieval was performed [13]. One hundred morphologically normal germinal vesicle oocytes were donated by 50 healthy women with normal ovarian reserve functions. The oocytes were aspirated transvaginally after COS. All the women had mature oocytes for ICSI, but they donated immature ones to our study. We obtained 50 germinal vesicle oocytes from 26 women aged 30.4 ± 5.5 years in the GnRH-a long protocol group and 50 germinal vesicle oocytes from 24 women aged 33.8 ± 5.6 years in the GnRH-ant protocol group. The oocytes were collected in a Quinn's Advantage Medium with HEPES (Sage, USA) supplemented with 20 % human serum albumin and then granulosa cells were removed from oocytes using mechanical and chemical (Hyaluronidase type 4, Sigma Aldrich, USA) methods.

After stripping off granulosa cells, we used an inverted microscope (Nikon, Tokyo, Japan) to monitor the maturity of the oocytes.

In the COS cycles, immature oocytes constitute up to 10-15 % of the retrieved oocytes. Germinal vesicle (GV) oocytes are immature oocytes whose maturation process have been stopped in the prophase of the first meiotic stage and are characterized by enlarged nucleus and absent of polar body. Germinal vesicle oocytes were individually transferred into RNase-free micro centrifuge tubes. Then, 30 μl of RLT buffer (Ambion, Austin, USA) was added to them. All samples were kept in a refrigerator at a temperature of –80°C until the time of the analysis. After the sampling, the pools of 50 germinal vesicle oocytes from the GnRH-a long protocol group and 50 germinal vesicle oocytes from the GnRH-ant protocol group were separately analyzed by qPCR.

RNA isolation, cDNA production and qPCR

ALLELEID 6.0 software was used for designing Exon-Junction primers. Molecular evolutionary genetics analysis (MEGA 4) software was also used for conducting sequence alignment. Oligo 6 Software was employed for the final assessment (Temperature/ Formation/False priming sites). Finally, we assessed primers in NCBI BLAST, as presented in Table 1.

Before isolating the RNA, the germinal vesicle oocytes were thawed within RLT buffer at room temperature and then pooled. To separate the RTL buffer from the pooled oocytes, they were then centrifuged at 12000 g for 3 minutes in order to extract total RNA, based on the standard protocol suggested by the manufacturer (Trizol, Invitrogen, USA). In order to remove genomic DNA contamination from the samples, the total RNA obtained from both groups was treated with DNase I (Fermentas, Sanktleon-rot, Germany). The total RNA concentration of the pooled germinal vesicle oocytes after treatment was 594 μg/ml for the GnRH-a long protocol group and 672 μg/ml for the GnRH-ant protocol group, determined by a Thermo Scientific Nano Drop 2000 Spectrophotometer. cDNA was synthesized according to manufacturer's instructions (Fermentas, Sanktleon-rot, Germany) using random hexamer primers.

We performed qPCR on the cDNA obtained from the pooled of germinal vesicle oocytes. Relative gene expression was calculated as the abundance ratio of each target gene to β-actin.

Quantitative real time PCR reactions were conducted in duplicates using a Roto- Gene Q instrument (Qiagen, German) with SYBR® Premix Ex Taq™ II master mix according to the procedure suggested by the manufacturer's instructions (Takara, Japan). The protocol for qPCR was initiated with a denaturing step at 95°C for 30 seconds, followed by 50 cycles of 2-step, real-time PCR under the following conditions: 5 seconds at 95°C for denaturation and 30 seconds at 59–60°C for annealing and extension.

No template control (NTC) was used as the negative control. The specificity of the PCR fragments was determined using melting curve analysis. All melting curves produced one peak for each of the PCR products.

Table 1 Oligonucleotide primer sequences used for qPCR in the present study

Gene name	Primer	Accession no.	T°C	Product size (bp)
GDF9		NM_005260.4	60	162
Sense	CCAGGTAACAGGAATCCTTC			
Antisense	GGCTCCTTTATCATTAGATTG			
BMP15		NM_005448.2	60	129
Sense	CCTCACAGAGGTATCTGGC			
Antisense	GGAGAGATTGAAGCGAGTTAG			
ATPase 6		YP_003024031.1	60	123
Sense	CTGTTCGCTTCATTCATTG			
Antisense	GGTGGTGATTAGTCGGTTG			
NAIP		NM_004536.2	60	184
Sense	GGAGTATTTGGATGACAGAAAC			
Antisense	TAGATTACCACTGGAGTCTTCC			
BUB1		NM_001278616.1	59	100
Sense	AAGGTCCGAGGTTAATCC			
Antisense	CACTGGTGTCTGCTGATAGG			
MADL2		NM_002358.3	60	169
Sense	CTTCTCATTCGGCATCAAC			
Antisense	ACACTTGTATAACCAATCTTTCAG			
CDC20		NM_001255.2	60	202
Sense	GATGTAGAGGAAGCCAAGATC			
Antisense	CCACAAGGTTCAGGTAATAGTC			
ATR		NM_001184.3	60	150
Sense	GATGCCACTGCTTGTTATG			
Antisense	CCACTCGGACCTGTTAGC			
ATM		NM_000051.3	60	107
Sense	GCATTACGGGTGTTGAAG			
Antisense	ATATAGAAGGACCTCTACAATG			
β.actin		NM_001101.3	60	90
Sense	CAAGATCATTGCTCCTCCTG			
Antisense	ATCCACATCTGCTGGAAGG			

Ethical considerations

The present study was approved by the ethics committee of Tehran University of Medical Sciences. The study was completely explained to the women, and informed consent was obtained before collecting germinal vesicles oocytes. The study was formally registered with the following code: IRCT 2014031112307 N3.

Statistical analysis

We used One-way ANOVA to compare quantitative variables between the two groups and chi-square for qualitative variables by SPSS version 16 (Chicago, IL, USA). The significance level was set at 0.05. The efficiency values given by the Linreg software and relative expression were calculated using the REST 2009 software (Qiagen, Hilden, Germany) [14], which is a standalone software tool used for estimating up and down regulation for gene expression studies. The $\Delta\Delta CT$ was obtained by finding the difference between the groups. The fold change was calculated as FC = $2^{-\Delta\Delta CT}$. For this purpose, β.actin was used as the reference gene for expression normalization.

Results

There were no significant differences in the age, hormonal profile, number of oocytes retrieved, infertility duration, and cause of infertility between the two groups (P > 0.05). However, the serum level of 17-beta estradiol on the day of hCG administration was higher in the GnRH-ant protocol group than in the GnRH-a long protocol group; however, this difference was not statistically significant, as presented in Tables 2 and 3.

Table 2 Mean (standard deviation) age, duration of infertility, number of oocytes retrieved, serum LH, FSH, TSH, PRL, AMH, and serum 17-beta estradiol in the GnRH-a protocol vs. GnRH-ant protocol group

Variable	GnRH-a long protocol (n = 26)	GnRH-ant protocol (n = 24)	Total (n=50)	P value
Age (yrs)	30.4 ± 5.5	33.8 ± 5.6	31.7 ± 5.7	0.100
Duration of infertility (yrs)	6.8 ± 3.5	4.6 ± 5.1	5.8 ± 4.5	0.086
Retrieved oocytes no.	11.0 ± 5.8	12.8 ± 8.3	11.8 ± 7.1	0.372
MII	6.2 ± 6.2	8.3 ± 6.3	7.2 ± 7.2	0.157
MI	1.8 ± 1.7	1.5 ± 1.6	1.6 ± 1.7	0.579
GV	2.1 ± 1.8	2.3 ± 1.8	2.2 ± 1.8	0.671
Deg.	0.8 ± 2.1	0.6 ± 2.1	0.7 ± 2.0	0.762
Serum 17 beta-estradiol (Pg/ml)*	5007.9 ± 8105	5988.3 ± 8110.6	5478.5 ± 8040.8	0.671
Serum LH (IU/L)	6.5 ± 2.9	5.5 ± 2.5	6.0 ± 2.8	0.256
Serum FSH (IU/L)	6.5 ± 2.5	6.3 ± 2.2	6.4 ± 2	0.706
Serum TSH (μIU/L)	3.0 ± 2.1	2.4 ± 1.1	2.7 ± 1.7	0.213
Serum PRL (ng/ml)	113.3 ± 186.2	107.0 ± 173.0	110.0 ± 178.2	0.902
Serum AMH (ng/ml)	5.0 ± 4.8	5.9 ± 5.6	5.4 ± 5.2	0.535

*On the day of hCG administration.
LH: luteinising hormone; FSH: follicle-stimulating hormone; TSH: thyroid-stimulating hormone; PRL: prolactin; AMH: anti-mullerian hormone.
MII: mature oocyte (Meiosis II); MI: immature oocyte (Meiosis I); GV: immature oocyte (Germinal Vesicle); Deg.: degenerative oocyte.

The present study showed that the expression levels of genes involved in the cytoplasmic maturity (*BMP15* and *GDF9*), antiapoptotic process *(NAIP)*, and adenosine triphosphate production *(ATPase 6)* in human GV oocytes were significantly higher in the GnRH-ant group versus in the GnRH-a group. ATPase 6, BMP15, and NAIP were significantly upregulated in the GnRH-ant group compared to the GnRH-a group with the fold change of 3.990 (SD ± 1.325), 6.274 (SD ± 1.542), and 2.156 (SD ± 1.443), respectively, (P value < 0.001). *GDF9* mRNA did not have any expression in the GnRH-a group; however, *GDF9* mRNA was expressed in the GnRH-ant group. These results are shown in Figure 1.

Finally, it was found that the genes involved in the DNA repairing, i.e. Ataxia telangiectasia and Rad3-related protein *(ATR)*, and Ataxia telangiectasia mutated *(ATM)*; and those involved in the cell cycle checkpoint, i. e. Bone morphogenetic protein 15 (*BUB1*), Mitotic arrest deficient-like 1 (*MAD2L1*), and Cell division cycle 20 (*CDC20*), did not have any expression in either group, as presented in Table 4.

Table 3 Distribution of the causes of infertility in the GnRH-a protocol vs. GnRH-ant protocol group

Variable	GnRH-a (%)	GnRH-ant (%)	P value
Cause of infertility			
● Male factor	16 (61.5)	9 (37.5)	
● Tubal factor	8 (30.8)	11 (45.58)	
● Unexplained	2 (7.7)	4 (16.7)	
Total	26.0 (100.0)	24.0 (100.0)	0.220

Discussion

Clinical studies have suggested similar pregnancy and live birth rates for both GnRH-a and GnRH-ant protocols [1,3,15-21], which has been further supported by some molecular studies [6-9]. Additionally, no significant morphological difference has been observed in the oocytes of the two groups after COS [22].

However, several advantages have been observed for the GnRH-ant protocol, including the fact that under this protocol, the endometrial receptivity is more similar to the natural cycle receptivity (in terms of endometrial chemokines and growth factors) [23]. In addition, when

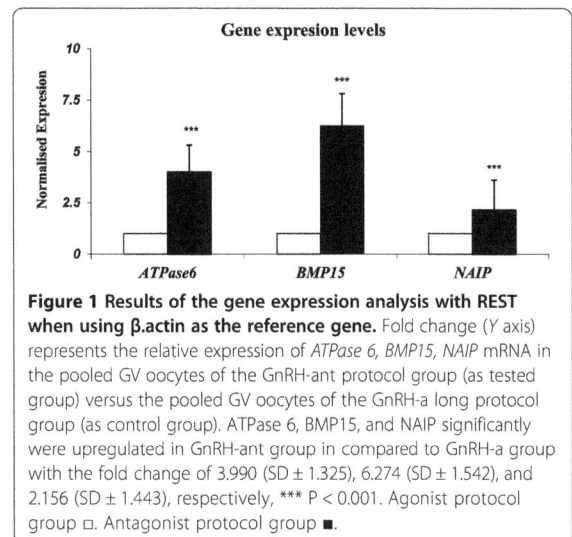

Figure 1 Results of the gene expression analysis with REST when using β.actin as the reference gene. Fold change (*Y* axis) represents the relative expression of *ATPase 6, BMP15, NAIP* mRNA in the pooled GV oocytes of the GnRH-ant protocol group (as tested group) versus the pooled GV oocytes of the GnRH-a long protocol group (as control group). ATPase 6, BMP15, and NAIP significantly were upregulated in GnRH-ant group in compared to GnRH-a group with the fold change of 3.990 (SD ± 1.325), 6.274 (SD ± 1.542), and 2.156 (SD ± 1.443), respectively, *** P < 0.001. Agonist protocol group □. Antagonist protocol group ■.

Table 4 The genes expression of germinal vesicle oocyte in GnRH agonist group compared with GnRH antagonist group

Gene symbol	Gene title	GnRH-a group		GnRH-anta group	
		Exist	Not exist	Exist	Not exist
Transforming growth factors					
GDF9	Growth differentiation factor 9		+	+	
BMP15	Bone morphogenetic protein 15	+		+	
Mitochondria					
ATPase6	Adenosine triphosphatase 6	+		+	
Antiapoptotic					
NAIP	Neuronal apoptosis inhibitory protein	+		+	
Cell cycle checkpoint markers					
BUB1	Budding uninhibited by benzimidazoles 1		+		+
MAD2L1	Mitotic arrest deficient-like 1		+		+
CDC20	Cell division cycle 20		+		+
DNA repair markers					
ATR	Ataxia telangiectasia and Rad3		+		+
ATM	Ataxia telangiectasia mutated		+		+
Reference gene					
B.actin	beta actin	+		+	

comparing GnRH-ant protocol and GnRH-a long protocols, the time of the appearance of the endometrial triple layer is statistically significant for the pregnancy rate only for the former protocol [24]. In addition to its safety and effectiveness, GnRH-ant allows for the flexibility of treatment in a wider range of women populations, including poor responders, women undergoing first-line controlled ovarian stimulation, and women diagnosed with polycystic ovarian syndrome. Therefore, the GnRH-ant protocol can be considered as a suitable alternative to the long agonist protocol, due mainly to its shorter duration of treatment and the need for fewer injections. Consequently, this leads to a significantly lower amount of administered gonadotropins, which most probably leads to improved women compliance [25]. We observed, for the first time, that the expression levels of genes involved in the cytoplasmic maturity, antiapoptotic process, and ATP production in human GV oocytes were significantly higher in the GnRH-anta group than in the GnRH-a group in COS.

As with other studies, in the present work, the same ovulation-triggering drug was used in the COS cycle for both groups; the only difference was the type of GnRH used for the two groups, which makes the present work different from the study of Hass et al. [26], in which oocyte cells were used for genetic evaluations.

The present study showed that the expression levels of genes involved in the cytoplasmic maturity, antiapoptotic process, and adenosine triphosphate production were significantly higher in the pooled oocytes of the women

in the GnRH antagonist group versus those of the women in the GnRH agonist group ($P < 0.001$). These results are shown in Figure 1.

ATPase 6 gene plays a critical role in ATP production by mitochondria. Deficiencies in the production of mitochondrial ATP can be linked to impaired oocyte fertilization, incomplete development of the embryo at later stages, and several other cellular and chromosomal disorders including errors in chromosomal segregation, lethal cytoplasmic defects, non disjunction disorders resulting in aneuploidy, and development failure of the sperm derived mitotic apparatus [27]. Therefore, the higher expression level of *ATPase6* in the pooled oocytes of the women in the GnRH-ant protocol group vs. those of the women in the GnRH-a long protocol group suggests that under the antagonist protocol, the mitochondrial activity may be more appropriate. In other words, higher-quality mitochondrial respiration and oxidative phosphorylation cascade occur in the oocytes of GnRH-ant group. The higher expression level of this gene and, in turn, higher energy production cause cell division spindles to form under better conditions [27].

Transforming growth factors beta *(TGF-ß)* are important paracrine growth factors that are secreted by the ovarian stroma or follicles surrounding the ovary, converting primordial follicles to primary ones. During folliculogenesis stages, oocytes secretion of *TGF-ß*, such as *BMP15* and *GDF9* [28], can regulate female fertility in several mammals [5,29,30]. *GDF9* and *BMP15* are responsible for transformation. They also cause the reproduction of granulosa cells under the influence of FSH, which mainly secrete estradiol [35]. Estradiol is required for the maturation of oocytes and development of embryo in vivo. Additionally, follicular atresia and granulosa cell apoptosis are inhibited by GDF9. Moreover, the proliferation, apoptosis, metabolism, and expansion of the cumulus oocyte complex are organized by the secretion of GDF9 and BMP15 [29].

According to the results from the present study, GDF9 and BMP15 are expressed in the pooled GV oocytes of the women in the GnRH-ant protocol group. Our study also showed that the expression level of GDF9 was higher than that of BMP15 in the antagonist group, which is consistent with the results of previous studies [30]. GDF9 gene was not expressed in the pooled GV oocytes of the women in the GnRH-a long protocol group. The higher expression of these genes in the pooled GV oocytes of the GnRH-ant protocol group could be due to the fact that in the GnRH-a long protocol, complete inhibition of gonadotropins occurs on the 2nd or the 3rd day of the current menstrual cycle. The study of Lainas et al. [36] indicated that the serum levels of E2, FSH, and LH hormones were significantly higher before administering OCP on the 2nd or the 3rd day of the pervious menstrual cycle when compared to the same day in the OCP plus GnRH-a long protocol, mainly due to the suppression of inner gonadotropin in this protocol (FSH: 5.8 vs. 3.6 IU/L; LH:5.6 vs. 1.2 IU/L; and E2: 30.5 vs. 12 pg/ml before and after using OCP/GnRH-a, respectively). This, however, does not occur in the GnRH-ant protocol. In the GnRH-ant protocol, the initial dose of GnRH-ant is administered on the 6th or the 7th day of the current menstrual cycle, which causes immediate inhibition of LH by influencing the GnRH receptors in the pituitary gland. Therefore, adequate follicle stimulation can be provided by a combination of exogenous FSH and endogenous LH secretion in early treatment [37]. In other words, administration of GnRH-ant protocol occurs in late follicular development (on the 5th or the 6th day of the gonadotropin stimulation when estradiol is increased).

NAIP is one of the members of the inhibitor of apoptosis protein (IAP) family. By regulating the caspase activity (inhibition of both caspase 3 and caspase 9), which is an important part of the apoptotic machinery, this gene can prevent apoptosis of granulosa cells during the ovarian folliculogenesis stages and can cause the follicles to develop from the primary stage to the graafian follicle [32]. In the oocyte, the expression of this gene can increase 2–4 times due to the effect of gonadotropin, which indirectly leads to oocyte survival [33,34]. After a thorough literature search, it was determined that the present study examined, for the first time, the expression level of NAIP in human oocytes. The higher level of the

expression of this gene in the pooled oocytes in the GnRH-ant protocol versus the pooled oocytes in the GnRH-a long protocol most likely suggests that the oocyte survival is improved by applying the former protocol.

In addition, in the present study, BUB1, MAD2L1, CDC20, ATR, and ATM genes did not have any expression in either group, which is most likely because that the oocytes used in the present work were germinal vesicle oocytes whose growth is arrested in the diplotene stage of the first meiotic prophase, as presented in Table 4.

ATR and ATM are a type of serine/threonine protein kinase. DNA double-strand breaks recruit and activate this serine/threonine protein kinase. This leads to the phosphorylation of several key proteins that are responsible for the initiation of DNA damage checkpoint activation, which finally results in cell cycle arrest, DNA repair, or apoptosis. ATM and ATR prevent premature chromosome condensation (PCC) until the DNA replication is completed [31].

In order to prevent premature separation of sister chromatids, MAD2L1 and BUB1, which in turn interact with CDC20 at check point activation, inhibit CDC20/APC [10]. Previous studies indicated that during the meiosis, BUB1, MAD2L1, and CDC20 had high expressions in the oocytes [28].

There are controversial findings regarding the difference in the serum levels of estradiol on the day of hCG administration between GnRH-ant and GnRH-a long protocols. Some studies have reported that the serum levels of estradiol on the day of hCG administration are significantly higher in the GnRH-a long protocol than in the GnRH-ant protocol [38]; other studies, however, have reported reverse findings [21,39-41]. In the present study, the serum levels of estradiol on the day of hCG administration were higher in the GnRH-ant protocol than the GnRH-a long protocol although the difference was not statistically significant, as presented in Tables 2. The serum level of estradiol is an indicator of the function of granulosa cells, suggesting that these cells have better performance in producing estradiol in the GnRH-ant protocol versus the GnRH-a long protocol.

Studies have indicated that the application of GnRH agonist protocol causes mid-cycle gonadotropine flares and ovarian hyperstimulation syndrome (OHSS), which is more observed in women with poly-cystic ovarian syndrome (PCOs). Therefore, the GnRH-ant protocol is a better choice than the GnRH-a protocol for ovarian stimulation in infertile women due to PCOs [1,4,25].

On the other hand, Li et al. [30] reported that the expression of GDF9 and BMP15 genes is necessary for the maturity of the oocyte cytoplasm; therefore, these two can be used as markers of oocyte quality in terms of its evolution. In addition, it was reported that in the oocytes of infertile women with PCOs, the expression level of GDF9 and BMP15 genes is lower than that of normal individuals, which can be the reason for the lowered quality of oocytes in these patients, which in turn leads to reduced fertility and the rate of success in IVF.

Therefore, since the results from the present study suggested higher expression level of these genes when GnRH-ant protocol is applied [Figure 1], this protocol seems to be a more appropriate choice for women with PCOs, because it can probably improve the expression of the aforementioned genes.

Although similar studies should be performed on the matured oocytes, but obtaining of donated mature oocytes (in vivo) is not ethically feasible for research purposes. On the other hand, the mature oocytes obtained from GV in vitro maturation is not appropriate for this purpose, mainly because studies have indicated that the in vitro culture conditions have adverse genetic and epigenetic impact on the growth of GV oocytes; therefore, this can prevent the researchers from observing the same findings. We suggest that future studies should be performed on donated mature oocytes which, together with the results of the present work, can help provide a broader molecular perspective in this field and make the most appropriate ovarian stimulation protocol.

Conclusions

Results from the present study indicated, for the first time, that in the germinal vesicle oocytes of women with normal ovarian function, the expression levels of genes involved in the cytoplasmic maturity (GDF9 and BMP15), antiapoptotic process (NAIP), and ATP production (ATPase 6) were significantly higher in the GnRH-anta protocol group than in the GnRH-a long protocol group. GDF9 mRNA did not have any expression in the GnRH-a group; however, GDF9 mRNA was expressed in the GnRH-ant group. Therefore, since the results from the present study suggested higher expression level of these genes when GnRH-ant protocol is applied, this protocol seems to be a more appropriate choice for women with PCOs, because it can probably improve the expression of the aforementioned genes.

Competing interest

The authors declare that they have no competing interests associated with this publication and there has been no significant financial support for this work that could have influenced its outcome.

Authors' contributions

FS H involving in the study design, data collection, and data analysis. N S, P E-Y, SMHN-M and F A-A involving in the study design. F A-A, B A and N S involving in data collection. SH A-B and R A involving in conducting the experiments, designing the primers, and analyzing the data. The manuscript was drafted by FS H, and all the other authors had intellectual contributions by critically reviewing the paper and leaving their comments. Finally, all the authors read and approved the final version of the manuscript.

Acknowledgments

The present study was funded by Deputy Ministry for Research, Tehran University of Medical Sciences (TUMS); grant no. 91-02-30-18324. The authors wish to thank all the oocyte donors. We would like to thank Dr. Masud Yunesian for helping with the study design and data analysis. We are also grateful to all the members of our ART team for their assistance during this study and to the staff of the Royan Institute for Reproductive Biomedicine and Stem Cell for carrying out the qPCR tests.

Author details

[1]Department of Anatomy and Reproductive Biology, School of Medicine, Tehran University of Medical Sciences, Tehran, Iran. [2]Departments of Histology, School of Medicine, Tehran University of Medical Sciences, Tehran, Iran. [3]Department of Obstetrics and Gynecology, Tehran Women General Hospital, School of Medicine, Tehran University of Medical Sciences, Tehran, Iran. [4]Department of Embryology at Reproductive Biomedicine Research Center, Royan Institute for Reproductive Biomedicine, ACECR, Tehran, Iran. [5]Lab director Assisted Conception Units, Laleh Hospital, Tehran, Iran and Madar Hospital, Yazd, Iran. [6]Department of Molecular Biology and Genetic Engineering, Stem Cell Technology Research Center, Tehran, Iran and Molecular Medicine Department, Biotechnology Research Center, Pasteur Institute of Iran, Tehran, Iran. [7]Department of Endocrinology and Female Infertility at Reproductive Biomedicine Research Center, Royan Institute for Reproductive Biomedicine, ACECR, Tehran, Iran. [8]Department of Physiotherapy, School of Rehabilitation of Tehran University of Medical Sciences, Tehran, Iran; Lab director Assisted Conception Unit, Tehran Women General Hospital, Tehran University of Medical Sciences, Tehran, Iran.

References

1. Marci R, Graziano A, Lo Monte G, Piva I, Soave I, Marra E, Lisi F, Moscarini M, Caserta D: GnRH antagonists in assisted reproductive techniques: a review on the Italian experience. Eur Rev Med Pharmacol Sci 2013, 17:853–873.
2. Nardo LG, Bosch E, Lambalk CB, Gelbaya TA: Controlled ovarian hyperstimulation regimens: a review of the available evidence for clinical practice. On behalf of the British Fertility Society P&P Committee. Hum Fertil (Camb) 2013, 16:144–150.
3. Johnston-MacAnanny EB, DiLuigi AJ, Engmann LL, Maier DB, Benadiva CA, Nulsen JC: Selection of first in vitro fertilization cycle stimulation protocol for good prognosis patients: gonadotropin releasing hormone antagonist versus agonist protocols. J Reprod Med 2011, 56:12–16.
4. Al-Inany HG, Youssef MA, Aboulghar M, Broekmans F, Sterrenburg M, Smit J, Abou-Setta AM: GnRH antagonists are safer than agonists: an update of a Cochrane review. Hum Reprod Update 2011, 17:435–435.
5. Orvieto R, Patrizio P: GnRH agonist versus GnRH antagonist in ovarian stimulation: An ongoing debate. Reprod BioMed Online 2013, 26:4–8.
6. Devjak R, Fon Tacer K, Juvan P, Virant Klun I, Rozman D, Vrtacnik Bokal E: Cumulus cells gene expression profiling in terms of oocyte maturity in controlled ovarian hyperstimulation using GnRH agonist or GnRH antagonist. PLoS One 2012, 7:e47106.
7. Kaya A, Atabekoglu CS, Kahraman K, Taskin S, Ozmen B, Berker B, Sonmezer M: Follicular fluid concentrations of IGF-I, IGF-II, IGFBP-3, VEGF, AMH, and inhibin-B in women undergoing controlled ovarian hyperstimulation using GnRH agonist or GnRH antagonist. Eur J Obstet Gynecol Reprod Biol 2012, 164:167–171.
8. Lavorato HL, Oliveira JB, Petersen CG, Vagnini L, Mauri AL, Cavagna M, Baruffi RL, Franco JG Jr: GnRH agonist versus GnRH antagonist in IVF/ICSI cycles with recombinant LH supplementation: DNA fragmentation and apoptosis in granulosa cells. Eur J Obstet Gynecol Reprod Biol 2012, 165:61–65.
9. Liu N, Ma Y, Li R, Jin H, Li M, Huang X, Feng HL, Qiao J: Comparison of follicular fluid amphiregulin and EGF concentrations in patients undergoing IVF with different stimulation protocols. Endocrine 2012, 42:708–716.
10. Gasca S, Pellestor F, Assou S, Loup V, Anahory T, Dechaud H, De Vos J, Hamamah S: Identifying new human oocyte marker genes: a microarray approach. Reprod Biomed Online 2007, 14:175–183.
11. Kahraman K, Berker B, Atabekoglu CS, Sonmezer M, Cetinkaya E, Aytac R, Satiroglu H: Microdose gonadotropin-releasing hormone agonist flare-up protocol versus multiple dose gonadotropin-releasing hormone

antagonist protocol in poor responders undergoing intracytoplasmic sperm injection–embryo transfer cycle. *Fertil Steril* 2009, **91**:2437–2444.

12. Roberto M, Donatella C, Vincenza D, Carla T, Antonio P, Massimo M: GnRH antagonist in IVF poor-responder patients: results of a randomized trial. *Reprod BioMed Online* 2005, **11**:189–193.

13. Ye H, Huang G-n, Zeng P-h, Pei L: IVF/ICSI outcomes between cycles with luteal estradiol (E2) pre-treatment before GnRH antagonist protocol and standard long GnRH agonist protocol: a prospective and randomized study. *J Assist Reprod Genet* 2009, **26**:105–111.

14. Pfaffl MW, Horgan GW, Dempfle L: Relative expression software tool (REST©) for group-wise comparison and statistical analysis of relative expression results in real-time PCR. *Nucleic Acids Res* 2002, **30**:e36–e36.

15. Luna M, Vela G, McDonald CA, Copperman AB: Results with GnRH antagonist protocols are equivalent to GnRH agonist protocols in comparable patient populations. *J Reprod Med* 2012, **57**:123–128.

16. Mekaru K, Yagi C, Asato K, Masamoto H, Sakumoto K, Aoki Y: Comparison between the gonadotropin-releasing hormone antagonist protocol and the gonadotropin-releasing hormone agonist long protocol for controlled ovarian hyperstimulation in the first in vitro fertilization-embryo transfer cycle in an unspecified population of infertile couples. *Reprod Med Biol* 2012, **11**:79–83.

17. Munoz M, Cruz M, Humaidan P, Garrido N, Perez-Cano I, Meseguer M: The type of GnRH analogue used during controlled ovarian stimulation influences early embryo developmental kinetics: a time-lapse study. *Eur J Obstet Gynecol Reprod Biol* 2013, **168**:167–172.

18. Nardo LG, Fleming R, Howles CM, Bosch E, Hamamah S, Ubaldi FM, Hugues JN, Balen AH, Nelson SM: Conventional ovarian stimulation no longer exists: Welcome to the age of individualized ovarian stimulation. *Reprod BioMed Online* 2011, **23**:141–148.

19. Prapas Y, Petousis S, Dagklis T, Panagiotidis Y, Papatheodorou A, Assunta I, Prapas N: GnRH antagonist versus long GnRH agonist protocol in poor IVF responders: a randomized clinical trial. *Eur J Obstet Gynecol Reprod Biol* 2013, **166**:43–46.

20. Pu D, Wu J, Liu J: Comparisons of GnRH antagonist versus GnRH agonist protocol in poor ovarian responders undergoing IVF. *Hum Reprod* 2011, **26**:2742–2749.

21. Yang S, Chen XN, Qiao J, Liu P, Li R, Chen GA, Ma CH: Comparison of GnRH antagonist fixed protocol and GnRH agonists long protocol in infertile patients with normal ovarian reserve function in their first in vitro fertilization-embryo transfer cycle. *Zhonghua Fu Chan Ke Za Zhi* 2012, **47**:245–249.

22. Cota A, Oliveira J, Petersen CG, Mauri AL, Massaro FC, Silva L, Nicoletti A, Cavagna M, Baruffi R, Franco JG Jr: GnRH agonist versus GnRH antagonist in assisted reproduction cycles: oocyte morphology. *Reprod Biol Endocrinol* 2012, **10**:33.

23. Haouzi D, Assou S, Dechanet C, Anahory T, Dechaud H, De Vos J, Hamamah S: Controlled ovarian hyperstimulation for in vitro fertilization alters endometrial receptivity in humans: protocol effects. *Biol Reprod* 2010, **82**:679–686.

24. Kuć P, Kuczyńska A, Topczewska M, Tadejko P, Kuczyński W: The dynamics of endometrial growth and the triple layer appearance in three different controlled ovarian hyperstimulation protocols and their influence on IVF outcomes. *Gynecol Endocrinol* 2011, **27**:867–873.25.

25. Copperman AB, Benadiva C: Optimal usage of the GnRH antagonists: A review of the literature. *Reprod Biol Endocrinol* 2013, **11**:20.

26. Haas J, Ophir L, Barzilay E, Yerushalmi GM, Yung Y, Kedem A, Maman E, Hourvitz A: Gnrh agonist vs hCG for triggering of ovulation–differential effects on gene expression in human granulosa cells. *PLoS One* 2014, **9**:e90359.

27. Lee SH, Han JH, Cho SW, Cha KE, Park SE, Cha KY: Mitochondrial ATPase 6 gene expression in unfertilized oocytes and cleavage-stage embryos. *Fertil Steril* 2000, **73**:1001–1005.

28. Assou S, Anahory T, Pantesco V, Le Carrour T, Pellestor F, Klein B, Reyftmann L, Dechaud H, De Vos J, Hamamah S: The human cumulus–oocyte complex gene-expression profile. *Hum Reprod* 2006, **21**:1705–1719.

29. Gode F, Gulekli B, Dogan E, Korhan P, Dogan S, Bige O, Cimrin D, Atabey N: Influence of follicular fluid GDF9 and BMP15 on embryo quality. *Fertil Steril* 2011, **95**:2274–2278.

30. Wei LN, Liang XY, Fang C, Zhang MF: Abnormal expression of growth differentiation factor 9 and bone morphogenetic protein 15 in

31. stimulated oocytes during maturation from women with polycystic ovary syndrome. *Fertil Steril* 2011, **96**:464–468.

31. Sancar A, Lindsey-Boltz LA, Unsal-Kaçmaz K, Linn S: Molecular mechanisms of mammalian DNA repair and the DNA damage checkpoints. *Annu Rev Biochem* 2004, **73**:39–85.

32. Verhagen AM, Coulson EJ, Vaux DL: Inhibitor of apoptosis proteins and their relatives: IAPs and other BIRPs. *Genome Biol* 2001, **2**:3009.3001–3009.3010.

33. Beug ST, Cheung HH: LaCasse EC. Korneluk RG: Modulation of immune signalling by inhibitors of apoptosis. Trends in immunology; 2012.

34. Smolewski P, Robak T: Inhibitors of apoptosis proteins (IAPs) as potential molecular targets for therapy of hematological malignancies. *Curr Mol Med* 2011, **11**:633–649.

35. Carlson BM, Brudon MC: *Human embryology and developmental biology*. St. Louis: Mosby; 1994.

36. Lainas TG, Petsas GK, Zorzovilis IZ, Iliadis GS, Lainas GT, Cazlaris HE, Kolibianakis EM: Initiation of GnRH antagonist on Day 1 of stimulation as compared to the long agonist protocol in PCOS patients. A randomized controlled trial: effect on hormonal levels and follicular development. *Hum Reprod* 2007, **22**:1540–1546.

37. Filicori M, Cognigni GE, Samara A, Melappioni S, Perri T, Cantelli B, Parmegiani L, Pelusi G, DeAloysio D: The use of LH activity to drive folliculogenesis: exploring uncharted territories in ovulation induction. *Hum Reprod Update* 2002, **8**:543–557.

38. Kara M, Aydin T, Aran T, Turktekin N, Ozdemir B: Comparison of GnRH agonist and antagonist protocols in normoresponder patients who had IVF-ICSI. *Arch Gynecol Obstet* 2013, **288**:1413–1416.

39. Lai Q, Zhang H, Zhu G, Li Y, Jin L, He L, Zhang Z, Yang P, Yu Q, Zhang S, XU JF, Wang CY: Comparison of the GnRH agonist and antagonist protocol on the same patients in assisted reproduction during controlled ovarian stimulation cycles. *Int J Clin Exp Pathol* 2013, **6**:1903–1910.

40. Li Y, Lai Q, Zhang H, Zhu G, Jin L, Yue J: Comparison between a GnRH agonist and a GnRH antagonist protocol for the same patient undergoing IVF. *J Huazhong Univ Sci Technolog Med Sci* 2008, **28**:618–620.

41. Taskin EA, Atabekoglu CS, Musali N, Oztuna D, Sonmezer M: Association of serum estradiol levels on the day of hCG administration with pregnancy rates and embryo scores in fresh ICSI/ET cycles down regulated with either GnRH agonists or GnRH antagonists. *Arch Gynecol Obstet* 2014, **298**:399–405.

14

Preparation, characterization and optimization of sildenafil citrate loaded PLGA nanoparticles by statistical factorial design

Elham Ghasemian[†], Alireza Vatanara[*†], Abdolhossein Rouholamini Najafabadi[†], Mohammad Reza Rouini[†], Kambiz Gilani[†] and Majid Darabi[†]

Abstract

Background and the aim of the study: The objective of the present study was to formulate and optimize nanoparticles (NPs) of sildenafil-loaded poly (lactic-co-glycolic acid) (PLGA) by double emulsion solvent evaporation (DESE) method. The relationship between design factors and experimental data was evaluated using response surface methodology.

Method: A Box-Behnken design was made considering the mass ratio of drug to polymer (D/P), the volumetric proportion of the water to oil phase (W/O) and the concentration of polyvinyl alcohol (PVA) as the independent agents. PLGA-NPs were successfully prepared and the size (nm), entrapment efficiency (EE), drug loading (DL) and cumulative release of drug from NPs post 1 and 8 hrs were assessed as the responses.

Results: The NPs were prepared in a spherical shape and the sizes range of 240 to 316 nm. The polydispersity index of size was lower than 0.5 and the EE (%) and DL (%) varied between 14-62% and 2-6%, respectively. The optimized formulation with a desirability factor of 0.9 was selected and characterized. This formulation demonstrated the particle size of 270 nm, EE of 55%, DL of 3.9% and cumulative drug release of 79% after 12 hrs. In vitro release studies showed a burst release at the initial stage followed by a sustained release of sildenafil from NPs up to 12 hrs. The release kinetic of the optimized formulation was fitted to Higuchi model.

Conclusions: Sildenafil citrate NPs with small particle size, lipophilic feature, high entrapment efficiency and good loading capacity is produced by this method. Characterization of optimum formulation, provided by an evaluation of experimental data, showed no significant difference between calculated and measured data.

Keywords: Sildenafil citrate, Nanoparticle, Optimization, Box-Behnken, Double emulsion

Background

Sildenafil is a selective inhibitor of phosphodiesterase enzyme type 5 (PDE-5) that effectively inactivates cyclic guanosine monophosphate (cGMP) and enhances the effect of nitric oxide [1]. This drug was primarily prescribed for angina pectoris and now is widely used for the treatment of erectile dysfunction [2]. Recently, PDE-5 inhibitors have been proposed to protect the endothelial function in human by selectively improving local blood flow [3]. Moreover, other complications like wound healing, diabetic gastropathy [4], Reynaud's phenomenon, respiratory disorders with ventilation/perfusion mismatch, congestive cardiac failure, hypertension and stroke have been widely studied with the hope that PDE-5 inhibitors can serve as novel promising treatment in such conditions. In addition, the selective and potent vasodilatory and antiproliferative effects of sildenafil on pulmonary vascular smooth muscle cells emphasize the importance of this drug in control of pulmonary artery pressure [4-6]. When sildenafil citrate (SC) is given orally, its bioavailability is relatively low (approximately 40%) in healthy subjects [7] because of the first pass metabolism. In addition, it exhibits a very short physiological half-life (about 3–4 hrs). Therefore repeated doses are required to sustain

* Correspondence: vatanara@tums.ac.ir
[†]Equal contributors
Pharmaceutics Department, Faculty of Pharmacy, Tehran University of Medical Sciences, Tehran, Iran

drug plasma level [8] that causes various side effects such as headache, flushing, dyspepsia and epistaxis [9].

Specially designed dosage forms that sustain levels of drug in the therapeutic window or local delivery of this drug into the site of action can be thus helpful [8,10]. Some published patents have reported that application of nano sized SC powder in formulation, shows faster onset of action, higher bioavailability and absorption than conventional dosage form [11-13]. Thus, nanoparticles (NPs) might improve the efficacy; reduce side effects and dosage of therapeutic agents [14]. Generally, nanocarrier systems provide advantages over conventional drug delivery systems such as protection of the entrapped drug from enzymatic destruction, sustained drug release, reduction of daily drug doses and side effects and cell targeting [15]. Consequently, biodegradable polymeric NPs have engrossed remarkable consideration as potential drug delivery devices in view of their applications in the controlled release of drugs [16]. poly(lactic-co-glycolic acid) (PLGA) is the most successfully used available biodegradable polymer due to its long clinical experience, desirable degradation characteristics and possibilities for sustained drug delivery [17]. This polymer is widely used in the production of NPs [18]. PLGA consists two endogenous monomers that are easily metabolized via the Krebs cycle and therefore, negligible systemic toxicity is associated with the use of PLGA for drug delivery [19]. Also, study of *in vitro* and *in vivo* cytotoxicity of PLGA nanoparticles highlighted the safety of biodegradable PLGA nanoparticles [20,21]. Selection of a particular method for preparation of NPs is usually determined by the solubility properties of the drug [22]. Double Emulsion Solvent Evaporation (DESE) technique is an effective method for encapsulation of hydrophilic compounds [23] and thus we selected this method to fabricate NPs, because of the polar properties of SC [24]. There are several variables in the DESE process that can affect the properties of the product. Response surface methodology (RSM) is a statistical method employed for the modeling and analysis of problems in which a response of concern is influenced by several variables and the goal is to optimize this response [25]. Application of such optimizing technique may be an efficient and economical method to gain the essential information and thus to understand the relationship between controllable independent variables and dependent variables or responses in terms of performance and quality [26].

Methods
Materials
PLGA, Resomer® RG503H, was acquired from Boehringer Ingelheim (Germany). Polyvinyl alcohol (PVA) (87−90% hydrolysis degree and molecular mass 30,000-70,000 g/mol) was purchased from Sigma Chemical Co. (USA). SC was purchased from Selleck Chemicals (USA). The organic solvents were supplied by Duksan (Korea).

Preparation of SC-loaded Nanoparticles
At the first, the drug was dissolved in warm distilled water (3 mg/ml) and emulsified in methylene chloride containing different amounts of PLGA. The emulsification was carried out using a probe sonicator set (Hielscher, Germany) at 80% of the energy output for 3 min. Then, the primary emulsion was added to 20 ml of double distilled water containing PVA and homogenized for 3 min in 20,000 rpm (IKA, Germany). Methylene chloride was eliminated by evaporation under reduced pressure using a rotary evaporator (Buchi, Switzerland). NPs were recovered by ultracentrifugation (Beckman Instruments, USA) at 100,000 g for 60 min at 25°C.

Experimental design
The effects of formulation variables on the NPs characteristics and optimization procedure were examined by employing a Box-Behnken design. The design and statistical analysis were performed by Design-Expert® V8 (DX8) Software for design of experiments (DOE). Experimental factors and factor levels were determined in preliminary studies. Studied responses which evaluated in this investigation, were the mass ratio of drug to PLGA (X_1), the volumetric ratio of water to solvent in primary emulsion (X_2) and the concentration of PVA (X_3) that classified to low, medium, and high values for the chosen variables as are described in Table 1. The evaluated studied responses were size (nm), entrapment efficiency (EE), drug loading (DL) and drug release in 1 hr and 8 hrs. The Box-Behnken design and observational data are shown in Table 2.

The quadratic non-linear model generated by design is in this form:

$$Y = A_0 + A_1X_1 + A_2X_2 + A_3X_3 + A_4X_1X_2 + A_5X_2X_3 + A_6X_1X_3 + A_7X_1^2 + A_8X_2^2 + A_9X_3^2 + E$$

In which Y is the measured response associated with each factor level combination; A_0 is an intercept; A_1-A_9 are the regression coefficients; X_1, X_2 and X_3 are the studied factors; X_1^2, X_2^2, X_3^2 are quadratic effects, $X_1X_2 + X_2X_3 + X_1X_3$ are interaction between variables and E is the error term [27].

Table 1 Factors and factor levels studied in a Box–Behnken experimental design

Factors		Levels		
		Low (−1)	Medium (0)	High (1)
X_1	D/P	0.05	0.13	0.2
X_2	W/O	0.25	0.38	0.5
X_3	%PVA	0.1	0.55	1

Table 2 Run parameters and responses for three-level three-factorial Box–Behnken experimental design

Runs order	D/P	W/O	PVA (%)	Size (nm)	EE (%)	DL (%)	Drug release in 1 hr	Drug release in 8 hrs
1	1	0	−1	291	35	6.3	70	72
2	0	0	0	241	43	5.3	62	68
3	−1	0	1	316	51	3.2	30	39
4	1	0	1	259	28	5.1	79	79
5	0	−1	−1	259	26	3.1	75	80
6	0	0	0	279	47	5.8	49	50
7	0	−1	1	260	16	2	80	92
8	0	1	−1	304	32	4	51	59
9	0	1	1	311	32	4.1	36	43
10	−1	1	0	301	49	2.4	54	62
11	1	−1	0	246	14	2.5	92	93
12	1	1	0	261	26	4.8	79	81
13	0	0	0	268	45	5.5	77	86
14	−1	0	−1	303	62	3	29	40
15	0	0	0	260	45	5.6	49	65
16	−1	−1	0	278	41	2	61	75
17	0	0	0	240	46	5.6	50	64

Physicochemical characteristics of NPs

Particle size

Mean hydrodynamic size (called z-average) and polydispersity index of the NPs were measured by photon correlation spectroscopy (Malvern, UK) at 25C. All the samples were diluted with double distilled water to create a suitable obscuration before analysis.

Determination of entrapped SC

The supernatant part of the centrifuged NP sample was carefully removed and examined to determine the amount of non-encapsulated drug. The precipitant was lyophilized, weighted, and then dissolved in a mixture of 3:2 of chloroform (a common solvent for PLGA) and water (a solvent for SC) by sonicating for one hour. Then, the undissolved fraction was removed by centrifugation. After that, a sample was taken from the aqueous phase to determine the amount of encapsulated SC. The drug incorporation efficiency was defined by the following formulas:

$$DL(\%) = \frac{\text{Mass of sildenafil in NPs}}{\text{The mass of NPs recovered}} \times 100$$

$$EE(\%) = \frac{\text{Mass of encapsulated sildenafil}}{\text{Mass of the total sildenafil}} \times 100$$

A reverse phase chromatography method was used for evaluation of SC using isocratic HPLC system (Waters, USA) and NucleoDur (5 μm, 25 cm) C_{18} column. The mobile phase consisted of acetonitrile and water (35:65, pH 4.0) at a flow rate of 1 ml/min with UV detection at 291 nm. The retention time was 5.6 min.

Differential scanning calorimetry (DSC)

A differential scanning calorimeter (Mettler Toledo, Switzerland) was used to evaluate the thermal behavior of all materials used in the NP formulations. The equipment was calibrated using indium. The samples (8 mg) were heated ranging 5–280°C at a scanning rate of 10°C/min in aluminum pans under nitrogen gas.

Scanning electron microscopy (SEM)

The surface morphology of NPs was assessed by a scanning electron microscope (Mira Tescan, Czech Republic). The Nanoparticles were spread on a stub and dried at 25°C and then spattered with gold using a sputter coater (BAL-TEC, Switzerland).

In vitro drug release studies

To predict the optimal formulation of NPs, the drug release of each formulation was studied in phosphate buffer (PBS) at pH 7.4 as dissolution medium. Briefly, 10 mg of each lyophilized NP formulation was dispersed in a screw-capped glass vial (50 ml) containing 40 ml of medium by shaking at 200 rpm and 37 ± 0.5°C in shaker incubator (LABOTEC, Germany). At predetermined time intervals (0, 0.5, 1, 2, 4, 8, 10, 12, 24 hrs) 1 ml of the dispersion was taken away and replaced with 1 ml of fresh PBS. The sample was centrifuged (Eppendorf, Germany) at 14,000 g for 30 min, and the supernatant was analyzed. All of the experiments were done in triplicate.

The release kinetics from optimal NPs was fitted on zero order, first order, Higuchi model, Korsmeyer–Peppas model and Hixson–Crowell model [28].

Results

NPs were successfully prepared by DESE method. The effects of formulation variables on the NP properties were evaluated and finally optimal NPs were proposed by design expert software. The characteristics of this formulation were compared to predicted values. In addition, release profile and release kinetics from optimal NPs were studied.

Particle size

SC loaded NPs sizes varied between 240 to 316 nm. Formulations displayed polydispersity index (PDI) of <0.5 which showed the narrow NP size distribution.

Analysis of data from ANOVA test exhibited that D/P and W/O ratios had significant effects on particle size ($p < 0.05$). Briefly, decrease in the D/P and increasing the W/O ratios resulted in the production of larger particles (Figure 1).

In size response, the reduced model showed better adjusted correlation coefficients than the primary model ($0.72 > 0.62$) with an F value of 8 ($p < 0.05$), which clearly indicated that the particle size and some variables were related. The reduced model for predicting size is presented in equation 1.

$$\text{Particle size} = +258.68 - 17.63*X_1 + 16.75*X_2 - 1.38*X_3 + 11.46*X_1^2 + 23.46*X_3^2 - 11.25*X_1*X_3 \tag{1}$$

The minimum particle size of 240 nm was achieved by operating the experiment at the midpoint of each independent variable. Analysis of independent factors showed that D/P and W/O ratios had effective impacts on particle size. There was no significant interaction between the studied factors.

Determination of entrapped SC

The EE of NPs in different formulations is represented in Table 2. Data analysis of this response proved the significant effect of all independent variables ($p < 0.05$) and an interaction between W/O ratio and the amount of PVA ($p < 0.05$). The quadratic model of Entrapment Efficiency followed equation 2.

$$\begin{aligned} EE = &+45.20 - 12.50*X_1 + 5.25*X_2 - 3.50*X_3 \\ &+ 2.40*X_1^2 - 15.10*X_2^2 - 3.60*X_3^2 \\ &+ 1.00*X_1*X_2 + 1.00*X_1*X_3 \\ &+ 2.50*X_2*X_3 \end{aligned} \tag{2}$$

Surface plots indicated that higher EE occurred in formulation with a W/O ratio about 0.38 and D/P ratios between 0.05-0.09. Also, PVA concentration was less effective than two other variables (Figure 2). The predictive model for DL is given in equation 3:

$$\begin{aligned} DL = &+5.56 + 1.01*X_1 + 0.71*X_2 - 0.25*X_3 - 0.77*X_1^2 \\ &- 1.87*X_2^2 - 0.39*X_3^2 + 0.48*X_1*X_2 - 0.35*X_1*X_3 \\ &+ 0.30*X_2*X_3 \end{aligned} \tag{3}$$

DL in NPs ranged between 2% and 6.3% (Figure 3); where, analysis of data by ANOVA showed that the D/P Ratio with an F value of 71.36 ($p < 0.05$) had the most important impact on DL and W/O ratios had a significant effect on this response ($p < 0.05$). Comparison of different formulations and surface plots revealed that formulations with the highest DL had the maximum D/P ratio of 0.2 and a W/O ratio of approximately 0.38.

In vitro drug release studies

To develop a formulation with acceptable release profile, drug release of each formulation was studied. Data of

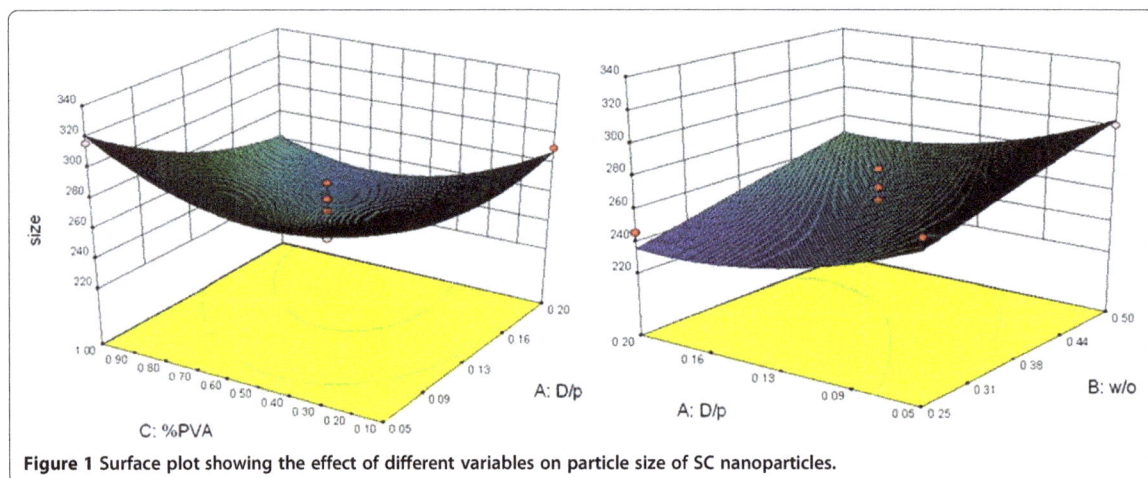

Figure 1 Surface plot showing the effect of different variables on particle size of SC nanoparticles.

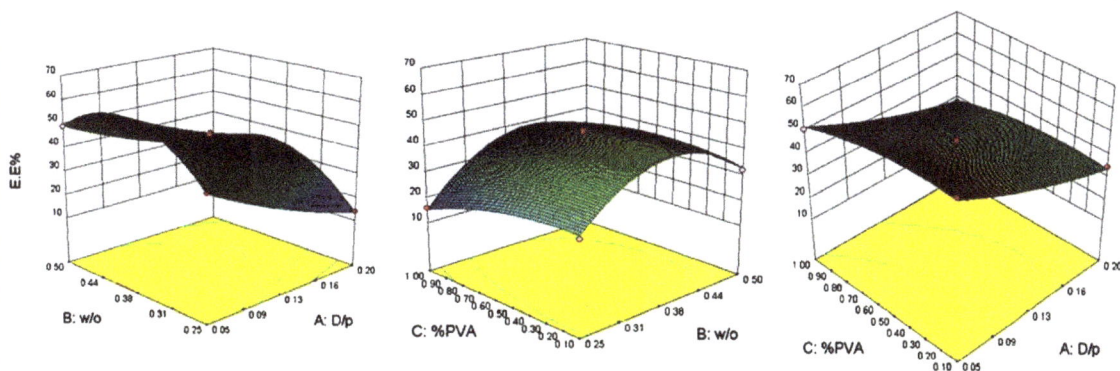

Figure 2 Three dimensional surface plots showing the effect of different variables on the %Entrapment Efficiency (EE) of SC nanoparticles.

release over the first hour of experiments were considered as a marker of burst effect and the amount of drug releasing in 8 hrs showed retardation efficiency over the time. Analysis of the data demonstrated that W/O and D/P ratios had significant influence on release profiles.

For predicting the release in 1 and 8 hrs, the linear model fitted as an effective one with data ($p < 0.05$) (equations 4–5).

$$\%Release\ 1\ hr = +60.18 + 18.25 * X_1 \\ - 11.00 * X_2 + 0.000 * X_3 \qquad (4)$$

$$\%Release\ 8\ hrs = +67.53 + 13.63 * X_1 \\ - 11.87 * X_2 + 0.25 * X_3 \qquad (5)$$

Data analysis showed that the D/P ratios with F values of 17.08 and 9.10 ($p < 0.05$) were the most important factors on the release of SC from NPs during 1 and 8 hrs, respectively (Figure 4). When the D/P ratio was minimized and W/O ratio was about 0.38, the formulation had the least burst release. On the other hand, this formulation could provide sustained release profile over the time.

Optimization

After confirming the polynomial equations relating the response and independent factors, in consequence of acceptable size of all formulations, the optimization model was constructed by combining the DL, EE and drug release in 1 hr responses. Optimization was performed by using a desirability function to obtain the levels of X_1, X_2 and X_3, which maximized EE, while minimizing drug release in 1 hr and targeting DL at 4%. Coefficients with p-value < 0.05 had a significant effect on the prediction efficacy of the model for the measured responses. Simultaneously, the formulation with W/O about 0.40, D/P of 0.06 and PVA about 0.50 conformed higher desirability. This formulation prepared and evaluated. Predicted and actual amounts of responses are compared and shown in Table 3. As seen in Table 3, excluding release in 1 h, the amount of responses for optimized formulation have lower than 10% difference with the predicted amount of Box-behnken design.

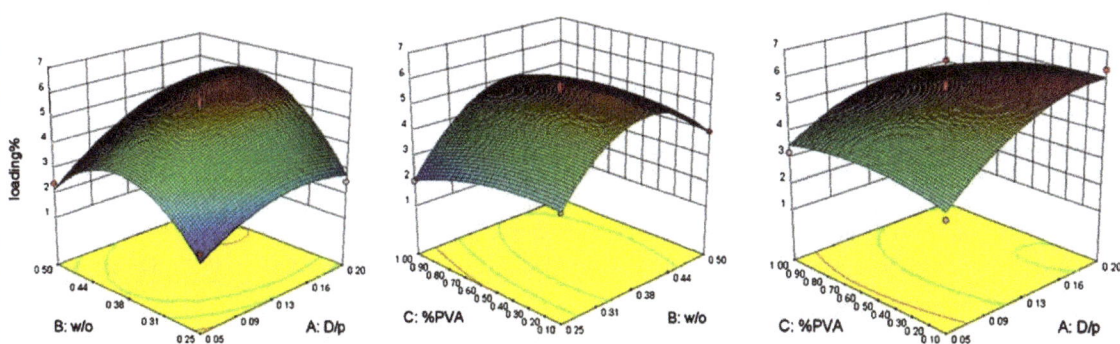

Figure 3 Three dimensional surface plots showing the effect of different variables on the %drug loading of SC nanoparticles.

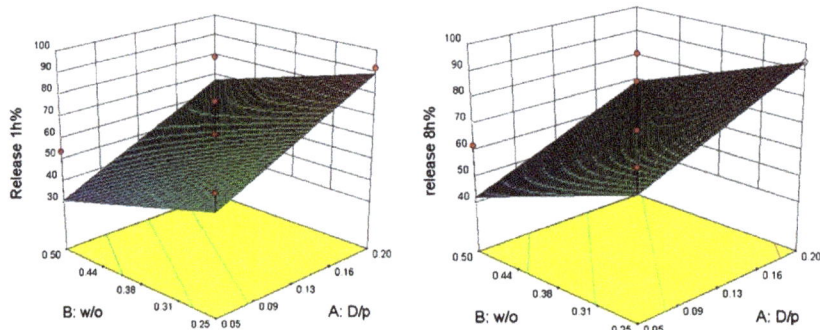

Figure 4 Three dimensional surface plots showing the effect of different variables on the release of drug from SC nanoparticles during 1 hr and 8 hrs.

Differential scanning calorimetry (DSC)

Thermal analysis is a supportive tool for determining the dispersion of the drug in polymeric materials. DSC thermograms of the pure drug, PVA, PLGA and SC-NPs are represented in Figure 5. The pure drug showed high endothermic peak indication of its melting peak at ~ 200°C which was absent in NPs.

Scanning electron microscopy (SEM)

SEM micrographs showed that uniform PLGA NPs were successfully prepared by using the DESE method. As shown in Figure 6, the PLGA nanoparticles were in spherical shapes and a smooth surface.

Release kinetics of optimal nanoparticles

Profile of release from optimal NPs is presented in Figure 7. *In vitro* drug release profiles of SLD from optimal PLGA NPs showed that the cumulative percentage of drug release was about 79% of drug content of the formulation in 12 hrs. The results support a burst release in the first one hour that followed by a sustained release over 12 hrs.

Release kinetics from the optimum formulation of NPs was compared to different kinetic models which showed that the best model fitted with data is the Higuchian equation (R^2: 0.95). This model explains the release of drug from an insoluble matrix time-dependently based on Fickian diffusion [29]. The release constant was computed from the slope of the suitable plots, and the regression coefficient was determined (Table 4). The plots and regression coefficient proved that after Higuchian

model, the best linearity followed by first-order kinetic (R^2: 0.91). The first order kinetics model can be described the drug dissolution of water-soluble drugs in porous matrices [30].

Discussion

Although the most applied method for encapsulation of hydrophilic drugs is DESE method, the low EE is usually a major problem. Experimental design methodology is an economic approach for extracting the maximum useful information from data. Applying this technique reduces the costs of experiments by saving time, materials and energy. Of course, optimization of NPs formulation is a complex procedure, which involves considering various parameters and their interactions. Due to increasing use of sildenafil in the treatment of pulmonary diseases and new indications proposed for this drug, preparation of optimum loaded NPs that release drug over the time can be potentially beneficial in the treatment of different pathological conditions.

Particle size and size distribution are important physicochemical properties that determine both uptake and biological fate of the particulate systems [31]. In the results, important effects of D/P and W/O ratios on size of NPs were confirmed. Production of NPs with higher polymer concentrations resulted in the formation of larger particles. In this manner, changing the diffusion rate of organic solvent through the interface could be proposed as a fundamental mechanism. In fact, increasing the amount of polymer or decreasing the volume of organic phase can potentially hinder the diffusion of solvent molecules

Table 3 Comparison of actual and predicted properties of optimized NPs

	Size (nm)	EE (%)	DL (%)	Release in 1 h (%)	Release in 8 hrs (%)
Predicted amount	270	58.9	4	41	90.8
Actual amount	250	55	3.9	30	85
Error (%)	7.4	6.6	2.5	26	6.4

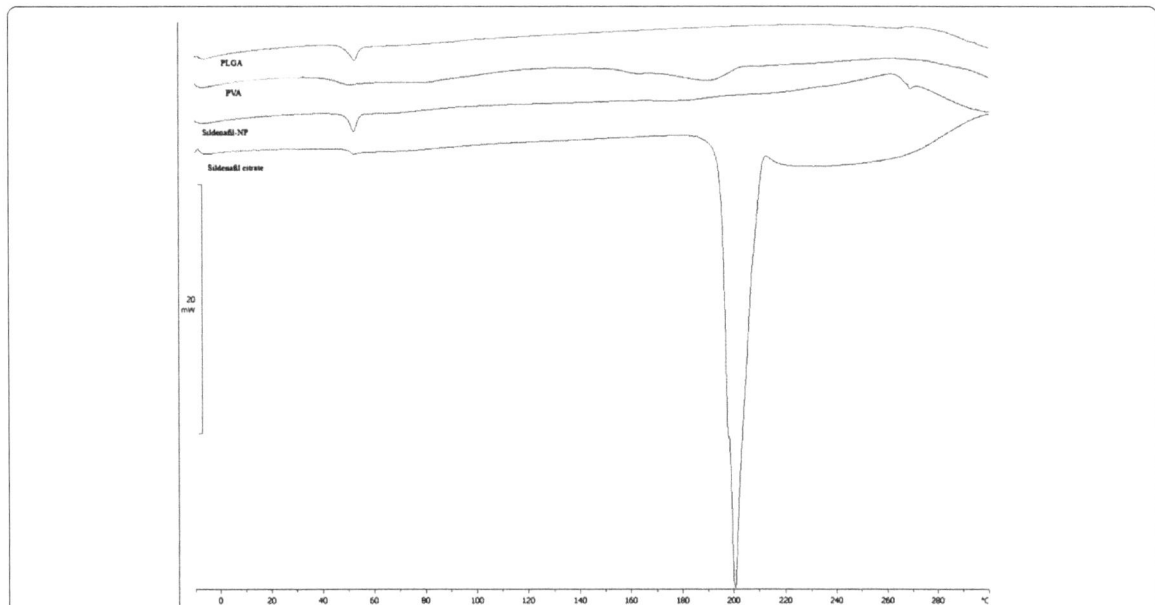

Figure 5 DSC thermogram of PLGA, PVA, Sildenafil citrate and Sildenafil-nanoparticles.

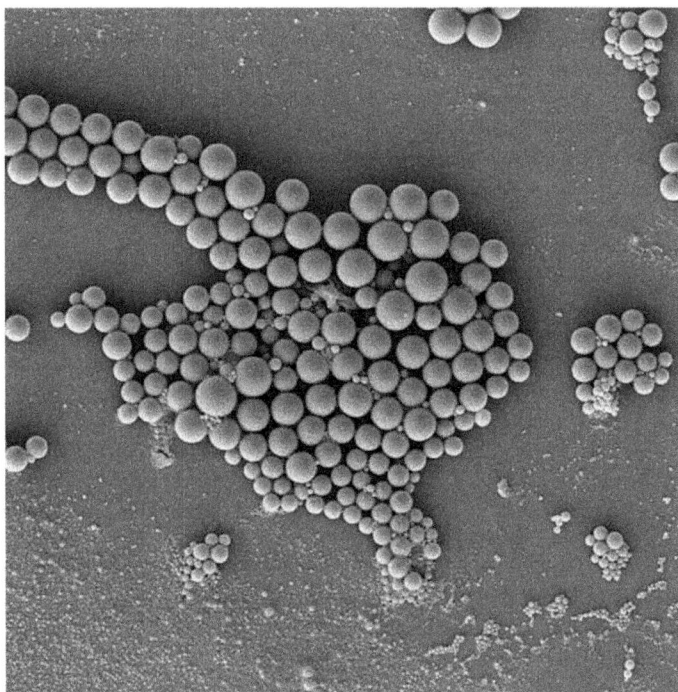

Figure 6 SEM micrograph showing the morphology of optimized PLGA-Sildenafil nanoparticles.

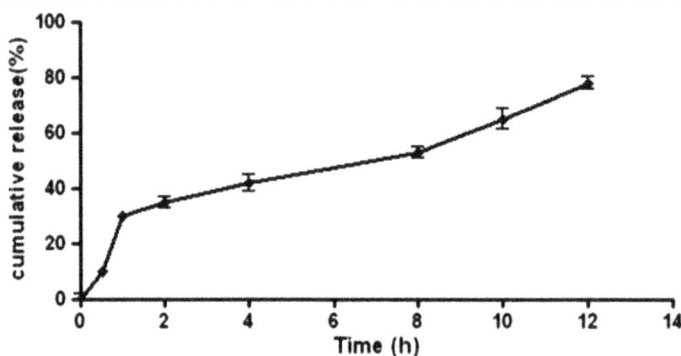

Figure 7 Profile of drug release from optimized SC nanoparticles.

through the polymeric chains [32]. Hence, formation of larger particles can be on account of two main factors: (a) the number of polymer chains per volume unit of solvent and (b) the viscosity of the solution [33]. As a result of applying a greater number of the polymeric chains per volume unit of solvent, diffusion of solvent into the aqueous phase becomes hard and causes the formation of aggregated and larger NPs, which is in agreement with previous reports [22,34]. On the other hand, it is more difficult for the viscous polymer solution to be broken up into smaller droplets during the formation of a second emulsion [35]. In this model, particle size reached to the minimum point when D/P and W/O ratios were about 0.13 and 0.36. Data analysis defined no significant effect of various PVA concentrations and this factor showed the minor influence on the particle size in this study. Of course, the presence of PVA as a surfactant is necessary to form stabilized NPs.

As mentioned in DESE method, the low EE of small and hydrophilic drug molecules into the polymer is an important challenge [36]. The water soluble nature of SC may be the cause of lower EE in higher D/P or W/O ratios. The higher EE values gained by the higher polymer contents can be explicated by the better coverage of drug molecules within the polymeric matrix [37]. In addition the initial amount of dissolved drug in the inner phase showed a great influence on EE. As the difference of drug concentrations between internal and external aqueous phase increases, the drug diffuses faster to the bulk aqueous phase during particle formation. In other words, higher DL values resulted in lower encapsulation efficiencies because of rapid partitioning of the drug between phases. So it can be claimed that DL and EE are strongly related responses [22,38]. In the formulations that the only changed parameter was W/O ratio, it seems that this factor had a dual effect. Although decreasing this ratio resulted in more efficiently covered aqueous droplets during first emulsion preparation, this larger amount of organic phase required much more

time to evaporate [38]. So the drug molecules had greater opportunity to escape from the inner to outer phase in formulations with higher W/O ratios (>midpoint). While the aqueous volume was kept constant, the enhanced viscosity of the polymer solution led to the formation of larger polymer/solvent droplets. Consequently, slower solidification of larger particles allowed more drug diffusion to the external phase, which again resulted in the lower entrapment of the drug into the NPs [39]. Moreover, employing higher concentrations of stabilizer in the external aqueous phase induced higher EE values.

The endothermic peak of SC disappeared in the thermogram of optimized drug loaded NPs, which indicated absence of crystalline drug in the NPs. So, it can be assumed that encapsulated drug was in an amorphous state or a molecular dispersion throughout the polymer matrix after fabrication of NPs [40].

SEM micrographs showed smooth surface and spherical shape of SC-NPs which can be explained by stability of primary emulsion that the polymer had adequate time to form the condense matrix around the drug molecules before particle formation [41].

All formulations were subjects of *in vitro* release studies. The release profiles exhibited an initial burst release during the first hour, followed by a sustained release pattern over 12 hrs. Surface response plots showed the influence of D/P and W/O ratios on drug release from NPs. The initial burst release was related to the degree of DL, where the minor burst effects were observed in lower DL values.

Table 4 Results of model fitting for optimized Sildenafil NPs

Models	Slope	R^2	Intercept
Zero order	0.002	0.772	0
First order	−0.106	0.925	4.496
Higuchi	21.44	0.950	0
Korsmayer-Peppas	0.51	0.860	3.044
Hixon-Crowell	0.187	0.656	2.264

It appears that at higher loading levels, more drug molecules might adsorb onto the surface of NPs, which contribute to the greater initial release. Actually during the first hour of release study, the large concentration gradient of the drug serves as the driving force for the diffusion. But during the next hours not only this gradient decreases but also it takes more time for SC molecules to diffuse via a path constructed from a series of interconnected pores and channels within the polymeric matrix. It is supposed that in formulations with lower polymer concentrations, the internal water droplets have a greater tendency to coalescence and thus more likely to make larger pores and less tortuous network. However, when the higher polymer concentrations are applied, a tighter structure is formed as a result of faster droplet coagulation during second emulsion formation and subsequent polymeric chain entanglement. In another research published recently on the formation of sildenafil-NPs, the sildenafil was incorporated as its water insoluble base into the PLGA-NPs by means of solvent evaporation method, whereas the most of the entrapped drug released during the first 90 min [42]. Fortunately, in the present study, the release profile of sildenafil citrate as a hydrophilic salt with better bioavailability [1], improved up to 12 hrs.

Conclusion

Comparing the actual and predicted responses indicated that surface response methodology is suitable to make optimization of SC NPs to produce a biphasic release pattern. These NPs can be utilized in the form of tablets or processed in the presence of inhalable sugars to form a dry powder for inhalation purposes. Further *in vivo* studies of SC NPs are recommended to determine whether oral, topical, transdermal and respiratory efficacies are created.

Although, providing SC in the form PLGA nanoparticles brings some advantages such as improvement in reaching many organs, tissues, and cells, the increased entrance into cells might fundamentally rises the chance of toxic effects. It is emphasized that changed size and surface area of the present nano form of sildenafil makes it prone to interact with various cellular components in various tissues. Therefore, future studies to collect the relationships between structure-size-efficacy-toxicity of the present nano form of sildenafil with special regard to portal of entry and target organ is crucial [43]. Additionally it would be nice to prove the safety of the new nano form of sildenafil in an appropriate biological system specially if the expectation is to use the new form of sildenafil for longer duration of time rather than its present single-dose indication in erectile dysfunction [44].

Competing interests

The authors declare that they have no competing interests.

Authors' contribution

All authors have contributed significantly to the research and preparation, design and final production of the manuscript and approve its submission.

Acknowledgments

Authors wish to thank Dr Atieh Sadat Tajalli Bakhsh who edited the article linguistically. This study was a PhD thesis of the first author and the study was financially supported by TUMS.

References

1. Jung SY, Seo YG, Kim GK, Woo JS, Yong CS, Choi HG: Comparison of the solubility and pharmacokinetics of sildenafil salts. *Arch Pharm Res* 2011, **34**:451–454.
2. Webb DJ, Freestone S, Allen MJ, Muirhead GJ: Sildenafil citrate and blood-pressure–lowering drugs: results of drug interaction studies with an organic nitrate and a calcium antagonist. *The Am J cardiol* 1999, **83**:21–28.
3. Rosano GM, Aversa A, Vitale C, Fabbri A, Fini M, Spera G: Chronic treatment with tadalafil improves endothelial function in men with increased cardiovascular risk. *Eur Urol* 2005, **47**:214–220. discussion 220–212.
4. Sharma R: Novel phosphodiesterase-5 inhibitors: current indications and future directions. *Indian J Med Sci* 2007, **61**:667–679.
5. Yildiz P: Molecular mechanisms of pulmonary hypertension. *Clin Chim Acta* 2009, **403**:9–16.
6. Farsaie S, Khalili H, Karimzadeh, Dashti-Khavidaki S: An old drug for a new application: potential benefits of Sildenafil in wound healing. *J Pharm Pharm Sci* 2012, **15**:483–498.
7. Fraisse A, Butrous G, Taylor MB, Oakes M, Dilleen M, Wessel DL: Intravenous sildenafil for postoperative pulmonary hypertension in children with congenital heart disease. *Intensive Care Med* 2011, **37**:502–509.
8. Elnaggar YS, El-Massik MA, Abdallah OY: Fabrication, appraisal, and transdermal permeation of sildenafil citrate-loaded nanostructured lipid carriers versus solid lipid nanoparticles. *Int J Nanomedicine* 2011, **6**:3195–3205.
9. McLaughlin VV, Archer SL, Badesch DB, Barst RJ, Farber HW, Lindner JR, Mathier MA, McGoon MD, Park MH, Rosenson RS, *et al*: ACCF/AHA 2009 expert consensus document on pulmonary hypertension: a report of the American College of Cardiology Foundation Task Force on Expert Consensus Documents and the American Heart Association: developed in collaboration with the American College of Chest Physicians, American Thoracic Society, Inc., and the Pulmonary Hypertension Association. *Circulation* 2009, **119**:2250–2294.
10. Shah V, Sharma M, Parmar V, Upadhyay U: Formulation of sildenafil citrate loaded nasal microsphers: an in vitro, ex vivo characterization. *Int J Drug Del* 2010, **2**:213–220.
11. Ryde TA, Hovey DC, Bosch HW: *Novel compositions of sildenafil free base. In Book Novel compositions of sildenafil free base (Editor ed.^eds.)*. City: Google Patents; 2004.
12. Filipcsei G, Otvos Z, Pongrácz K, Darvas F: Nanostructured Sildenafil base, its pharmaceutically acceptable salts and co-crystals, compositions of them, process for the preparation thereof and pharmaceutical compositions containing them. In *Book Nanostructured Sildenafil base, its pharmaceutically acceptable salts and co-crystals, compositions of them, process for the preparation thereof and pharmaceutical compositions containing them*. City: Google Patents; 2010.
13. Ryde TA, Hovey DC, Bosch WH: Novel compositions of Sildenafil free base. In *Book Novel compositions of Sildenafil free base*. City: EP Patent; 2008. 1,658,053.
14. Chidambaram M, Manavalan R, Kathiresan K: Nanotherapeutics to overcome conventional cancer chemotherapy limitations. *J Pharm Pharm Sci* 2011, **14**:67–77.
15. Ungaro F, d'Angelo I, Miro A, La Rotonda MI, Quaglia F: Engineered PLGA nano- and micro-carriers for pulmonary delivery: challenges and promises. *J Pharm Pharmacol* 2012, **64**:1217–1235.
16. Soppimath KS, Aminabhavi TM, Kulkarni AR, Rudzinski WE: Biodegradable polymeric nanoparticles as drug delivery devices. *J Control Release* 2001, **70**:1–20.
17. Makadia HK, Siegel SJ: Poly Lactic-co-Glycolic Acid (PLGA) as Biodegradable Controlled Drug Delivery Carrier. *Polymers (Basel)* 2011, **3**:1377–1397.

18. Zou W, Liu C, Chen Z, Zhang N: Studies on bioadhesive PLGA nanoparticles: a promising gene delivery system for efficient gene therapy to lung cancer. *Int J Pharm* 2009, **370**:187–195.

19. Danhier F, Ansorena E, Silva JM, Coco R, Le-Breton A, Preat V: PLGA-based nanoparticles: an overview of biomedical applications. *J Control Release* 2012, **161**:505–522.

20. Mura S, Hillaireau H, Nicolas J, Le-Droumaguet B, Gueutin C, Zanna S, Tsapis N, Fattal E: Influence of surface charge on the potential toxicity of PLGA nanoparticles towards Calu-3 cells. *Int J Nanomedicine* 2011, **6**:2591–2605.

21. Semete B, Booysen L, Lemmer Y, Kalombo L, Katata L, Verschoor J, Swai HS: In vivo evaluation of the biodistribution and safety of PLGA nanoparticles as drug delivery systems. *Nanomedicine* 2010, **6**:662–671.

22. Lamprecht A, Ubrich N, Hombreiro Perez M, Lehr C, Hoffman M, Maincent P: Influences of process parameters on nanoparticle preparation performed by a double emulsion pressure homogenization technique. *Int J Pharm* 2000, **196**:177–182.

23. Cohen-Sela E, Chorny M, Koroukhov N, Danenberg HD, Golomb G: A new double emulsion solvent diffusion technique for encapsulating hydrophilic molecules in PLGA nanoparticles. *J Control Release* 2009, **133**:90–95.

24. Badwan AA, Nabuls L, Al-Omari MM, Daraghmeh N, Ashour M: Sildenafil Citrate. In *Analytical Profiles of Drug Substances and Excipients. Volume 27.* Edited by Harry GB. Amman, Jordan: Academic Press; 2001:339–376.

25. Prakobvaitayakit M, Nimmannit U: Optimization of polylactic-co-glycolic acid nanoparticles containing itraconazole using 2(3) factorial design. *AAPS PharmSciTech* 2003, **4**:E71.

26. Neumann D, Merkwirth C, Lamprecht A: Nanoparticle design characterized by in silico preparation parameter prediction using ensemble models. *J Pharm Sci* 2010, **99**:1982–1996.

27. Nazzal S, Khan MA: Response surface methodology for the optimization of ubiquinone self-nanoemulsified drug delivery system. *AAPS PharmSciTech* 2002, **3**:E3.

28. Basu S, Mukherjee B, Chowdhury SR, Paul P, Choudhury R, Kumar A, Mondal L, Hossain CM, Maji R: Colloidal gold-loaded, biodegradable, polymer-based stavudine nanoparticle uptake by macrophages: an in vitro study. *Int J Nanomedicine* 2012, **7**:6049–6061.

29. Higuchi T: Mechanism of sustained-action medication. Theoretical analysis of rate of release of solid drugs dispersed in solid matrices. *J Pharm Sci* 1963, **52**:1145–1149.

30. Dash S, Murthy PN, Nath L, Chowdhury P: Kinetic modeling on drug release from controlled drug delivery systems. *Acta Pol Pharm* 2010, **67**:217–223.

31. Shavi GV, Kumar AR, Karthik A, Naseer M, Aravind G, Praful BD, Reddy MS, Udupa N: Novel paclitaxel nanoparticles: development, in vitro anti-tumor activity in BT-549 cells and in vivo evaluation. *J Control Release* 2010, **148**:e119–e121.

32. Zhang J, Fan Y, Smith E: Experimental design for the optimization of lipid nanoparticles. *J Pharm Sci* 2009, **98**:1813–1819.

33. Galindo-Rodriguez S, Allemann E, Fessi H, Doelker E: Physicochemical parameters associated with nanoparticle formation in the salting-out, emulsification-diffusion, and nanoprecipitation methods. *Pharm Res* 2004, **21**:1428–1439.

34. Beck-Broichsitter M, Kleimann P, Gessler T, Seeger W, Kissel T, Schmehl T: Nebulization performance of biodegradable sildenafil-loaded nanoparticles using the Aeroneb Pro: formulation aspects and nanoparticle stability to nebulization. *Int J Pharm* 2012, **422**:398–408.

35. Mahboubian A, Hashemein S, Moghadam S, Atyabi F, Dinarvand R: Preparation and in-vitro evaluation of controlled release PLGA microparticles containing triptoreline. *Iranian J Pharm Res* 2010, **9**:369–378.

36. Tewes F, Munnier E, Antoon B, Ngaboni Okassa L, Cohen-Jonathan S, Marchais H, Douziech-Eyrolles L, Souce M, Dubois P, Chourpa I: Comparative study of doxorubicin-loaded poly(lactide-co-glycolide) nanoparticles prepared by single and double emulsion methods. *Eur J Pharm Biopharm* 2007, **66**:488–492.

37. Guhagarkar SA, Malshe VC, Devarajan PV: Nanoparticles of polyethylene sebacate: a new biodegradable polymer. *AAPS PharmSciTech* 2009, **10**:935–942.

38. Yang Y, Chung T, Ng N: Morphology, drug distribution, and in vitro release profiles of biodegradable polymeric microspheres containing protein fabricated by double-emulsion solvent extraction/evaporation method. *Biomaterials* 2001, **22**:231–241.

39. Das MK, Rao KR: Evaluation of zidovudine encapsulated ethylcellulose microspheres prepared by water-in-oil-in-oil (w/o/o) double emulsion solvent diffusion technique. *Acta Pol Pharm* 2006, **63**:141–148.

40. Jelvehgari M, Nokhodchi A, Rezapour M, Valizadeh H: Effect of formulation and processing variables on the characteristics of tolmetin microspheres prepared by double emulsion solvent diffusion method. *Indian J Pharm Sci* 2010, **72**:72–78.

41. Meng FT, Ma GH, Liu YD, Qiu W, Su ZG: Microencapsulation of bovine hemoglobin with high bio-activity and high entrapment efficiency using a W/O/W double emulsion technique. *Colloids Surf B Biointerfaces* 2004, **33**:177–183.

42. Beck-Broichsitter M, Schmehl T, Gessler T, Seeger W, Kissel T: Development of a biodegradable nanoparticle platform for sildenafil: formulation optimization by factorial design analysis combined with application of charge-modified branched polyesters. *J Control Release* 2012, **157**:469–477.

43. Mostafalou S, Mohammadi H, Ramazani A, Abdollahi M: Different biokinetics of nanomedicines linking to their toxicity; an overview. *Daru* 2013, **22**: 21(1):14.

44. Pourmand A, Abdollahi M: Current opinion on nanotoxicology. *Daru* 2012, **15**: 20(1):95.

15

Epidural administration of neostigmine-loaded nanofibers provides extended analgesia in rats

Masoomeh Yosefifard and Majid Hassanpour-Ezatti[*]

Abstract

Background: In this study, neostigmine-loaded electrospun nanofibers were prepared and then their efficacy and duration of analgesic action were studied after epidural administration in rats by repeated tail flick and formalin tests.

Methods: The neostigmine poly vinyl alcohol (PVA) nanofibers were fabricated by electrospinning methods. The nanofibers (1 mg) were injected into the lumbar epidural space (L5-L6) of rats (n = 6). Cerebrospinal fluid samples of rats were collected 1, 5 and 24 hours after injection and then were sampled once weekly for 4 weeks. Free-neostigmine concentration was measured in the samples spectrophotometrically. Rat nociceptive responses were evaluated by repeated tail-flick and formalin tests for 5 weeks after the nanofibers (1 mg) injection. Locomotor activity of rats was measured in the open-field at the same period.

Results: The cerebrospinal fluid concentration of free neostigmine reached 5 μg/ml five hours after injection and remained constant until the end of the experiments. The tail-flick latency of treated rats was significantly (p < 0.01) increased and remained constant up to 4 weeks. Pain scores of the rats in both phases of formalin test were significantly (p < 0.01) reduced during the same periods, Epidural injection of the nanofibers had no effect on locomotor activity of rats in an open-field.

Conclusions: Our results indicate that the neostigmine nanofibers can provide sustained release of neostigmine for induction of prolonged analgesia after epidural administration. High tissue distribution and penetration of the nanofibers in dorsal horn can increase thermal and chemical analgesia duration without altering locomotor activity in rats for 4 weeks.

Keywords: Neostigmine, Nanofibers, Analgesia, Epidural, Electrospinning

Background

Recently, researchers have been employing new techniques to improve both the efficacy and duration of analgesic effect of some drugs. Epidural administration of neostigmine could reduce pain in patients with uncontrolled pain [1]. It has been reported that intrathecally administered neostigmine could also provide effective analgesia in both phases of formalin test in rat [2]. Although, in clinical studies intrathecal neostigmine infusion is used for induction of prolonged analgesia in chronic patients [3], the application of a catheter for drug infusion would increase the risk of infection in patients and also requires complicated surgery. An alternative procedure for increasing the duration of neostigmine action after epidural injection is its combination with other drugs [4]. However, this method might induce side effects such as nausea, vomiting, sedation and respiratory depression in patients. It is shown that elevation of endogenous acetylcholine level at spinal cord synapses mediate neostigmine analgesia following epidural injection [5]. Also, intrathecal co-administered of neostigmine with local anesthetic can increase its duration of action [6]. Liposomal neostigmine for epidural application is another approach being used for control release of neostigmine, but unfortunately this formulation has short duration of action [7]. In recent years, incorporation of drugs in electrospun nanofibers has been used for making sustained and controlled-release drugs; Tseng and coworkers could fabricate lidocaine biodegradable nanofiber and showed a sustain delivery of lidocaine into the epidural space in rats [8]. On the other hand, it has been shown that intratecal administration of a dose of an analgesic drug could

* Correspondence: hassanpour@Shahed.ac.ir
Department of Biology, Sciences School, Shahed University, Tehran, IRAN

produce different results in the tail-flick and formalin tests [9]. Therefore, scientists compared the epidural or intrathecal anesthetic efficacy of same doses of an analgesic compound with two kinds of nociceptive stimulus such as tail flick and formalin test. Thus, it is certain that the selected dose of the drug is effective for different kinds of pain.

The aims of present study were: (1) fabrication of neostigmine-loaded poly vinyl alcohol (PVA) nanofibers by electrospinning methods; (2) *in-vitro* evaluation of neostigmine release from the nanofibers; (3) assessment of free-neostigmine concentration in the cerebrospinal fluid of rats after the nanofiber injection for 4 weeks; and (4) evaluation of the efficacy and duration of analgesia in thermal and chemical pain model by consecutive tail-flick and formalin test during 5 weeks after the injection of nanofibers.

Materials and methods
Chemical
Neostigmine methylsulfate was obtained as a gift sample from the laboratory of Dr. Sayyed Omid Ranaei Syadat, Tehran, Iran. In our experiment, all chemicals were of analytical grade purchased from Sigma-Aldrich.

Preparation of nanofibers using electrospinning
The neostigmine-loaded poly vinyl alcohol nanofibers were prepared according to the procedure of Arecchi et al. [10]. Briefly, poly vinyl alcohol solution was prepared by dissolving 6 gram of poly vinyl alcohol powder in 100 ml of deionized water. The mixture was slowly heated to 95°C for 8 hours. To compensate for the loss of water due to evaporation during heating and stirring, deionized water was added to the solution to return it to the original volume. Thus, the final concentration of poly

vinyl alcohol in solution was kept at 6 wt% [10]. Neostigmine 1.25% (w/w) was dissolved in double distilled deionized water and was added to the poly vinyl alcohol solution and stirred for 25 minutes before electrospinning. For preparing neostigmine-loaded electrospinning nanofibers, the 6% PVA solutions were mixed by volumetric ratios of 50:50 with neostigmine solution. Then, the mixture was pumped at a constant rate using a syringe pump toward a needle tip. The utilized electrical potential for electrospinning was 25 kV and the distance between the collector and the needle tip was 15 cm. The electrospinning was performed at room temperature and the resulting neostigmine-loaded nanofibers were collected on an aluminum foil. The schematic figure of electrospinning set up is shown in Figure 1. Then, the nanofibers were incubated at 150°C for 5 minutes, treated with ethanol for 1 hour and dried overnight at room temperature [11]. Final neostigmine-loaded nanofibers contained %1.25 (w/w) neostigmine/poly(vinyl alcohol). Finally, the structure of free and neostigmine-loaded nanofibers was studied using scanning electron microscopy.

In vitro Acetylcholinesterase (AChE) inhibition assay by nanofibers containing different ratios of neostigmine/poly (vinyl alcohol)
The measurement of AChE inhibitory activity of neostigmine released from the nanofibers was carried out in a vial using spectrophotometric method proposed by Ellman et al. [13]. The percent of AChE inhibition was compared among the nanofibers that were made from different proportions of poly vinyl alcohol (5, 6, 7, 8%w/w) and contained different concentrations of neostigmine (0.000125 and 0.00125w/w). Acetylcholinesterase, AChE (E.C 3.1.1.7) was expressed with the baculovirus system

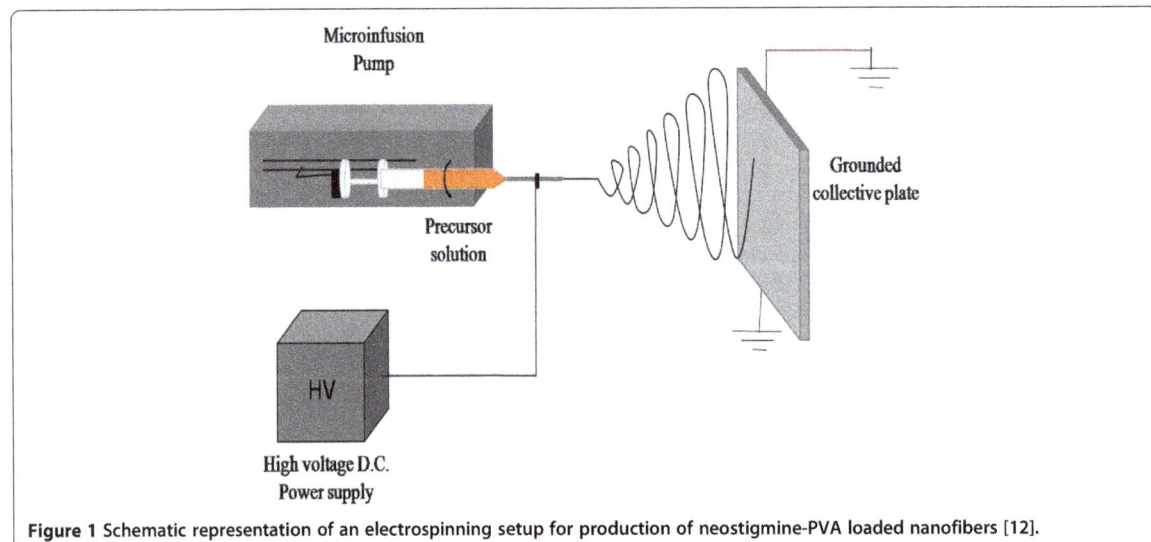

Figure 1 Schematic representation of an electrospinning setup for production of neostigmine-PVA loaded nanofibers [12].

[14]. A typical run consisted of 5 μL of AChE solution at final assay concentrations of 0.03 U/mL; 200 μL of 0.1 M phosphate buffer (pH 7.4); 5 μL of DTNB at a final concentration of 0.3 mM, prepared in 0.1 M phosphate buffer (pH 7.4) with 0.12 M of sodium bicarbonate. Then, the nanofibers containing neostigmine were added to each mixture reaction (1 mL) in vials, vortexed for 1 min, and then centrifuged rapidly at 16 000 g for 1 min. The intensity of the yellow solution in the resulting supernatants were determined spectrophotometrically at 412 nm every 5 min, three times consecutively. Percent of remaining activity of AChE was determined after incubation with the neostigmine-loaded nanofibers which were fabricated by different concentrations of poly vinyl alcohol and loaded with different doses of neostigmine.

Encapsulation efficiency and in vitro release
To determine the encapsulation efficiency, 10 mg of the neostigmine-loaded nanofibers were stored in 1 ml of PBS (pH 7.4). The solution was incubated for 1 min at 37°C. At 5 min intervals, a sample was withdrawn and centrifuged at 16,000 g for 10 min. The precipitated samples were taken and resuspended in 10 ml fresh release medium to keep a complete sink condition and placed back to the shaker. The supernatant solution was retained for HPLC analysis. A mixture of acetonitrile and ammonium acetate (75:25 v/v) was added to the solution after the PBS had been removed. The resulting solution was analyzed using HPLC, in which a C-18 column was used and the mobile phase was delivered at a rate of 1 ml/min. One hundred microliters of sample was injected by an autosampler and the column effluent was detected at 248 nm.

Morphologies of electrospun nanofibers
The surface morphology of the nanofibers was observed by scanning electron microscopy (S-4800, Hitachi, Japan). The free poly vinyl alcohol and neostigmine-loaded nanofibers were placed on a stage and sputter-coated with carbon.

Animals
Adult male Sprague–Dawley rats (200–250 g) were purchased from Razi Institute of Iran. The rats were kept at 22°C, 12 hour night/day cycle, and received tap water and food *Ad libitum*. The present study followed the ethical guidelines for investigation of experimental pain in conscious animals as well as the Institutional Animal Ethical Committee of Shahed University, formed under Committee for Purpose of Control and Supervision of Experiments on Animals (CPCSEA, Reg. No. PRC-115), approved by the pharmacologic protocols [15].

The experimental groups
The experimental groups consisted of six rats. Rats were divided into: (a) control group in which, the rats received epidural injection of 5 μl normal saline solution; (b) sham group in which, the rats were treated with epidural injection of 1 mg poly vinyl alcohol nanofibers and flushed by 5 μl saline solution; (c) neostigmine-loaded nanofiber group in which, the rats were treated with epidural injection of neostigmine-loaded nanofibers (1 mg) and flushed by 5 μl saline solution. Epidural injection was done at L5-L6 intervertebral space.

Lumbar epidural injection of the neostigmine-loaded nanofibers
Rats were anesthetized briefly with ether and shaved at the lower back, then placed in the prone position with lower back elevated and flexed ventrally. A lumbar puncture was performed at L5–L6 intervertebral space, perpendicular to the skin, using a 30-gauge needle attached to a 50-μl Hamilton syringe. A catheter of a PE10 polyethylene tube, which was pre-filled with 1 mg neostigmine-loaded nanofibers isolated from 5 μl of saline using a small air bubble, was placed into the needle and advanced 4 cm from the tip of the needle up to the lumber enlargement, which was confirmed by a tail-twitch. The nanofibers were slowly injected and flushed with saline. Three minutes later, the catheter and the needle were respectively removed.

Methylene blue injections
Pilot experiments were performed to evaluate the spread of injected solution in the spinal subarachnoid space. Using the same technique and injection volumes described above, the rats received spinal injections of 5 μl methylene blue 1 mg/ml solution. The area of spread of the methylene blue was examined upon animal necropsy 10 min after intrathecal injections. Besides, all intrathecal solutions contained 5% methylene blue and the included data were only from the animals in which intrathecal placement was confirmed postmortem.

CSF sampling
CSF samples were collected based on procedures described by Haddadi et al. Rats anesthetized by i.p. injection of a mixture of ketamine (80 mg/kg) and xylazine (10 mg/kg) [16]. Then, each rat was placed in a stereotaxic apparatus and its neck was flexed so that a 29-gauge needle could be lowered between the base of the skull and the first cervical vertebra into the cisterna magna. Needle placement was verified by drawing a small amount of CSF into the needle and observing the clear CSF in the polyethylene tube connecting the needle to a 100 μl syringe (Hamilton). CSF (50 μl) was collected in polypropylene test tubes that were put immediately on dry ice and then stored at −80°C until the determination of neostigmine concentration. Samples of CSF of rats were taken 1, 5 and 24 h after the injection of neostigmine nanofibers. The sampling procedure continued once a week for 4 weeks.

Measurement of neostigmine concentration in CSF of rats

Neostigmine concentration in CSF sample of rats (n = 6) was estimated by ultraviolet visible spectrophotometer at 261 nm (Shimadzu UV-1700, Japan) [17]. Aqueous standard solutions of neostigmine methylsulfate were prepared in phosphate buffer (pH 7.4) and their absorbance was measured by applying the same procedures. The method was validated with respect to precision and linearity. To determine the precision of the method, neostigmine concentration in CSF samples was analysed six times a day (intra-day precision) and during six continuous days (inter-day precision). The linearity of measurement was evaluated by analyzing different concentrations of the standard solution of neostigmine. Beer-Lambert's concentration range was found to be 0.01-0.001 μg/ml [17].

Behavioral tests

In the present study, two methods were simultaneously used for evaluating anesthetic effect of a single dose of neostigmine-loaded nanofibers against thermal and chemical types of nociceptive stimuli after epidural injection. Some scientists have claimed that the analgesic effect due to the activation of cholinergic mechanisms also depends on the experimental pain model that is utilized for its evaluation [18].

Tail-flick test

The repeated tail-flick method was used for measuring the analgesic responses of rats after epidural treatment with the neostigmine-loaded nanofibers to a high intensity thermal nociceptive stimulus. Some researchers have also suggested that changes in tail-flick latency may be interpreted in terms of central sensitization and that the repeated tail-flick latency might be considered as a useful marker of chronic nociception [19]. Thus, the tail-flick latencies were repeatedly measured in rats before and on 1st, 15th and 21st days after epidural injection based on the methods proposed by Kríz et al. [19]. The average time interval between the onset of light stimuli and the tail-flick response was measured and defined as tail-flick latency. Since the test should be conducted in triplicates, the tail was marked in three places: proximal, middle, distal. The intensity of radiant heat was adjusted to establish the baseline latencies for 3–5 seconds. The heat stimulus was discontinued after 20 seconds to avoid tissue damages. (Cut off point = 20 s). Each rat was tested 3 times with a 3-second interval. Data were expressed as mean ± SEM (n = 6).

Formalin test

The formalin test is usually used for evaluation of anti-nociceptive drugs which are administrated intrathecally against the high intensity of chemical pain stimulus. In order to avoid interaction of both techniques' effects on the same animals, it is better to evaluate the formalin test at least 7 days after the tail-flick test, because the tail-flick test has no impact on the formalin test results after this period [20]. Therfore, in this study the formalin test was performed 7 days after the tail flick test. In practice, formalin (2.5%, 50 μl) was injected subcutaneously into the intraplantar surface of different feet of rats after treatment with nanofibers. Then, the rats were gently placed in plexiglass chambers. The pain behavior within the first 15 min of intraplantar formalin injection was recorded as the early phase scores, while the pain behavior between 20 and 60 min of the formalin injection was recorded as the late phase. The behavioral rating scale was as follows: 0 = the injected paw is not favored; 1 = the injected paw rests lightly on the floor and little or no weight is placed on it; 2 = the injected paw is elevated and is not in contact with any surface; 3 = the injected paw is licked, bitten and shaken. Pain scores were calculated by using this formula:

$$\text{Pain score} = 0T0 + 1T1 + 2T2 + 3T3/\text{Time block(s)}$$

where T0-T3 is the number of seconds spent in each of the behavioral categories. All tests were conducted between 9:00 AM and 5:00 PM. Pain scores were expressed as mean ± SEM. A probability of p < 0.01 was considered significant.

Measurement of locomotor activity in open field

Locomotor activity was measured using an open field test. The rats were individually placed in one corner of the open field (100 × 100 × 48 cm). Movement of each rat in the field during 15 min of testing session was recorded. After 15 min, the rat was removed to the home cage, and the open field area was cleaned. The total distance and the average velocity of each rat in the field were recorded.

Statistical analyses

The results were expressed as mean ± S.E.M., and statistical significance was evaluated by a two-way repeated measure analysis of variance (ANOVA) followed by Bonferroni tests. The statistical significance criterion (P-value) was 0.05. All data calculations and statistical analyses were done by using Prism version 5 (GraphPad Software Inc., San Diego, CA).

Results

Morphology of electrospun nanofibers

According to the SEM micrograph shown in Figure 2, electrospun free poly vinyl alcohol nanofibers (A) and the neostigmine-loaded nanofibers (B) were circular in cross-section with an average diameter ranging from 500 nm up to 1,000 nm. The drug encapsulation in vesicular-like reservoirs along the nanofibers was confirmed by the scanning electron microscopy.

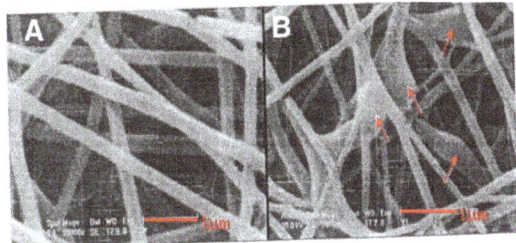

Figure 2 The Scanning electron microscope photomicrograph of Polyvinyl Alcohol nanofibers before (A) and after neostigmine loading (B). In this figure the arrows show the loading position of neostigmine in the core of nanofibers. Magnification: 20,000 × .

In vitro AChE inhibition

The percent of AChE inhibition changed with proportions of PVC (Figure 3A) and the concentration of neostigmine (Figure 3B) that were used in fabrication of the loaded-nanofibers. All neostigmine-loaded nanofibers contained some levels of inhibitory activity against AChE. However, the nanofibers containing 6% poly vinyl alcohol and 0.00125w/w neostigmine showed more effective inhibitory effect on AChE activity compared to others in vitro.

Verification of epidural injection

The spread of methylene blue dye into the epidural space indicated that the dye was only distributed in lumbar segments of rat spinal cord (Figure 4).

Neostigmine concentration in CSF of rats

The time course of neostigmine concentrations in CSF is shown in Figure 5. The results of this study showed that

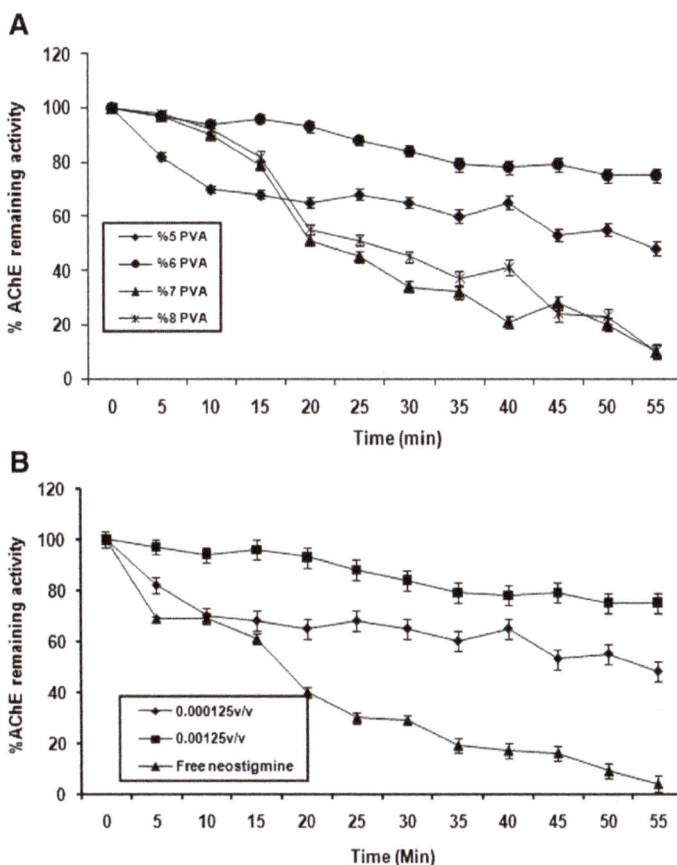

Figure 3 Percentage activity remaining during inhibition of acetylcholinesterase after addition of nanofibers. (A) The measurement of acetylcholinesterase activity following addition of the nanofibers were fabricated with different proportions of poly vinyl alcohol and neostigmine (0.00125 v/v); **(B)** the acetylcholinesterase activity after addition of the neostigmine nanofibers that fabricated by %6 PVA and two different concentrations of neostigmine (pH = 7/4, 22°C).

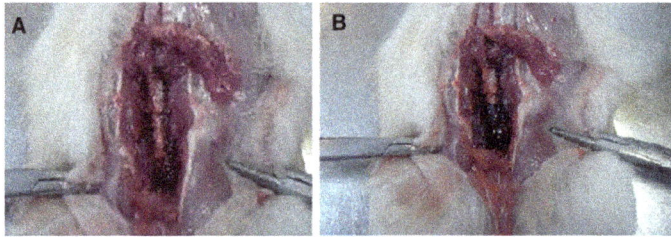

Figure 4 Verification of injection site and evaluation the distribution of methylene blue injected into the epidural space. (A) The exposed lumbar spinal cord region of control rats and **(B)** drug extension evaluation by epidural injection of 50 μL 1% methylene blue.

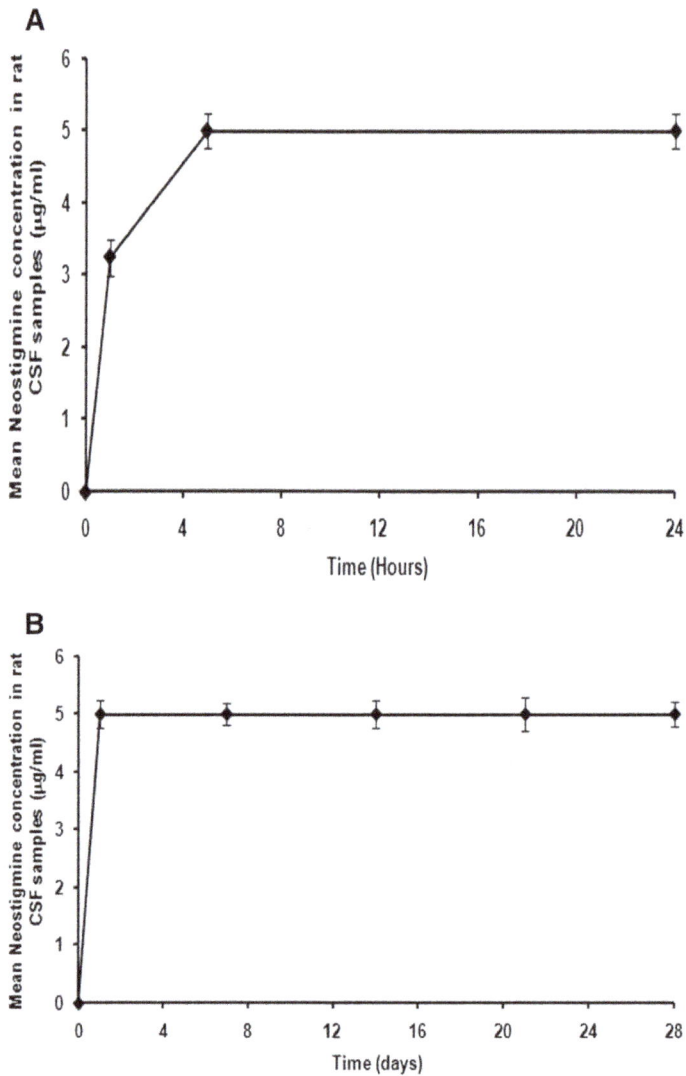

Figure 5 Measurement of neostigmine concentration in CSF in rats. CSF concentrations of neostigmine were measured, **(A)** up to 24 hours and **(B)** for 4 weeks after epidural injection of neostigmine loaded nanofibers. Values presented are means ± SEM.

neostigmine concentrations in CSF were significantly increased from baseline to a maximum concentration (5 ± 0.1 µg/ml) during 5 hours after epidural administration (Figure 5-A). The concentration of free neostigmine in CSF of rats remained constant at 5 ± 0.1 µg/ml during 4 weeks after injection of the nanofibers (Figure 5-B).

Formalin test

The epidural administration of neostigmine-loaded nanofibers decreased the pain score significantly ($p < 0.001$) in early (Figure 6A) and late (Figure 6B) phases of the formalin test in rats for five weeks after injection of the neostigmine nanofibers.

Tail-flick test

The duration of analgesia after epidural injection of neostigmine-loaded nanofibers is shown in Figure 7. The

tail-flick latency of rats was significantly ($p < 0.01$) increased and remained stable for four weeks after injection of the neostigmine nanofibers.

Locomotor activity in open-field

The mean traveling distance (Figure 8A) and the velocity (Figure 8B) of rats in the open-field in 7, 14 and 21 days post-injection were not affected by epidural administrations of the nanofibers in comparison with the sham group.

Discussion

The results of the present investigation revealed that neostigmine was successfully loaded into the poly vinyl alcohol nanofibers using the electrospinning technique. The SEM images confirmed the incorporation of neostigmine in the nanofibers. As seen in Figure 2, no drug crystals

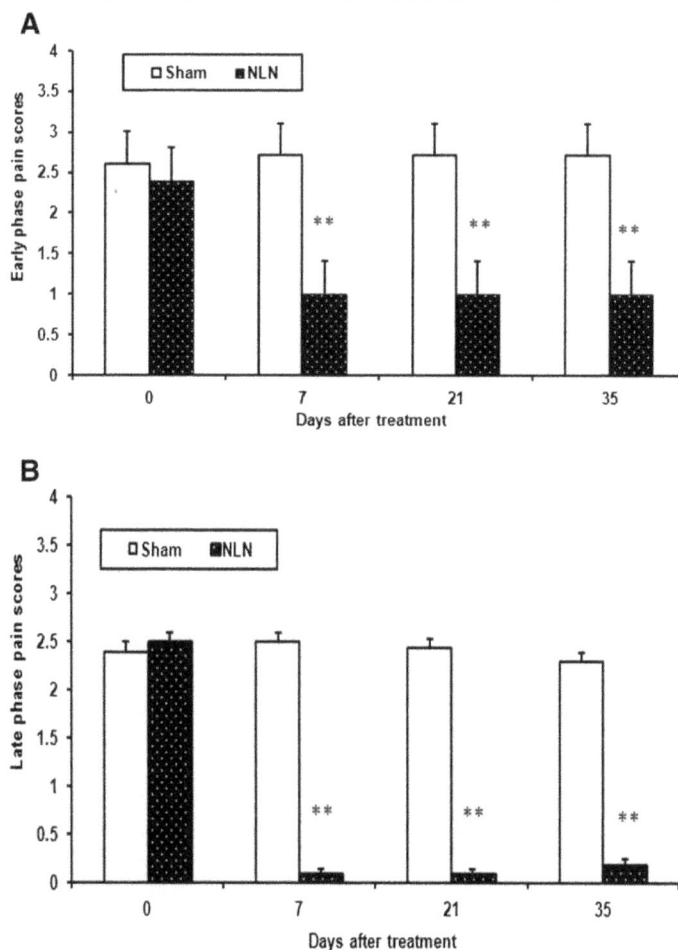

Figure 6 The effect of epidural injection of neostigmine loaded nanofibers (NLN) on the cumulative nociceptive scores of rats in the early phase (A) the late phase (B) of formalin test. Sham group treated with free PVA nanofibers (Mean ± SEM, n = 6, **p < 0.01, Repeated-two way ANOVA followed by Bonferroni test).

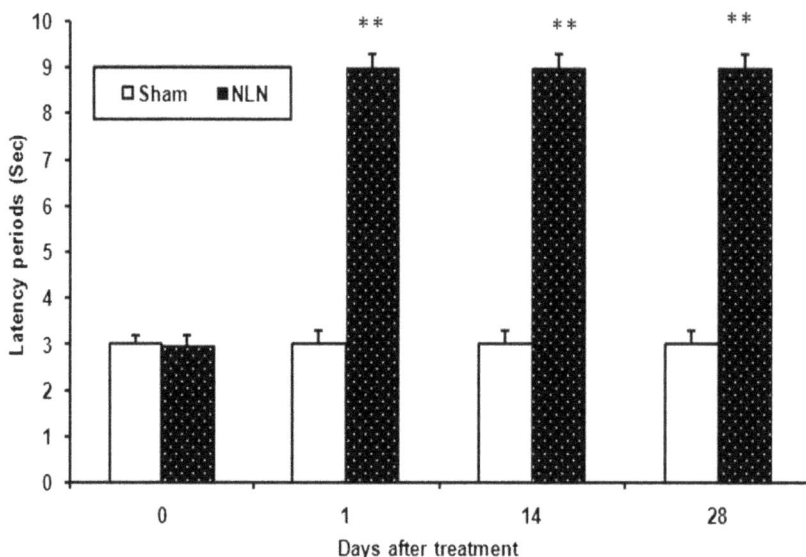

Figure 7 Effect of epidural neostigmine loaded nanofibers (NLN) administration on tail-flick latencies of rats (Mean ± SEM, n = 6, **p < 0.01, repeated two way ANOVA followed by Bonferroni test), Sham group treated with epidural free PVA nanofibers.

were detected by electron microscopy on the surface or outside of the loaded nanofibers. The electrospinning technique has been already used effectively to produce other drug-loaded nanofibers. The poly vinyl alcohol nanofibers have proven their performance in controlled release of antinociceptive drugs [21]. PVA nanofibers prepared by electrospinning technique also provide a suitable matrix for sustain release of drugs based on available evidence [22]. Therefore, it seems that the electrospinning method and poly vinyl alcohol nanofibers are appropriate choices for encapsulation of neostigmine.

The in vitro study of AChE inhibition after injection of the nanofibers indicated that the neostigmine released from the nanofibers can inhibit AChE effectively and the loading of neostigmine within the nanofibers did not compromise the inherent of AChE inhibitory activity. The results of enzyme activity assay also indicated that

the change in the ratio of PVA- neostigmine can influence the amount of neostigmine release and percent of AChE inhibition. Measurement of neostigmine concentrations in cerebrospinal fluid (CSF) has suggested that the profile of the neostigmine release from the loaded nanofibers follows a biphasic pattern characterized by an initial fast release during 5 hours and following sustained release phase. A similar biphasic behavior has also been reported for ethyl cellulose nanofibers fabricated by using electrospinning process [23]. This form of drug release is an ideal situation for the rapid relief of symptoms which optimizes the therapy and avoids repeated administration for the patients' convenience. Furthermore, the researchers treated the nanofibers with ethanol in order to reduce the drug release rate. It is reported that the burst release of drug from nanofibers was eliminated after treatment with alcohol. In practice, the use of

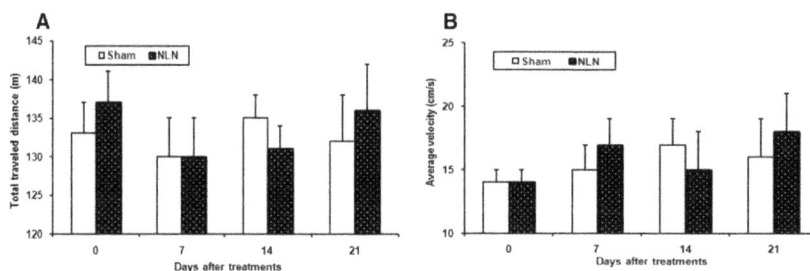

Figure 8 Measurement of rats total traveled distance (A) and average velocity (B) for 3 weeks after epidural injection of neostigmine loaded nanofibers (NLN). Sham group treated with free PVA nanofibers (Mean ± SEM, n = 6, **p < 0.01, Repeated-two way ANOVA followed by Bonferroni test).

such drug-loaded nanofibers for spinal cord drug delivery can increase the duration of drug efficacy. For example, Schmidt and co-workers enhanced epidural liposome-encapsulated hydromorphone's duration of analgesia action from 2 to 72 hours in rats [24]. Based on the above reports, a combination of all these mechanisms can provide explanation for stable concentration of neostigmine in in vitro situation.

The results of the present study indicated that the thermal pain threshold was increased in rats after single epidural injection of the neostigmine-loaded nanofibers and persisted for as long as 28 days. Consecutive formalin test in rats also showed that the pain scores decreased in both phases and remained stable up to 35 days after injection. The early phase response of the formalin test was considered to be the result of direct effects of formalin on nociceptive fibers. It may be modulated by cholinergic spinal inhibitory interneurons [25]. The late phase was caused by tissue damage as well as inflammation and reflecting a state of central sensitization. Park and co-workers demonstrated that intratecal administration of atropine, a muscarinic antagonist, could decrease rat hindpaw persistent pain after formalin injection into the hindpaw [26]. Moreover, the intrathecal injection of neostigmine could reduce the pain in both phases of the formalin test.

The high sensitivity of tail flick technique for measurement of pain threshold after manipulation of spinal cholinergic system has been reported [27]. In addition, consecutive evaluation of tail-flick latency was considered as a marker of chronic nociception. Comparing the antinociceptive effect of the neostigmine loaded nanofibers in these two pain models showed that the effective analgesic dose of neostigmine was chosen for pain relief in our experiments.

In support of the present findings it can be said that after being release from nanofibers, the free neostigmine increased the level of endogenous acetylcholine at dorsal horn of spinal cord. Following mechanisms have been proposed to explain the anti-nociception action of acetylcholine at the dorsal horn level. It is shown that acetylcholinesterase inhibition increased acetylcholine level at spinal cord and then it caused (i) the activation of presynaptic nicotinic acetylcholine receptors and decrease in glutamate release from C-fiber terminals in the dorsal horn [28]; (ii) the inhibition of presynaptic release of glutamate from primary afferent axons by stimulation of GABAergic interneurons via activation of muscarinic acetylcholine receptors [29]; (iii) the stimulation of the nicotinic acetylcholine receptors on GABA-ergic inhibitory interneurons that triggered the firing of spinothalamic pain transmission neurons [30]; and (iv) the reduction of neuroinflammation by blocking microglial cell activity via stimulation of the nicotinic receptors

[31]. Furthermore, neostigmine could stimulate GABA release from dorsal horn neurons [32] and its stimulatory effect on GABA release continued even after drug clearing from the CSF [33]. All of these mechanisms can play a significant role in effective analgesia induced by epidural application of neostigmine nanofibers.

In addition, loading of drugs in nanostructures increased its tissue penetration power [34], which probably makes them activate more inhibitory interneurons in deeper layers of dorsal horn of spinal cord. This property could provide an additional advantage for neostigmine-loaded nanofibers.

Comparison of the present findings with previous results [3,35] showed that the duration of analgesia after administration of the neostigmine-loaded nanofiber was longer than all previous neostigmine-containing mixture in animal or human studies. A relation was shown between concentrations of a drug in cerebrospinal fluid and its analgesic effect [36]. It can be concluded that the loaded amount of neostigmine in the nanofibers was sufficient to produce and maintain a relatively constant concentration of free neostigmine in CSF for induction of long-term analgesia. Also, the low rate of drug biotransformation in CSF could be another possible factor to increase the duration of neostigmine effect after epidural injection [37].

In spite of the free neostigmine side effects on locomotor activity after epidural administration in human [38], injection of the neostigmine-loaded nanofibers had no adverse effects on rats. Furthermore, the epidural administration of neostigmine-loaded nanofibers did not significantly alter locomotor activity in rats. Probably, the lack of side effects is due to the restricted release of neostigmine from nanofibers in dorsal horn of spinal cord. In support of this idea, it was shown that no adverse effects were noted after the epidural administration of neostigmine when the drug spread was restricted into lower part of the spinal cord [39].

Conclusion

In this study, electrospun polyvinyl alcohol nanofibers were used as a controlled release matrix for the incorporation of neostigmine. The findings suggested that the nanofibers made from poly vinyl alcohol can easily be loaded with neostigmine. The SEM image confirmed loading of drug in nanofibers. The lumbar epidural administration of the nanofibers can reduce acute and chronic thermal and chemical pain in rats for 5 weeks. Also, its application had no significant effect on locomotor activity of rats.

Abbreviations

AChE: Acetylcholinesterase; PBS: Phosphate Buffer Saline; CSF: Cerebrospinal Fluid; NLN: Neostigmine Loaded Nanofibers.

Competing interests
The authors declare that they have no competing interests.

Acknowledgments
The authors would like to thank Dr. Sayyed Omid Ranaei for her preparation of neostigmine nanofibers.

References

1. Mahajan R, Grover VK, Chari P: **Caudal neostigmine with bupivacaine produces a dose-independent analgesic effect in children.** *Can J Anaesth* 2004, 51:702–6.

2. Yoon MH, Choi JI, Kwak SH: **Characteristic of interactions between intrathecal gabapentin and either clonidine or neostigmine in the formalin test.** *Anesth Analg* 2004, 98:1374–1379.

3. Jain A, Jain K, Bhardawaj N: **Analgesic efficacy of low-dose intrathecal neostigmine in combination with fentanyl and bupivacaine for total knee replacement surgery.** *J Anaesthesiol Clin Pharmacol* 2012, 28:486–490.

4. Owen MD, Ozsarac O, Sahin S, Uckunkaya N, Kaplan N, Magunaci I: **Low-dose clonidine and neostigmine prolong the duration of intrathecal bupivacaine-fentanyl for labor analgesia.** *Anesthesiology* 2000, 92:361–366.

5. Greig NH, Utsuki T, Ingram DK, Wang Y, Pepeu G, Scali C, Yu QS, Mamczarz J, Holloway HW, Giordano T, Chen D, Furukawa K, Sambamurti K, Brossi A, Lahiri DK: **Selective butyrylcholinesterase inhibition elevates brain acetylcholine, augments learning and lowers Alzheimer beta-amyloid peptide in rodent.** *Proc Natl Acad Sci U S A* 2005, 102:17213–17218.

6. Kumar P, Rudra A, Pan AK, Acharya A: **Caudal additives in pediatrics: a comparison among midazolam, ketamine, and neostigmine coadministered with bupivacaine.** *Anesth Analg* 2005, 101:69–73.

7. Grant GJ, Piskoun B, Bansinath M: **Intrathecal administration of liposomal neostigmine prolongs analgesia in mice.** *Acta Anaesthesiol Scand* 2002, 46:90–94.

8. Tseng YY, Liao JY, Chen WA, Kao YC, Liu SJ: **Biodegradable poly ([D, L]-lactide-co-glycolide) nanofibers for the sustainable delivery of lidocaine into the epidural space after laminectomy.** *Nanomedicine (Lond)* 2014, 9:77–87.

9. Lv S1, Yang YJ, Hong S, Wang N, Qin Y, Li W, Chen Q: **Intrathecal apelin-13 produced different actions in formalin test and tail-flick test in mice.** *Protein Pept Lett* 2013, 20:926–231.

10. Arecchi A1, Mannino S, Weiss J: **Electrospinning of poly (vinyl alcohol) nanofibers loaded with hexadecane nanodroplets.** *J Food Sci* 2010, 75:N80–88.

11. Kenawy ER, Abdel-Hay FI, El-Newehy MH, Wnek GE: **Controlled release of ketoprofen from electrospun poly (vinyl alcohol) nanofibers.** *Mater Sci Eng A* 2007, 459:390–396.

12. Welcome Z, Wu H, Nyairo E, Rogers C, Dean D, Wekesa K, Gunn K, Villafane R: **Cytotoxicity and cell adhesion properties of human mesenchymal stem cells in electrospun nanofiber polymer scaffolds.** *Int J Adv Biotec Bioinform* 2012, 1:41–47.

13. Ellman GL, Courtney KD, Andres V Jr, Feather-stone RM: **A new and rapid colorimetric determination of acetylcholinesterase activity.** *Biochem Pharmacol* 1961, 7:88–95.

14. Chaabihi H, Fournier D, Fedon Y, Bossy JP, Ravallec M, Devauchelle G, Cérutti M: **Biochemical characterization of *Drosophila melanogaster* acetylcholinesterase expressed by recombinant baculoviruses.** *Biochem Biophys Res Commun* 1994, 203:734–742.

15. Zimmermann M: **Ethical guidelines for investigations of experimental pain in conscious animals.** *Pain* 1983, 16:109–110.

16. Haddadi R, Nayebi AM1, Farajniya S, Brooshghalan SE, Sharifi H: **Silymarin improved 6-OHDA-induced motor impairment in hemi-parkisonian rats: behavioral and molecular study.** *Daru* 2014, 22:38–46.

17. Thatte AA, Kadam RJ, Pramila T, Bhoi UA, Deshpande KB: **Development, validation and application of UV spectrophotometric method for the determination of oseltamivir phosphate in bulk and pharmaceutical dosage.** *Int J ChemTech Res* 2011, 3:569–573.

18. Prado WA, Gonçalves AS: **Antinociceptive effect of intrathecal neostigmine evaluated in rats by two different pain models.** *Braz J Med Biol Res* 1997, 30:1225–1231.

19. Kríz N, Yamamotová A, Tobiás J, Rokyta R: **Tail-flick latency and self-mutilation following unilateral deafferentation in rats.** *Physiol Res* 2006, 55:213–20.

20. Afolabi AO, Mudashiru SK, Alagbonsi IA: **Effects of salt-loading hypertension on nociception in rats.** *J Pain Res* 2013, 6:387–392.

21. Taepaiboon P, Rungsardthong U, Supaphol P: **Drug loaded electrospun mats of poly(vinyl alcohol) fibres and their release characteristics of four model drugs.** *Nanotechnology* 2006, 17:2317–2329.

22. Yu DG, Zhu LM, White K, Branford-White C: **Electrospun nanofiber-based drug delivery systems.** *Health* 2009, 1:67–75.

23. Li C, Wang ZH, Yu DG, Williams GR: **Tunable biphasic drug release from ethyl cellulose nanofibers fabricated using a modified coaxial electrospinning process.** *Nanoscale Res Lett* 2014, 9:258–268.

24. Schmidt JR, Krugner-Higby L, Heath TD, Sullivan R, Smith LJ: **Epidural administration of liposome-encapsulated hydromorphone provides extended analgesia in a rodent model of stifle arthritis.** *J Am Assoc Lab Anim Sci* 2011, 50:507–512.

25. Yu D, Thakor DK, Han I, Ropper AE, Haragopal H, Sidman RL, Zafonte R, Schachter SC, Teng YD: **Alleviation of chronic pain following rat spinal cord compression injury with multimodal actions of huperzine A.** *Proc Natl Acad Sci U S A* 2013, 110:E746–55.

26. Park P, Schachter S, Yaksh T: **Intrathecal huperzine A increases thermal escape latency and decreases flinching behavior in the formalin test in rats.** *Neurosci Lett* 2010, 470:6–9.

27. Lograsso M, Nadeson R, Goodchild CS: **The spinal antinociceptive effects of cholinergic drugs in rats: receptor subtype specificity in different nociceptive tests.** *BMC Pharmacol* 2002, 2:20–29.

28. Young T, Wittenauer S, McIntosh JM, Vincler M: **Spinal alpha3beta2 nicotinic acetylcholine receptors tonically inhibit the transmission of nociceptive mechanical stimuli.** *Brain Res* 2008, 1229:118–124.

29. Cai YQ, Chen SR, Han HD, Sood AK, Lopez-Berestein G, Pan HL: **Role of M2, M3, and M4 muscarinic receptor subtypes in the spinal cholinergic control of nociception revealed using siRNA in rats.** *J Neurochem* 2009, 111:1000–1010.

30. Rashid MH, Ueda H: **Neuropathy-specific analgesic action of intrathecal nicotinic agonists and its spinal GABA-mediated mechanism.** *Brain Res* 2002, 953:53–62.

31. Shytle RD, Mori T, Townsend K, Vendrame M, Sun N, Zeng J, Ehrhart J, Silver AA, Sanberg PR, Tan J: **Cholinergic modulation of microglial activation by alpha 7 nicotinic receptors.** *J Neurochem* 2004, 89:337–343.

32. Baba H, Kohno T, Okamoto M, Goldstein PA, Shimoji K, Yoshimura M: **Muscarinic facilitation of GABA release in substantia gelatinosa of the rat spinal dorsal horn.** *J Physiol* 1998, 508:83–93.

33. Perucca E: **Extended-Release Formulations of Antiepileptic Drugs: Rationale and Comparative Value.** *Epilepsy Curr* 2009, 9:153–157.

34. Khanbabaie R, Jahanshahi M: **Revolutionary Impact of Nanodrug Delivery on Neuroscience.** *Curr Neuropharmacol* 2012, 10:370–392.

35. Yoon MH, Park HC, Kim WM, Lee HG, Kim YO, Huang LJ: **Evaluation for the interaction between intrathecal melatonin and clonidine or neostigmine on formalin-induced nociception.** *Life Sci* 2008, 83:845–850.

36. Natalini CC: **Plasma and cerebrospinal fluid alfentanil, butorphanol, and morphine concentrations following caudal epidural administration in horses.** *Ciência Rural* 2006, 36:1436–1443.

37. Suto T, Obata H, Tobe M, Oku H, Yokoo H, Nakazato Y, Saito S: **Long-term effect of epidural injection with sustained-release lidocaine particles in a rat model of postoperative pain.** *Br J Anaesth* 2012, 109:957–967.

38. Alkan M, Kaya K: **Postoperative analgesic effect of epidural neostigmine following caesarean section.** *Hippokratia* 2014, 18:44–49.

39. Omais M, Lauretti GR, Paccola CAJ: **Epidural morphine and neostigmine for postoperative analgesia after orthopedic surgery.** *Anesth Analg* 2002, 95:1698–1701.

Commercialization of biopharmaceutical knowledge in Iran; challenges and solutions

Nasser Nassiri-Koopaei[1], Reza Majdzadeh[2*], Abbas Kebriaeezadeh[1,3*], Arash Rashidian[4], Mojtaba Tabatabai Yazdi[5], Saharnaz Nedjat[2] and Shekoufeh Nikfar[1,3]

Abstract

Background: The objective of this study was to investigate the application of the university research findings or commercialization of the biopharmaceutical knowledge in Iran and determine the challenges and propose some solutions.

Results: A qualitative study including 19 in-depth interviews with experts was performed in 2011 and early 2012. National Innovation System (NIS) model was employed as the study design. Thematic method was applied for the analysis. The results demonstrate that policy making, regulations and management development are considered as fundamental reasons for current commercialization practice pattern. It is suggested to establish foundation for higher level documents that would involve relating bodies and provide them operational guidelines for the implementation of commercialization incentives.

Conclusions: Policy, regulations and management as the most influential issue should be considered for successful commercialization. The present study, for the first time, attempts to disclose the importance of evidence input for measures in order to facilitate the commercialization process by the authorities in Iran. Overall, the NIS model should be considered and utilized as one of the effective solutions for commercialization.

Keywords: Knowledge translation, Biopharmaceutical research, Facilitators and barriers

Introduction

Biotechnology science has proven to be a fast growing source of new technologies and innovative medicines for the pharmaceutical industries during the recent decades [1]. Biopharmaceuticals is presenting itself as the future promise for the safer, targeted and curative medicines opening the scope for treatment of rare and incurable health conditions [2]. New pharmaceutical companies are emerging with a portfolio of biotechnology drug candidates, while the current market leaders are transforming their pipelines to biotechnology derived lead compounds. The specific feature of biotechnology, in general, in being based largely on academic and university researches renders the commercialization of research finding substantial importance [3]. The sufficient research budgets and innovation commercialization expertise to remains

as an ever growing issue to be addressed [4]. Speculating the Iranian Pharmaceutical market, which has been substantially growing during past two decades, demonstrates that medical expenditures has increased as part of overall health system costs [5-7]. There are a satisfactory number of research institutes in the biopharmaceutical field in Iran, but the number of biopharmaceutical companies has been limited to few ones. One possible explanation for the perceived gap between research and production might be the malfunction of the commercialization practice. In the fields, including biopharmaceuticals, where an essential part of knowledge creation takes place in universities and research institutes, the fruitful application of the knowledge needs a transformation process, which involves inventing uses for new scientific ideas and making products or services possible out of them [8,9]. Many universities have persuaded their academic staff and researchers to commercialize their findings and have established university-industry cooperation offices to potentiate these activities, but these mere initiatives are not adequate tools for assuring commercialization prosperity [10]. Very few research finding have been successful enough to turn into

* Correspondence: rezamajd@tums.ac.ir; kebriaee@tums.ac.ir
[2]Knowledge Utilization Research Centre and School of Public Health, Tehran University of Medical Sciences, Tehran, Iran
[1]Department of Pharmacoeconomics and Pharmaceutical Administration, Faculty of Pharmacy, Tehran University of Medical Sciences, Tehran, Iran
Full list of author information is available at the end of the article

commercialized products [4]. Moreover different goals and terminology wielded in academic and industrial contexts, a function of translation to render the two sides a dual comprehension capability is required. So prior to a simple transfer of knowledge, we need an active mechanism making the newly formed knowledge understandable and available for the various technical contexts [11]. Biopharmaceutical industry, among the other high tech ones, encounters with the growing and uncertainty inherent in technological changes, difficulties in handling forthcoming changes due to the immaturity of the industry and the shortage of intrinsic management skills. In addition, dependent on the well-established pharmaceutical and chemical industries, biopharmaceutical industry needs to be assisted with introducing its developing products into market place [12]. All these issues render knowledge translation a substantial importance. In Iran, biopharmaceutical researches have a remarkable history; from when Pasteur and Razi institutes were established in 1919 and 1930, respectively [13]. Recently, more research institutes and academic groups have been engaged in biopharmaceutical research. Some biopharmaceutical corporations have been founded in early previous decade. The number has grown but some experts believe that this capacity can be further potentiated. University-industry relationship has been a topic of concern in Iran. To date some steps have been taken to strengthen such a relation, but outcomes might not fulfill the primary goals. In the present study we aim at investigating the commercialization of the biopharmaceutical knowledge in Iran and determining the barriers and then proposing facilitations possible to further strengthen university knowledge utilization.

Methods

The present qualitative study, in 2011 and early 2012, was carried out on some groups: biopharmaceutical professionals, policy makers and some activists involved in the industry, a purposive sampling method was admitted and included 19 in-depth interviews. Ethics Committee approval was received for the study from Tehran University of Medical

Sciences research deputy. Involvement in research and development, science and technology or drug policy making level, industrial and business background were considered while defining the subgroups of the study. The study's subgroups are shown in Table 1. Researchers were selected from the faculty members of Tehran University of Medical Sciences and Pasteur institute of Iran. Both the academic organizations possess biopharmaceutical department, conducting researches and offer PhD degrees in pharmaceutical biotechnology. These instruction and research organizations have great background in the biopharmaceuticals in Iran and the most important biopharmaceutical companies in Iran have derived from these institutes. In-depth interviews were held with all the participants in the study. Interviews and discussions on the questions listed in Table 2 were done until the point of saturation. Totally 19 individual in-depth interviews, each lasting for 0.5 to 1.5 h, were conducted. Data gathering on the research output of the research organizations were done, regarding the outcome of the current status of putting research into action in two important research institutes. In this study, term definition was as follows: linking research to action or knowledge translation has been considered as the collection of activities that range from 'designing the research question up to application of its results with the aim of improving health and healthcare services [14] and technology commercialization is the process of bringing technical innovation to the marketplace. In the study, the barriers and solutions of knowledge translation in the biopharmaceutical sector have also been studied. Due to the active role of the researcher as a researcher at the department of pharmaceutical biotechnology at the faculty of pharmacy, Tehran University of Medical Sciences, the interviewer became a research fellow observer for the Tehran University of Medical Sciences as a typical example of Iranian research institutes being analyzed in this study [15]. Some interviewees function simultaneously or have background in different positions such as academic staff, industry shareholder and manager or policy making

Table 1 The groups interviewed in the study on 'Commercialization of biopharmaceutical knowledge in Iran'

Group	Subgroup's characteristics	Individuals interviewed
Researcher and academics	Researchers in units under MOHME's authority	Academic staff and researchersfrom Tehran University of Medical Sciences, Pasteur institute, Tehran university, Shahed university
	Researchers in units under authority of Ministry of science and technology	
Policy makers	Pharmaceutical market managers and policy makers in FDO and related organizations	MOHME's Deputy of Research and Technology, Ex-director general of deputy of Food and Drug, Office of health technology at MOHME, Office of research development at MOHME, Office of biological products at FDO, Feasibility study manager at the Ministry of Industry, mine and commerce, Governmental Insurance company manager, Chancellor of faculty of pharmacy, Biopharmaceutical production unit managers, industrial factories
	Research managers and policy makers in MOHME and related organizations	
Biopharmaceutical Industry experts	Experts in the biopharmaceutical industry	

MOHME, Ministry of Health and Medical Education.

Table 2 Questions to conduct the in dept interviews

Question
1 What is your perspective on commercializing university research findings in the field of biopharmaceutical knowledge in Iran?
2 What are the main challenges in commercialization of university research findings in the field of biopharmaceutical knowledge in Iran? How do you assess them?
3 What do you propose to meet these challenges? And what will be the ideal situation of biopharmaceutical knowledge commercialization in Iran?

that causes the lack of separation in the sample through different groups.

Data analysis

The in-depth interviews were documented by a note taker and audio-recorded. Qualitative analysis was performed through the thematic method; the documented interviews and their transcripts were studied several times by the interviewer. Thereafter thematic coding process was done on the interviews and their transcripts by the interviewer while other members of the team regarded the themes and the categories were extracted [15].

Table 3 Categories and codes extracted from the in dept interviews

No.	Category	Code
1	Policy making, regulations and management development	Policy making, legislation and management procedure reform
		Reform in authorities
		Transparency
		Concentration in policy making and legislation
		Stability
		Management challenges
		Market control and expansion policies
		Standards setting
		Control and auditing regulations
		Facilitating regulations
		Prioritization
2	Investment and financial contribution	Financial support management and targeting
		Private sector capacity use
		Private investment
3	Improving the research capability	Purposeful research
		Research and education system reform
4	Extending the relations	Scientific, technological and trade relations
		Interaction between the authorities and consistent approach
		International relations
5	Human resource development	Instruction and evaluation
		Provocation and leading
		HR pyramid development
6	Encouraging the entrepreneurship	Entrepreneurial training and culture
		Commercialization and entrepreneurial facilitation
		Professional commercialization and entrepreneurial services
7	Industrial manufacturing capacity	Knowledge and corporation management
		Pharmaceutical industry renewal and amendment
8	Promoting values (attitudes) and the public culture	Providence
		Cooperation, perseverance and lack of exaggeration
		National production support
		Innovation and risk taking

Results

The eight categories extracted in the study were policy making, regulations and management development, investment and financial contribution, improving the research capability, human resource development, encouraging the entrepreneurship, industrial manufacturing capacity, promoting the social culture and values and extending the relations (Table 3). These categories were extracted while the National Innovation System model was admitted as the cornerstone for the structure of thematic analyses and formulation of categories. In each sector the challenges and barriers are presented and then the facilitations possible.

Policy making, regulations and management development
Challenges

According to the topics noticed by the interviewees, the most critical factors affecting the commercialization of the biotechnology in Iran lie within this category, as expressed by all. One of the academic staff said:

"We have everything but one; that is management!"

In the past twenty years, a great amount of policies have been made to promote biotechnology commercialization but there has been no organized structure to monitor and document their outcomes. Short term decisions to react to day-by-day issues have been prevalent. Prioritization in the national needs has been lacking. Nearly all experts agreed that management practice and method has slowed down the process by obscure protocols, extensive bureaucracy, outdated technology, lacking predefined and clear workflow and very long period to acquire new knowledge impeded smooth progress. Moreover, standards and criteria for performance were not well defined or lacking. Planning and defining targets did not comply with scientific principles of management and in most cases based on personal preferences. One manager at a science park said that:

"Incubators are managed through personal preferences without any performance criteria."

Legislation has not followed specific methodology and practice. Most interviewees emphasized that:

"Introduction of intellectual property law should be regarded as a basement factor."

Conflicting regulations, very late legislation, ambiguous and interpretable regulations and regulations opposing the overall national laws and policies were among the most vital issues noted. On the other hand the authorities in charge of the pharmaceutical sector engaged themselves

in the medicine supply rather than control and auditing, that could endanger serious quality improvement by abating the competition in the market. Transparency was stressed as the underpinning reason for a substantial portion of secrecy among researchers, malfunction of the granting system and conflict of interest in the whole pharmaceutical sector. Moreover lack of assurance to implementation of regulations in practice vigorously damaged public trust, in spite of decentralized decision making, especially in granting. Regarding the unorganized manner under which supports are offered, conflicting decisions in distinct institutions, conflict of interest and consecutive management changes, dispensed policy making renders the entrepreneurial context unstable and undesirable for investment. Some interviewees believe that strict market control, pricing policy, generic medicine scheme and confinement deteriorates market power of companies. In this regard one policy maker said:

"The government of Iran had better withdraw itself from medicine supply."

Definition of standards attracts great attention in the experts as management practices are not well controlled and the outcomes do not serve any feedback for any corrective actions. Some criteria for the scientific board promotion, as explained earlier, appear to create obstacles for innovative researches.

Solutions

Introduction of responsible management into the pharmaceutical sector without conflict of interest and in a stable situation was suggested. Using the course of action adopted by pioneering countries while accommodating to the local circumstances and taking advantage of domestic or international consultants can be suitable. Successes and losses pursuit and causation would be a solution. One of the industrial activists said:

"No one knows where others have gone; we progress by try and error."

Determining the national priorities and broadcasting them for all the researchers was proposed. Intellectual property right regulations were regarded as a substantial need for the productive researches, since protected rights, as the driver for efforts to do innovative researches, warrants the ultimate possible profits. Stability in the management and enforcement of the regulations and policies should be assured by the government. Briefly, management practices, regulation and policy making must be revised.

Investment and financial contribution

Challenges

Financial support plays an undeniable role in conduction of purposeful research. Nevertheless, noted by most interviewees, the current flow of monetary support would not suffice further growth and assist the researches through to commercialization, except that more resources in a consistent manner be underway. Terms and conditions under which the supports are allocated is a point of controversy since there are not any transparent and predetermined procedure approved for the granting and some conflicts of interest, of course, exist. An academic staff said:

"Research budget undergoes great lobbies and suffers from conflict of interest and personal tastes."

Venture capitalist funds are neither present nor functioning properly in Iran. Almost all interviewees emphasized the supportive and facilitating role of such funds. Publishing articles has turned to the pervasive outcome of most the researches, a fact that has been criticized by a great number of research and development experts. Patenting as an alternative would better be introduced to the Iranian scientific society, especially biopharmaceuticals and other high tech fields to help them protect their research findings for probable future commercialization which needs financial contribution. Another issue, as specified by nearly all interviewee groups, which could open the way up to the commercialization and knowledge translation, is privatization in the biopharmaceutical sector. Industrialists agreed that the few presently functional corporations are private and almost all entrepreneurs prefer establishing private ones to prevent tackling the governmental bureaucratic management style. Efforts should focus on capital marketing within the private sector to attract more investment to the newly formed science based companies. One of the industrialists said:

"There is a great deal of money nested in the private sector seeking the opportunity to enter the field."

Solutions

So revising the resource allocation policies and earmarking them to more efficient universities and institutes and simultaneously to research priorities appointed by a joint collaboration between researchers and industrialists are strictly recommended. Financial support from patenting remains to be considered. A growing amount of grants are being awarded to the researchers especially in larger universities. One of the academic staff said:

"The government should direct its money correctly to the most efficient parts."

Improving the research capability

Challenges

Increasing the number of researches and improving its content was regarded as necessary that are both applicable and purposeful in nature. Such types of researches need good research planning by the institution management. Those researches should include all fields relating to the biopharmaceutical sciences such as cellular and molecular biology, microbiology, genetic engineering and process engineering that involve facilitated communications between those disciplines. Basic sciences constitute a pivotal part of the knowledge needed in the biopharmaceutical industry which is somehow ignored. Prioritization in the biopharmaceutical sector according to the domestic market needs would aid the better research topic and field selection. In spite of the speedy movement of the universities in the world towards knowledge generation and turning that knowledge to wealth, Iranian universities are struggling with the ambiguity of role and mission and have not redirected their work flow toward that aim yet. One researcher said:

"Our universities wonder how to act; human resource production or research or commercialization."

Assuming the structural and management practice modification, universities can consolidate dynamism and dexterity in electing to research novel and high tech disciplines. Most interviewees complained about the low amount of research budget. A pharmaceutical biotechnologist added:

"With the current funds we are going nowhere!"

Solutions

Most universities in Iran are pursuing the human resource training goals and recently have fortunately paid attention to the research. In this regard, universities must redefine their mission and vision. Redefining and redirecting the research budgets should be considered. Searching for new financial sources especially from the private sector was deemed as a feasible solution. A technology policy maker holds that:

"We can let the private sector to establish its research institutes and substitute the governmental bodies.

Human resource (HR) development

Challenges

Most interviewees emphasized that both the quantity and quality of the graduates should be regarded; proposing a national or sector-wide qualification system. Although some level of disagreement was observed in the interviewees on the qualifications of the HR, some regulators and policy makers stated that the present graduates are well trained and qualified but some others, most of whom rooted in academia, expressed that qualified and experienced graduates are few in quantity in comparison to the needs. One of the interviewees engaged in policy making believed that:

"There is quite enough number of biotechnology experts in Iran and they should be appropriately assigned and recruited."

While another interviewee as an academic staff, held that:

"We have not adequate quantity and quality workers and experts in the biotechnology industry, albeit a growing number of higher education students graduate every year."

There was remarkable agreement on the following issues, although some interviewees did not express if they were for or against. Pharmacy curriculum revision seems necessary, incorporating the fundamentals of pharmaceutical biotechnology as well as the industrial and downstream processing aspects and the fields mentioned earlier. Education system reform should also introduce more applied and experimental training rather than pure ones, a matter that is regarded as a deleterious problem with the trainings offered in the universities. Designing and establishing auxiliary courses to complement the content of pharmacy training with emphasis on the industrial and entrepreneurial aspects are necessary. Researchers welfare is another factor that can affect the proper research performance in the universities.

Solutions

Training more and more number of students to conduct research on the biopharmaceutical issues is an important need, a prevalent thought among the interviewees. Guiding the students for their career is a must. Applied and purposeful research is denoted as one of the most influential factors on the commercialization in Iran. One academic staff said:

"Our students amaze in their career and most of them have no plan to how to select their research field."

Leading the researchers toward the national priorities may be regarded as remarkable choice for redirecting the research. Providing incentives for applied researches as performed currently by the Iranian Nanotechnology Initiative Council (INIC), is deemed to be efficient a way.

A researcher on the academic policies said:

"Continuous training and knowledge improvement by the researchers and the industrial work fellows including managers and research and development (R&D) staff is some task that could be accomplished by the universities, as well as involvement in the technology transfer process."

Encouraging the entrepreneurship
Challenges

Learning commercial thinking seems scarce and sporadic among the scientific society in Iran that may derive from the social attitude toward wealth. One policy maker as well as an academic staff said:

"In general the rich are regarded as negative and pursuing such morale equates accepting levels of stigmatization."

On the other hand some regulations had previously restricted researchers from establishment of science based companies, but recently revoked. Offering the courses and trainings relevant to entrepreneurship presently is lacking in the pharmacy and other disciplines education curriculum, even in primary and elementary schools. Designing and facilitating the procedures for commercialization was stated by nearly all the interviewees to be of substantial criticality. Presently there are no defined structures or organizations responsible for fostering the commercialization process and researchers have to personally seek some supports. One biotechnologist stated that:

"There are no paved ways to commercialization; the way is so rough that withdrawal is by far wiser."

The role of the existing incubators and science and technology parks are somehow ambiguous and undefined. These entrepreneurial centers function less efficiently however successful progenitors do exist. Providing specific services to the researchers seeking ways for supplying their services needs through specialized corporations is absent currently, albeit an efficient example exists within the Nanotechnology Network of Iran. Unspecialized function of the incubators and science and technology parks in the defined fields render them non professional and inefficient, for example Tehran University of Medical Sciences has established its incubator (pharmaceutical product development center) as a specialized incubator. Think tanks, commercialization consultation centers and idea evaluation centers are absent. As mentioned earlier, the commercialization and entrepreneurial activity in the biopharmaceutical sector depends upon the national economic growth. So, further growth in biopharmaceutical sector is subject to macroeconomic policies. An industrialist said:

"In comparison, most countries experiencing considerable biotechnology growth, also experience high economic growth rates."

Solutions

Commercialization and entrepreneurship advocacy can contribute to more extended efforts by the researchers and students through to the goal. One policy maker said:

"We have not learned entrepreneurship in the schools and feel stranger with that concept."

Establishing offices dedicated to entrepreneurial facilitations in universities would put a breakthrough to the present situation. Management practices revision as mentioned in the first part is recommended by the experts. Active pathways for informing the researchers about the policies and regulations in concordance with introducing further transparency in the management are suggested.

Industrial manufacturing capacity
Challenges

The pharmaceutical industry is mainly possess by the government and its related bodies, most companies are outdated ones and should undergo renewal and reconstruction to cope with continuously tightening current good manufacturing practice (cGMP) requirements and can hardly absorb new technologies that may be ascribed partly to management practices applied and production capabilities. However the few biopharmaceutical companies are private. Not sufficient are the experienced, well educated and innovative middle and top level managers in the industry. Knowledge and technology management, organizational excellence models, innovation friendly atmosphere are not frequent in the industry but some movements have formed recently. An academic staff with industrial experience said:

"Managers in the biopharmaceutical industry are, most, not science and technology oriented enough to attract innovation."

Strategic alliances and clusters are new to the industry. However uncompetitive domestic market hinders quality improvement.

Solutions

Biopharmaceutical industry as the direct interface between biopharmaceutical innovation and the market requires attention. Privatization of the industry and the total economy is a necessity. An industrialist said:

"Till the economy is ruled by the government no major outbreak in the pharmaceutical and bio industry is probable."

Biopharmaceutical industry human resources should also be well replaced and trained.

Promoting values and the public culture
Challenges

Cultural factors are important items that determine the background and context for entrepreneurial activity in the society, as emphasized by most academic staff and policy makers.
One academic staff stressed that:

"Nowadays most researchers prefer rather short term and fast resulting fields. Long term investment has not yet been prevalent and most investors prefer fields with immediate profitability, which can hinder the vital R&D time and long term investment."

Some research policy makers believed that:

"Policy makers, on the other hand, should follow and foresee the trends in the industry and research field to prepare for the situations coming forth as well as the researchers and industrial activists."

Being bound to team work culture was shown to be a key issue that could render the current research capacity more efficient and fruitful. This issue is not so prevalent in the universities and research institutes. Most interviewees shed light on the fact that team work is a must:

"We should oblige ourselves to team work, an ignored necessity."

Values like perseverance, lack of egoism, not exaggerating the achievements, team work and international cooperation are necessary for the whole system; as most interviewees mentioned. Industrial activists, especially, pointed at some basic cultural determinants like consuming the national products and self esteem in the provision of the domestic market needs and meanwhile focusing efforts towards export of science based and high technology products that should be fixed in the whole society of the country. Another considerable aspect, mentioned iteratively by the academic staff, is the promotion of innovation and the need for change in the student and researchers attitudes. Regarding the fundamental impact of seeking innovation on the commercialization and applicability of the researches being conducted, one can comprehend the influence of people looking for new products and process on the overall economic growth in the biopharmaceutical sector. One of the policy makers stated that:

"We, naturally, try to copy and imitate others efforts; not looking for being different."

Policy makers and industrial activists stated that risk taking and continuous improvement among the managers is drastically not evident, a matter that negatively affects the organizational development especially in the high technology fields. Evidence based policy and decision making, as proposed by most interviewees, is capable of lessening a great deal of issues.

Solutions
Providence and long term thinking in the research and development should be incorporated. Perseverance in the applied fields of research helps the commercialization process. "Management by values (MBV) principles" in the organizations such as universities and small and medium-sized enterprises (SMEs) can also promote the entrepreneurial motions.

Cultural modifications require the involvement of top level bodies responsible for the public culture to act properly. Being free of any obligations for the selection of the study discipline is somehow approached as the basic element to allow the researchers function properly. One policy maker said:

"Most students have to achieve ambitions and wishes of their parents."

Innovative ideation can promote novel and modern research areas and technologies for the biopharmaceutical industry.

Extending the relations and communications
Challenges
Miscellaneous efforts in the universities and contemporary efforts in the industry are being done but not cooperating to synergize the expenditure and time. Approach toward scientific and technological cooperation among the activists from both sides must be modified and the false self sufficiency be exchanged by the interactionism. Brokering is neglected in the Iranian biopharmaceutical industry as well as other industries. One of the industrialists said:

"We approach the brokers as negative characters while they can help us."

Communication with the pioneering sources including outstanding universities, international biopharmaceutical companies and consultancy incorporations are not expanded as much as needed. Most experts but especially industrialists laid stress on the scientific communications to extrapolate biotechnology commercialization advocacy among the researchers. Relations between the authorities and policy making and regulatory bodies were perceived as cornerstone aspect for the biopharmaceutical commercialization that functions unsatisfactorily. Adopting consistent and stable policies within different authorities specifically on the manufacturing policies is an important challenge, although firm centralization in legislation and policy making is presently applied. It was regarded as a crucial point that international relations of the country drastically influenced the whole economy and as a sector, the biopharmaceutical industry. A science and technology policy maker cited:

"We cannot restrict ourselves in the national borders; since, today, the product and raw material market is an international one."

Scientific communications with developed countries, regional and international organizations relating to biotechnology, entering commercial and industrial treaties with pioneers, extending the market beyond the national and local boundaries, among others, are all heavily overshadowed by the extent to which the international relations may protrude.

Solutions
Well managed university and biopharmaceutical industry relation was mentioned as an obligation. Interaction and partnership in research among scientists from different fields relating to the biopharmaceutical industry was deemed to be helpful. Some academic staff stressed that:

"There are so many research problems that can be solved only through scientific cooperation."

As the literature on knowledge translation denotes, active characterization and probing into the real knowledge and technology needs can make remarkable assistance to the commercialization process, a role which may be played satisfactorily by the brokers. Training in fields like commercial management and international marketing can also notably contribute to further extend the relations. Technology transfer might be perceived as a suitable choice for making up the delay in the knowledge and technology creation by the research institutes. One policy maker stated that:

"We can compensate our lag in biotechnology by transferring the critical technologies."

Discussion
Biotechnology as a fast growing source of new technologies and innovative, safer, targeted and curative medicines

for the pharmaceutical industries has obtained attention [1]. Biopharmaceuticals accounts for an increasing part of the expenditure on the pharmaceuticals. The specific feature of biotechnology, in general, in being based largely on academic and university researches renders the commercialization of research findings substantial importance. There are a satisfactory number of research institutes in the biopharmaceutical field in Iran, but the number of biopharmaceutical companies has been limited to few ones. One possible explanation for the perceived gap between research and production might be the malfunction of the commercialization practice [8,16]. All interviewees perceived university research finding commercialization as necessary as the researches conducted in the biopharmaceutical field [17,18]. They expressed that expending research budget on researches that were not to be applicable and help the country solve any problem, is of no significance, a situation referred to as valley of death for research. There was consensus on these facts: there are no adequate research budgets and grants while private sector is so weak, purposeful and applied researches are rare, commercialization underpinned no structured and organized system, communications in/outside the sector and international ones dose not fulfill the requisites, entrepreneurial facilitations and knowledge is shortcoming and cultural basis is lacking [19]. Amendment and revision in policies, regulation and organizational management, as the most critical issue expressed, in relating grounds such as research, communications, entrepreneurial and commercialization procedures must be considered [20]. Moving towards free market and economic privatization was mentioned, requiring the lessened involvement of the government in medicine market. Regarding the complex and multi faceted nature of the commercialization process and to gather the more of the stakeholder's approaches toward the topic for provision of a policy making aid and not testing hypotheses, a qualitative method was chosen to discover and develop more detailed body of knowledge on the issue [21,22]. Sampling was based on the stakeholders engaged in a purposeful way, while, perhaps naturally, the formal positions held influenced their responding pattern and attitudes, particularly those serving as policy makers and top level managers of the governmental authorities, as qualitative methodology presupposes. However, very few studies have specifically investigated the biopharmaceutical commercialization process in developing countries [23]. Various background types like industrialists, policy making and researchers focused on different aspect of the commercialization process. Technical biotechnology issues, pricing policy and market competition regards were emphasized by the industrialists while policy makers mainly highlighted the social and public benefits for higher quality and moderate price and researchers underlined grants and entrepreneurial aspects

[24]. Although some experts who were involved in more than one background like research and industry entered the study, a fact that eased the inter profession interpretation. However, each background potentiated some approaches to some extent, especially in the industrialists. We tried to include the most comprehensive informant society of the research and industry and policy making sides, however, some conflicts of interest and bias were noted and cared. Governmental interventions on the medicine market control, pricing and policy making raised some disagreements, which the impact of the interviewee position was evident on. Different data gathering methodologies fairly increased the data accuracy and trustworthiness by triangulation of data sources [25] as well as the construct validity of the present study [26]. Ireland et al. [27] have studies different new biotechnology firms and developed a conceptual model to delineate how they had organized business and science issues. They have concluded that the successful firms could have balanced their scientific and business issues. Terziovski et al. [28] have investigated management practices and strategies that are critical for successful commercialization in the biotechnology industry. They have also specifies the challenges faced by the biotechnology industry in human resources, financial issues, entrepreneurial and business skills and supply chain linkages, however they have focused on the industry rather than the university. Markman et al. [29] studied the factors that could affect the speed of university technology to the market. They found some factors that influenced technology commercialization in the university side of the commercialization process. They shed light on the capabilities and resources available for the university technology transfer offices (UTTOs) and their impact on the commercialization speed. Fontes [12] has studied the role that biotechnology spin-offs could play in the commercialization of the knowledge produced by the research organizations (ROs). It was shown that these spin-offs can be regarded as alternatives for technology transfer offices. The present study tries to provide a comprehensive approach into the commercialization of biopharmaceutical knowledge. Major barriers and challenges in the successful commercialization process in Iran were identified and the most influential factors for overcoming the challenges were introduced. The results imply that national innovation system can be respected as a suitable model to go for investigating the barriers and providing facilitators for commercialization practice [30-33].

Conclusion

The present study tries to discover the major factors that influence the commercialization of the biopharmaceutical knowledge and propose processes for moving research to marketplace. As the nature of qualitative study denotes, results derived from one situation could hardly be extrapolated to other ones, but some general issues can be highlighted. Management practices, regulations particularly on the intellectual property right and policy making affects the entire commercialization process even the research as the antecedent. Financial support for the researches is a factor that can facilitate commercialization [18]. Globally, few university researches after long time may be commercialized; therefore quantity and quality of the researches and their applicability may be respected. Human resource management plays an important role in the biopharmaceutical industry, as a high tech field especially training the HR. Entrepreneurial facilitations can encourage the researchers for commercialization [34]. Cultural factors like trust and team work influence whole the process [35]. University-industry and international relations can affect the applicability of the researches and knowledge transfer, while noticing the disadvantages of university-industry relation [36]. Such a study that goes through this issue for the first time can open the way for further studies that specifically investigates each factor. Nearly all the interviewees stated that the commercialization process has been facilitated deeply during recent years, but there are others to do to achieve what is desired. Iran as a developing country can be regarded as a pattern for other developing countries while specific local situations being kept in mind. We can conclude here that the further potentiation of the national innovation system can vitally facilitate the commercialization of biopharmaceutical knowledge.

Consent

Written consent was obtained from the interviewees for tape recording the interviews and the publication of this report.

Abbreviations
NIS: National Innovation System; MOHME: Ministry of Health and Medical Education; HR: Human Resource; INIC: Iranian Nanotechnology Initiative Council; R&D: Research and Development; cGMP: Current Good Manufacturing Practice; MBV: Management by Values; SMEs: Small and Medium-sized Enterprises; UTTOs: University Technology Transfer Offices; ROs: Research Organizations.

Competing interests
The authors declare that they have no competing interests.

Authors' contributions
NNK conceived and implemented the strategy, performed the interviews and data analysis and drafted the paper, RM conceived the strategy of study and supervised the project, AK revised the strategy and supervised the project, AR gave consultation on study design and qualitative methodology and edited the draft, MTY gave consultation on biopharmaceutical industry, SN gave consultation on designing the study and qualitative methodology, SN gave consultation on the study implementation and edited the draft. All authors read and approved the final manuscript.

Acknowledgements
The authors are thankful to the Research and Technology Deputy of Ministry of Health and Medical Education and researchers who entered the study from research institutes, universities and biopharmaceutical companies.

Author details
[1]Department of Pharmacoeconomics and Pharmaceutical Administration, Faculty of Pharmacy, Tehran University of Medical Sciences, Tehran, Iran. [2]Knowledge Utilization Research Centre and School of Public Health, Tehran University of Medical Sciences, Tehran, Iran. [3]Pharmaceutical Policy Research Center, Faculty of Pharmacy, Tehran University of Medical Sciences, Enqelab Square, Tehran, Iran. [4]Knowledge Utilization Research Centre and Department of Health Management and Economics, School of Public Health, Tehran University of Medical Sciences, Tehran, Iran. [5]Department of Pharmaceutical Biotechnology, Faculty of Pharmacy, Tehran University of Medical Sciences, Tehran, Iran.

References
1. Hulse JH: Biotechnologies: past history, present state and future prospects. *Trends Food Sci Tech* 2004, **15**:3–18.
2. Kayser O, Warzecha H: *Pharmaceutical Biotechnology: Drug Discovery and Clinical Applications.* John Wiley-VCH verlag: Weinheim; 2012.
3. Friedl KE: Overcoming the "valley of death": mouse models to accelerate translational research. *Diabetes Technol Ther* 2006, **8**(3):413–414.
4. Powers JB: Commercializing academic research: Resource effects on performance of university technology transfer. *J Higher Educ* 2003, **74**(1):26–50.
5. Kebriaeezadeh A, Nassiri-Koopaei N, Abdollahias A, Nikfar S, Nafiseh Mohamadi: Trend analysis of the pharmaceutical market in Iran; 1997–2010; policy implications for developing countries. *DARU* 2013, **21**(1):52.
6. Nikfar S, Kebriaeezadeh A, Dinarvand R, Abdollahi M, Sahraian MA, Henry D, Akbari Sari A: Cost-effectiveness of different interferon beta products for relapsing-remitting and secondary progressive multiple sclerosis: decision analysis based on long-term clinical data and switchable treatments. *DARU* 2013, **21**(1):50.
7. Nikfar S, Kebriaeezadeh A, Majdzadeh R, Abdollahi M: Monitoring of National Drug Policy (NDP) and its standardized indicators; conformity to decisions of the national drug selecting committee in Iran. *BMC Int Health Hum Rights* 2005, **5**(1):5.
8. Lichtenthaler U, Lichtenthaler E, Frishammar J: Technology commercialization intelligence: organizational antecedents and performance consequences. *Technol Forecast Soc Change* 2009, **76**:301–315.
9. Hashemi Meshkini A, Kebriaeezadeh A, Dinarvand R, Nikfar S, Habibzadeh MG, Vazirian I: Assessment of the vaccine industry in Iran in context of accession to WTO: a survey study. *DARU* 2012, **20**:19.
10. Szelényi K, Goldberg RA: Commercial funding in academe: examining the correlates of faculty's use of industrial and business funding for academic work. *J Higher Edu* 2011, **82**(6):775–799.
11. Clarysse B, Tartari V, Salter A: The impact of entrepreneurial capacity, experience and organizational support on academic entrepreneurship. *Res Policy* 2011, **40**(8):1084–1093.
12. Fontes M: The process of transformation of scientific and technological knowledge into economic value conducted by biotechnology spin-offs. *Technovation* 2005, **25**:339–347.
13. Davari M, Walley T, Haycox A: Pharmaceutical policy and market in Iran: Past experiences and future challenges. *J Pharm Health Serv Res* 2011, **2**(1):47–52.
14. Majdzadeh R, Sadighi J, Nejat S, Shahidzade Mahani A, Gholami J: Knowledge Translation for Research Utilization: design of a Knowledge Translation Model at Tehran University of Medical Sciences. *J Contin Educ Health Prof* 2008, **28**(4):270–277.
15. Patton MQ: *Qualitative research and evaluation methods.* Thousand Oaks, CA: Sage Publications; 2001.
16. Goldfarb B, Henrekson M: Bottom-up versus top-down policies towards the commercialization of university intellectual property. *Res Policy* 2003, **32**(4):639–658.
17. Onyeka CJ: Biotechnology commercialisation in universities of developing countries: a review of the University of Ibadan. *Nigeria. J Commer Biotechnol* 2011, **17**(4):293–300.
18. Olivieri NF: Patients' health or company profits? The commercialisation of academic research. *Sci Eng Ethics* 2003, **9**(1):29–41.
19. Meyers AD, Pruthi S: Academic entrepreneurship, entrepreneurial universities and biotechnology. *J Commer Biotechnol* 2011, **17**(4):349–357.

20. Gilsing VA, van Burg E, Romme AGL: Policy principles for the creation and success of corporate and academic spin-offs. *Technovation* 2010, **30**(1):12–23.

21. Hall ZW, Scott C: University-industry partnership. *Science* 2001, **291**(5504):553.

22. Kharabaf S, Abdollahi M: Science growth in Iran over the past 35 years. *J Res Med Sci* 2012, **17**(3):1–5.

23. De Luca LM, Verona G, Vicari S: Market orientation and R and D effectiveness in high-technology firms: an empirical investigation in the biotechnology industry. *J Prod Innovat Manag* 2010, **27**(3):299–320.

24. Bureth A, Pénin J, Wolff S: Start-up creation in biotechnology: lessons from the case of four new ventures in the upper rhine biovalley. *IJIM* 2010, **14**(2):253–283.

25. Tashakkori A, Teddlie C: *Handbook of mixed methods in social and behavioral research*. Thousand Oaks, CA: Sage Publications; 2002.

26. Yin RK: *Case Study Research: Design and Methods*. Thousand Oaks, CA: Sage Publications; 2002.

27. Ireland DC, Hine D: Harmonizing science and business agendas for growth in new biotechnology firms: case comparisons from five countries. *Technovation* 2007, **27**:676–692.

28. Terziovski M, Morgan JP: Management practices and strategies to accelerate the innovation cycle in the biotechnology industry. *Technovation* 2006, **26**(5–6):545–552.

29. Markman GD, Gianiodis PT, Phan PH, Balkin DB: Innovation speed: transferring university technology to market. *Res Policy* 2005, **34**(7):1058–1075.

30. Larijani B, Majdzadeh R, Delavari AR, Rajabi F, Khatibzadeh S, Esmailzadeh H, Lankarani KB: Iran's health innovation and science development plan by 2025. *Iran J Public Health* 2009, **38**(SUPPL. 1):13–16.

31. Bérard C, Delerue H: A cross-cultural analysis of intellectual asset protection in SMEs: the effect of environmental scanning. *J Small Bus Enterprise Dev* 2010, **17**(2):167–183.

32. Eisenberg RS: Patent costs and unlicensed use of patented inventions. *Univ Chic Law Rev* 2011, **78**(1):53–69.

33. Bagheri SK, Moradpour HA, Rezapour M: The Iranian patent reform. *World Pat Inf* 2009, **31**(1):32–35.

34. Jain S, George G, Maltarich M: Academics or entrepreneurs? Investigating role identity modification of university scientists involved in commercialization activity. *Res Policy* 2009, **38**:922–935.

35. Fiedler M, Welpe IM: Commercialisation of technology innovations: an empirical study on the influence of clusters and innovation networks. *Int J Technol Manag* 2011, **54**(4):410–437.

36. Kumar MN: Ethical conflicts in commercialization of university research in the post-bayh-dole era. *Ethics Behav* 2010, **20**(5):324–351.

17

Generation of stable ARE- driven reporter system for monitoring oxidative stress

Paria Motahari[1], Majid Sadeghizadeh[1*], Mehrdad Behmanesh[1], Shaghayegh Sabri[2] and Fatemeh Zolghadr[1*]

Abstract

Background: NF-E2-related factor2 (Nrf2)-antioxidant response element (ARE) signaling pathway is the major defensive mechanism against oxidative stress and is up regulated by specific antioxidants and oxidants to comprise the chemoptotective response. Detection of ARE-activating compounds helps to develop new drugs and identify/quantify the tension range of the oxidants.
Important reasons promoting this work are high throughput, rapid and inexpensive experiments relative to the in vitro studies for ARE-Nrf2 pathway monitoring of chemicals and environmental samples.

Methods: In this study hepatoma Huh7 reporter cell line was generated which contains a luciferase gene under the control of an ARE. This is the first example of ARE construct containing one copy of extended consensus response element. The cells were treated with hydroquinone (HQ) and p-benzoquinone (BQ) (oxidative stress inducers) and the antioxidant, curcumin.

Results: The luciferase activity was induced in a concentration-dependent manner in a concentration range of 1–2 μM for BQ and HQ. Curcumin was also validated as an ARE inducer in concentration above 10 μM. In addition, this reporter cell line provides a rapid detection as early as 4 h to respond to the ARE inducers.

Conclusion: It is a powerful tool for the sensitive and selective screening of chemicals, drugs and environmental samples for their antioxidant and oxidant activities.

Keywords: Antioxidants, Nrf2-ARE, Oxidative stress, Reporter cell line

Background

Monitoring compounds on pathways of interest to provide insight into the molecular mode of action to evaluate the possible toxicity is required in modern medicine. Furthermore, the lack of information about the cellular signaling pathways of drugs is a weakness in clinical treatment. Recently in vitro studying of pathways involved in genotoxic responses is developed to determine whether specific compounds affecting particular pathways [1]. Due to environmental issues, antioxidant and oxidant response pathway has attracted much more attention [2]. Reactive oxygen species (ROS) are highly unstable molecules; interfering with the normal cell function by trigging cascade of oxidative stress pathways. Defensive system in response to oxidative tension turns multifarious of signaling pathways on to

protect the cells [3]. Mounting evidence demonstrated that human genome consists of protective genes acting through the enhanced sequence known as the ARE in their promoter region. Metabolization by the ARE mechanism is one of the common responses, which is also induced by the certain groups of antioxidants to confer guard against oxidative tension [4]. The regulation of these genes is performed by Nrf2 transcription factor (NF-E2-related factor2). Heterodimerized Nrf2 along with other factors including Jun and small Maf proteins binds to the ARE leading to the expression of ARE target genes [5].

The aim of this study was to establish a sensitive, stable ARE reporter cell line, using a luciferase gene under the transcriptional control of one copy of the ARE core sequence of the human NQO1 promoter (NAD (P) H: quinoneoxidoreductase) (one of the Nrf2 target genes) and it was carried out using immortalized cells derived from human liver. The reporter cell line was challenged with a range of compounds, to evaluate the ARE activation potential in the

* Correspondence: sadeghma@modares.ac.ir; zolghadr@modares.ac.ir
[1]Faculty of Biological Sciences, Department of Molecular Genetics, School of Biological Sciences, Tarbiat Modares University, Jalal Ale Ahmad Highway, PO Box 14115–111, Tehran, Iran
Full list of author information is available at the end of the article

engineered cell line. The reporter cell line is sensitive enough to screen chemicals with toxicity risk and drugs with antioxidant activity related to the activation potency of the ARE signaling pathway.

Methods

Chemicals

Fetal bovine serum (FBS) was purchased from Invitrogen/Life Technologies (Carlsbad, CA, USA). BQ, HQ, dimethyl sulfoxide (DMSO) were the products of Sigma-Aldrich (St. Louis, USA). Curcumin was purchased from Merck KGaA (Darmstadt, Germany) with a purity of 95 %.

Cell culture and condition

The human hepatoma Huh7 cell line was purchased from National Cell Bank, Pasteur Institute of Iran and were grown in Dulbecco's modified Eagle's medium (DMEM) (Invitrogen/Life Technologies,Carlsbad, CA, USA). Cells were supplemented with 10 % fetal bovine serum, 100 U/mL penicillin, and 100 mg/mL streptomycin (Invitrogen/Life Technologies, Carlsbad, CA, USA). Cells were grown at 37 °C in a humidified atmosphere of 5 % carbon dioxide. Cells tripsinized/sub cultured every 2 to 3 days.

Oligonucleotides

The NQO1 ARE was originally described by Li and Jaiswal in a 5′-TCG AGA TGC AGT CAC AG**T GAC TCA** GCA GAA TCT GA-3′ and 3′-CTA CGT CAG TGT CAC TGA GTC GTC TTA GAC TAG CT-5′ nucleotides sequences (Activator protein 1 (AP1) binding site is shown in bold) [6]. ARE oligonucleotides were commercially synthesized through *XhoI-HindIII* restriction sites at either ends (oligonucleotides were synthesized by Bioneer (Daejeon, South Korea). The synthetic oligonucleotides were annealed, phosphorilated, purified on a 12 % polyacrylamide gel and cloned at the *XhoI-HindIII* sites of pGL4.26 using standard protocols. The orientation and sequences of this element were confirmed by sequencing of the plasmids.

Chemicals exposure

Sterile stock solutions of BQ, HQ and curcumin were prepared in DMEM just before use. Briefly, Cells were seeded at a density of 2×10^5 per well in 24-well microtiter plates, and incubated until cells reached 70–80 % confluence. Following overnight recovery, the culture medium was replaced by the fresh DMEM supplemented with antibiotics along with a range of chemical concentrations in triplicate for 4 h, 6 h, 8 h and 24 h to estimate the luciferase shortest induction time.

Cell viability assay

Cell viability was assessed by methylthiazoltetrazolium (MTT) assay (Sigma-Aldrich, St Louis, USA) according

to the manufacturer's instruction. Briefly, cells (1×10^4) were cultured overnight in a 96-well plate. Afterwards, the medium of each well was replaced by 200 μL fresh medium plus 50 μL of the MTT solution (5 mg/mL in PBS). The plates were incubated at 37 °C for 4 h. The absorbance being proportional to cell was subsequently measured at 570 nm in each well using an enzyme-linked immunosorbent assay plate reader (Bio-RAD 680, USA). All experiments were performed in triplicate, and the relative cell viability (%) was calculated as a percentage relative to the untreated control cells.

Development of an ARE luciferase-reporter

The ARE-luciferase reporter plasmids were generated using the pGL4.26-minimal promoter vector (Promega, UK, Southampton, United Kingdom) containing a minimal TATA promoter upstream of the firefly luciferase gene. Double-stranded oligonucleotides ligated into the pGL4.26 [minP]. Consequently, TOP10 competent cells were transformed with the recombinant DNA for amplification. Engineered vector contains one copy of ARE sequence that have been inserted, in head-to-tail orientation, through *XhoI-HindIII* restriction sites upstream of the promoter-luc + transcriptional unit (Fig. 1). Eight positive clones were sequenced using the RV primer.

Huh7-1x-ARE-luc reporter-gene assay

Huh7 cells were seeded in 24-well plates at a density of 2×10^5 cells per well and grown overnight. Consequently, the cells were transiently transfected with the recombinant reporter plasmids. The plasmid pGL4.26 without the ARE piece, was considered to control the performance of the construction. Transfection was done by LipofectAMINE 2000 (Invitrogen, Carlsbad, CA, USA) reagent in triplicate according to the manufacturer's instructions. Following transfection the culture medium was replaced

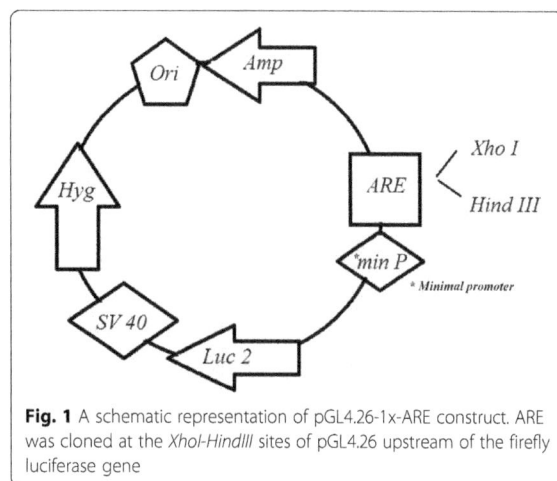

Fig. 1 A schematic representation of pGL4.26-1x-ARE construct. ARE was cloned at the *XhoI-HindIII* sites of pGL4.26 upstream of the firefly luciferase gene

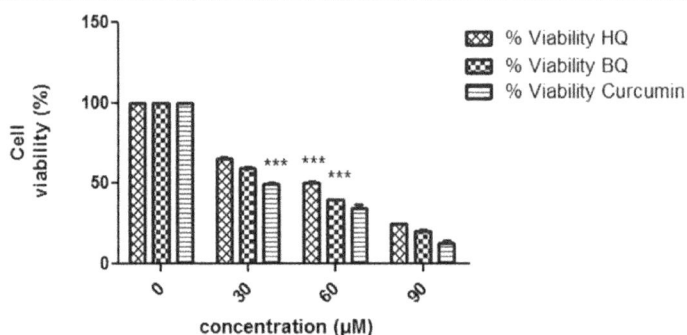

Fig. 2 Toxicity of HQ, BQ and curucmin to human hepatoma (Huh7) cells. Huh7 cells were cultured with different doses for 24 h as indicated in the Methods. Left column represents the percentage of cell viability treated with chemicals. Data showed LD50 values of 60 μM HQ and 45 μM BQ and 30 μM curucmin for Huh7 cells. Notes: Data expressed as mean ± SD; ***, p <0.001 compared to nontreated cells

24 h later with the fresh growth medium containing 10, 20, 30 μmol/L HQ which was prepared immediately before each experiment. Cells were left for 24 h to respond the oxidative stress inducers, and then the firefly luciferase activities in their lysates were monitored.

Luciferase assay
Luciferase assays were performed following the manufacturer's instruction (Promega). Cells were washed twice with phosphate buffered saline (PBS). Each well received 75 μl lysis buffer (Promega, UK, Southampton, United Kingdom) after removing PBS. Cell lysates were harvested and spin for 5 min. The cell lysates (50 μl) were added to 100 μl luciferase assay reagent (Promega, UK, Southampton, United Kingdom). Luciferase bioluminescence measurements were performed at room temperature using a luminometer (Sirius tube Luminometer, Berthold Detection System, Germany). Activity was expressed as relative light units (RLU) emitted from total assays and it was calculated versus background activity.

Generation of stable ARE-driven reporter cell line
The Huh7-1x-ARE-luc containing the hygromycin selectable marker was stably transfected into the Huh7 cells using the LipofectAMINE 2000 reagent. According to the LD50 value transfected cells were selected using 450 μM hygromycin (Invitrogen/Life Technologies, CA, USA) in the media for 4 to 5 weeks. The hygromycin-resistant clones were isolated and screened by measuring their basal and inducible luciferase activity at different concentration of HQ and BQ. Positive clones, which showed high inducible luciferase activity, were passaged and maintained in growth medium containing 450 μM hygromycin for further analysis.

Statistical analysis
All experiments were conducted in triplicate, and the results were expressed as mean ± SD (standard deviation). One-way analysis of variance (ANOVA) was used to assess the statistical analysis, and p <0.05 was considered to be significant. Data was analyzed using Microsoft Excel software and GraphPad InStat software.

Results
Cytotoxic studies
Data from MTT assay clearly showed LD50 values of 60 μM HQ and 45 μM BQ and 30 μM curucmin for huh7 cells and demonstrated higher levels of either BQ, HQ or curucmin inhibits cell metabolism of Huh7 cells. (Fig. 2)

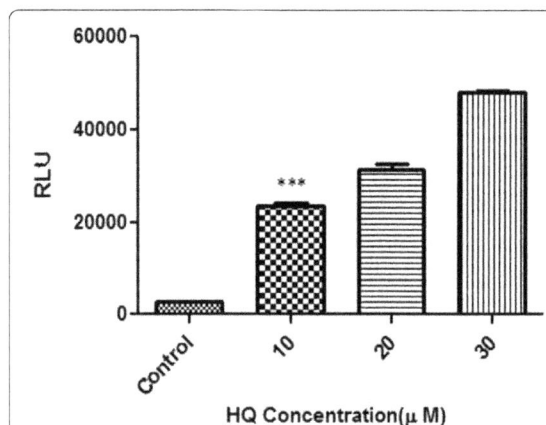

Fig. 3 Luciferase reporter activity in transiently transfected Huh7-1x-ARE-luc cells. Recombinant cells were seeded overnight in 24 well plates at 2×10^5 cells per well. Cells were incubated with increasing concentration of HQ (10, 20, and 30 μM). After 24 h of treatment, luciferase activity was assessed by measuring luciferase activity in cell lysates. Control cells (which lacks any ARE) failed to induce luciferase activity. Notes: Data expressed as mean ± SD; ***, p <0.001 compared to control

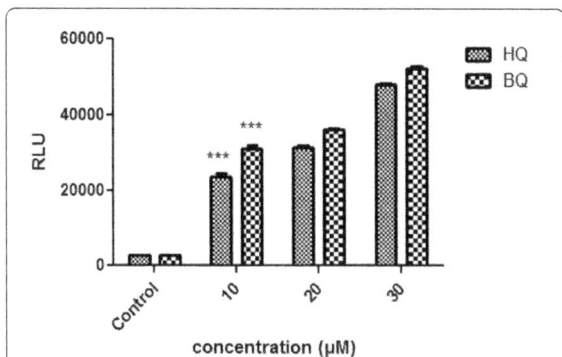

Fig. 4 ARE inductions in stable transfected Huh7 exposed to HQ and BQ (10, 20, and 30 μM). Luciferase activity was measured after 24 h. The numbers in the left column represent the relative luciferase activities. Luciferase activity was increased following treatment with increasing concentrations of oxidative stress inducers. Each bar shows the mean ± SD; ***, $p < 0.001$ compared to control

Transient transfection and analysis of luciferase reporter gene activity

Prior to stable transfection, ARE responsiveness of the plasmid pGL4.26-1x-ARE-luc was confirmed in transient transfection experiments and it was found that stimulation of ARE could induce expression of luciferase in these cells (Fig. 3). HQ treatment of Huh7 cells transfected with pGl4.26-luc (which lacks any ARE) failed to induce luciferase activity, whereas a significant induction of luciferase activity was observed in cells transfected with pGl4.26 -1x-ARE-Luc. HQ (10 μM) caused an approximately 11-fold increase in luciferase activity compared to the negative control during 24 h of exposure ($p < 0.001$).

Generation of a stable ARE reporter cell line and oxidative stress induction assay

The pGL4.26-1x-ARE-luc plasmid containing the hygromycin selectable marker was stably transfected into Huh7

cells. Cells were selected for ARE inducibility in media containing 450 μM hygromycin for 4 weeks (according to the hygromycin LD50, data are not shown). Stable clones were isolated and screened by measuring their inducible (obtained by treatment with 10, 20 and 30 μM BQ, HQ) luciferase activities as described before. As mentioned in Fig. 4 luciferase activity was increased following treatment with different dosage of oxidative stress inducers ($p < 0.001$).

No changes in the ARE responsiveness of Huh7-1x-ARE-luc cells were measured over eight passages and after multiple rounds of storage in liquid nitrogen and re-culture.

Dose dependent of luciferase induction by oxidative stress inducers in the recombinant cell line

When it was proved that the recombinant cells were sensitive to ARE stimuli treatment, the dose dependent effects of inducers on this cell line was investigated. In this regard cells were incubated with increasing concentrations of BQ and HQ. Inducers stimulated luciferase activity in a dose dependent manner, with maximal stimulation reached at 60 μM of HQ and 50 μM of BQ (Fig. 5). Furthermore a minimum luciferase activity (around 2.5 fold increases) was seen following treatment with 1 μmol/L BQ and ~ 2.4 fold by 2 μmol/L HQ ($p < 0.05$).

Shortest induction validation

Induction of luciferase activity by BQ and HQ was also time dependent; it increased 6-fold after four hours, 7.3-fold after eight hours, 9.1-fold after twelve hours of treatment with 10 μmol/L HQ and reached 10-fold after 24 h of treatment with the same dose of HQ. The luciferase induced significantly after 4 h as the shortest induction time ($p < 0.001$). The time course of induction of luciferase by 10 μM of HQ and BQ in recombinant cell lines is shown in Fig. 6.

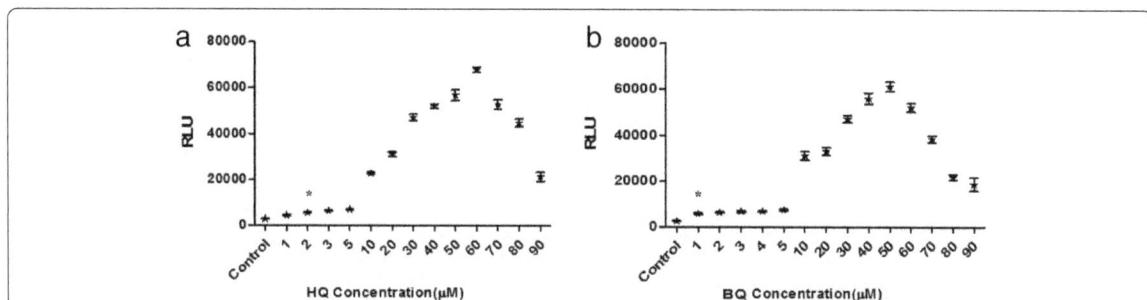

Fig. 5 Induction of luciferase activity in a dose-dependent manner. Cells were incubated with increasing concentration of HQ(**a**) and BQ(**b**). Maximal stimulation reached at 60 μM of HQ and 50 μM of BQ. Around 2.5 fold increases luciferase activity was seen following treatment with 1 μmol/L BQ and ~ 2.4 fold by 2 μmol/L HQ. The results are presented as the mean ± SD; *, $p < 0.05$, as determined by one way ANOVA, compared with the corresponding no treated control

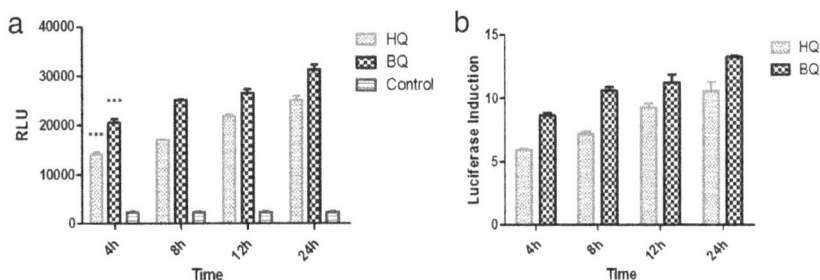

Fig. 6 The time course of luciferase activity induction. The Recombinant cell line was incubated with HQ and BQ (10 μM) at 37 °C for the indicated time after which luciferase activity in cell lysates was measured as described under the "Methods" section. Luciferase activity was expressed as (**a**) RLUs or (**b**) as a percent of the luciferase induction by HQ and BQ in recombinant Huh7 cell line. The luciferase induced significantly after 4 h as the shortest induction time. Each bar shows the mean ± SD; ***, $p < 0.001$ compared to control

Huh7- 1x-ARE-luc sensitivity to antioxidants

Huh7-1x-ARE-luc cells were subsequently assessed to examine whether recombinant cells would also respond to compounds with antioxidant activity through ARE mediated activation. In this regard, luciferase activity induction was tested after recombinant cell line treatment with curcumin (diferuloylmethane or 1-7-bis (4-hydroxy-3-methoxyphenol)-1,6-heptadiene-3,5-dione). ARE induction by curcumin in recombinant cells was observed after incubation for 24 h, and the induction effects were detected at 10 μM concentrations of curcumin ($p < 0.001$)(Fig. 7). In contrast, low concentration of curcumin did not induce luciferase activity.

Discussion

Possible threat of food and environmental compounds to human health through elevation of oxidative stress level shows the importance of ARE induction monitoring after exposure with suspected compounds. Studying Nrf2-ARE signaling pathway of drugs and natural compounds with antioxidant activity gives target information to discover novel drug-protein relationship [7].

In this study a stable ARE- reporter cell line was generated; it provides a good model system to screen and identify chemicals as ARE inducers and explores induced pathway of natural and synthetic antioxidants. The engineered cell line called Huh7-1x-ARE-luc, contained the 31 nucleotides core promoter of human NQO1 (Nrf2 targeted gene) ARE, which is used to direct expression of luciferase. Primitive investigation showed a necessary core sequence of ARE as a sufficient sequence to mediate induction [6]. Further nucleotide sequence analysis in the human NQO_1 gene ARE (hARE) revealed the requirement for perfect AP1 and imperfect AP1 elements arranged in inverse orientation at the interval of three base pairs and a GC box for optimal expression. Huh7-1x-ARE-luc contains AP1 binding site (5′-TGACTCA-3′) and imperfect AP1 (5′-ACTG ACG-3′) and nucleotides GCA (GC box) located within the human ARE considered to be responsible for more transcription of the respective genes [8]. The stable cell line have the benefit of high correlation with Nioi new reported ARE sequence (5′-gagTcA**C** aGTgAGt**C**ggCAaaatt-3′) which two cytosine (shown in bold) residues are substituted with two 'n' residues [9]. Thus far no other ARE cell lines have been shown to match with the new reported sequence and just limited to TMAnnRTGAYnnnGCRWWW core promoter. This cell line has the potential to be a unique tool because it is the first example which has used huh7 cell line. The main advantages of using HuH7 cell line for research is that, sharing several characteristics of normal hepatocyte. These cells offer stable phenotype, reproducibility and cheaper to culture, which make them useful for in vitro drug safety analysis [10]. Human hepatoma Huh-7 cell line is a proper model system to study liver metabolism and toxicity of xenobiotics; and the detection of antitoxic

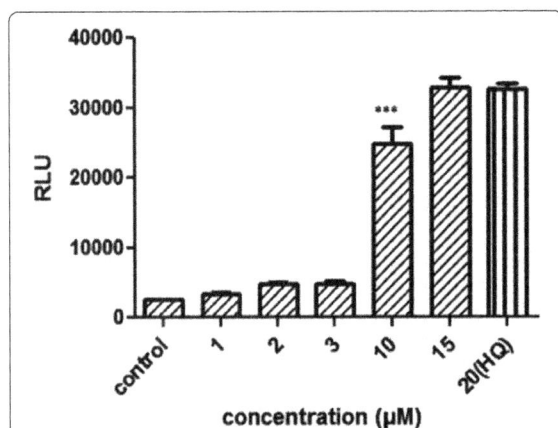

Fig. 7 ARE induction in Huh7-1x-ARE-luc after exposure to 1, 2, 3, 10, 15 μM of curcumin. Briefly, Cells (2×10^5) were cultured overnight in a 24-well plate. Luciferase activity was measured 24 h after exposure to different concentration of curcumin. (***, $p < 0.001$)

agents [11]. One characteristic of Huh7 cells that makes them attractive for use them in toxicity studies is the expression of drug metabolizing enzymes. These cells display the functional activities of various carbohydrate-metabolizing enzymes and represent an alternative model system for drug efficacy or toxicity studies related to the liver-specific genes induction [12]. In vitro liver cell line are increasingly used for the toxicological studies due to the central role of the liver in chemical transforming and clearing.

The performance of this assay was evaluated using HQ and BQ as oxidative stress inducers and curcumin as a compound with antioxidant activity. HQ and BQ are metabolites which derived from benzene biotransformation in liver and have been shown to produce reactive oxygen species; and causing oxidative stress [13]. Furthermore, a number of protective mechanisms; via the ARE are induced in response to HQ and BQ cytotoxicity [14, 15]. So these are a good choice to challenge the construct to explore sensitivity. The responsiveness of this stable cell line to BQ and HQ is in the 1–2 μM range, which would imply sufficient sensitivity; because the reporter gene expression in pGL4 vectors are increased compared with the other vectors. Even though other studies show that 1 μM of HQ could induce NQO1 activity and less concentration (0.1 μM) could not induce NQO1 [14].

It is shown that luciferase activity in Huh7-1x-ARE-luc cells is dose dependent, this cell line gives a ~ 26 fold increase in reporter gene activity in the presence of 60 μM of HQ and an approximate 25 fold increase in luciferase activity by a 50 μM dose of BQ as the oxidative stress inducers. According to the LD50 values (The LD50 of HQ and BQ following a 24-h exposure was approximately 60 μM and 45 μM, respectively) maximal detection depends on the toxicity. Previously, a stable reporter MCF7 (human breast adenocarcinoma cell line) cell line was generated. The reporter construct contained eight copies of ARE containing promoter sequence from mouse gsta1 and gave 50-fold induction according to the treatment with 50 μmol/L t-BHQ [2]. In this study it is shown that single copy of ARE is sufficient to confer responsiveness for a sensitive detection.

As demonstrated, ARE expression reflected by luciferase reporter is in a time-dependent manner. To examine the shortest period induction, luciferase activities were analyzed in 4 h, 8 h, 12 h and 24 h. These experiments revealed that Huh7-1x-ARE-luc could stimulate a small, but apparent induction of luciferase activity as early as 4 h after treatment as a rapid detection.

The construct was also validated with curcumin, a polyphenol yellow pigment in the rhizome of *Curcuma longa Linn* (Zingiberaceae) [16], which is reported to induce Nrf2 in HUh7 human hepatoma cells to exert antioxidant effect [17]. As Rachana Garg and his collogues showed in mice treated with curcumin the level of NQO1 expression increased due to nuclear translocation of Nrf2 and then association with ARE sequences [18]. According to this information, reporter cell line was challenged with curcumin. Huh7-1x-ARE-luc is induced by 10 μM of curcumin. It was demonstrated that less concentration of curcumin could not induce luciferase expression via ARE induction; maybe due to the fact that the antioxidant activity of curcumin through ARE is dose dependent. In this regard, other experiments also revealed that concentration above 10 μM of curcumin increased the expression of genes involved in ARE-Nrf2 pathway in renal epithelial cell [19].

Conclusion

In vitro assays are becoming more attractive as screening tools because they are rapid, and they have the potential to reduce the number of animals needed for chemical testing. Stably transfected cell lines offer several advantages in comparison to other in vitro systems. They are an excellent aid in defining the mechanism of unknown compounds [20]. Huh7-1x-ARE-luc assay demonstrated the values of an in vitro screen for a battery of tests to examine ARE inducers like oxidative stress stimuli and natural/chemical agents with antioxidant activity. It is a reproducible and reliable in vitro assay that measures the activation of the ARE via a luciferase reporter gene.

Abbreviations
ARE: Antioxidant response element; BQ: p-benzoquinone; HQ: Hydroquinone; NQO1: NAD (P) H dehydrogenase [quinone] 1; Nrf2: NF-E2-related factor 2.

Competing interests
The authors declare that they have no competing interests.

Authors' contributions
PM carried out molecular and cell bioassay studies and drafted the manuscript. MS participated in the design of the study and helped to draft the manuscript. MB participated in the design of the study. SS helped to draft the manuscript. FZ conceived of the study, and participated in its design, data collection, and analysis and helped to draft the manuscript. All authors read and approved the final manuscript.

Author details
[1]Faculty of Biological Sciences, Department of Molecular Genetics, School of Biological Sciences, Tarbiat Modares University, Jalal Ale Ahmad Highway, PO Box 14115–111, Tehran, Iran. [2]Department of Medical Genetics, School of Medical Sciences, Tarbiat Modares University, Tehran, Iran.

References
1. Linden SC, Bergh ARM, Vught-Lussenburg BMA, Jonker LRA, Teunis M, Krul CAM, et al. Development of a panel of high-throughput reporter-gene assays to detect genotoxicity and oxidative stress. MUTAT RES-GEN TOX EN. 2014;760:23–32.
2. Wang X, Hayes J, Wolf C. Generation of a stable antioxidant response element-driven reporter gene cell line and its use to show redox-dependent activation of nrf2 by cancer chemotherapeutic agents. Cancer Res. 2006;66:10983–94.
3. Lyakhovich VV, Vavilin VA, Zenkov NK, Menshchikova EB. Active defense under oxidative stress. The antioxidant responsive element. Biochemistry. 2006;71:962–74.

4. Rushmore T, Morton M, Pickett C. The antioxidant responsive element. Activation by oxidative stress and identification of the DNA consensus sequence required for functional activity. JBC. 1991;266(18):11632–9.

5. Kaspar JW, Niture SK, Jaiswal AK. Nrf2:INrf2 (Keap1) signaling in oxidative stress. Free Radic Biol Med. 2009;47(9):1304–9.

6. Li Y, Jaiswal A. Regulation of human NAD(P)H:quinone oxidoreductase gene. Role of AP1 binding site contained within human antioxidant response element. J Biol Chem. 1992;267:15097–104.

7. Apic G, Ignjatovic T, Boyer S, Russell R. Illuminating drug discovery with biological pathways. FEBS Lett. 2005;579(8):1872–7.

8. Xie T, Belinsky M, Xu Y, Jaiswal AK. ARE- and TRE-mediated regulation of gene expression. Response to xenobiotics and antioxidants. J Biol Chem. 1995;270(12):6894–900.

9. Nioi P, McMahon M, Itoh K, Yamamoto M, Hayes JD. Identification of a novel Nrf2-regulated antioxidant response element (ARE) in the mouse NAD(P)H:quinone oxidoreductase 1 gene: reassessment of the ARE consensus sequence. Biochem J. 2003;374(Pt 2):337–48.

10. Gómez-Lechón MJ, Tolosa L, Donato MT. Cell-based models to predict human hepatotoxicity of drugs. Rev Toxicol. 2014;31:149–56.

11. Krelle AC, Okoli AS, Mendz GL. Huh-7 Human Liver Cancer Cells: A Model System to Understand Hepatocellular Carcinoma and Therapy. JCT. 2013;4:606–31.

12. Choi S, Sainz Jr B, Corcoran P, Uprichard S, Jeong H. Characterization of increased drug metabolism activity in dimethyl sulfoxide (DMSO)-treated Huh7 hepatoma cells. Xenobiotica. 2009;39(3):205–17.

13. Zolghadr F, Sadeghizadeh M, Amirizadeh N, Hosseinkhani S, Nazem S. How benzene and its metabolites affect human marrow derived mesenchymal stem cells. Toxicol Lett. 2012;214(2):145–53.

14. Moran JL, Siegel D, Ross D. A potential mechanism underlying the increased susceptibility of individuals with a polymorphism in NAD(P)H:quinone oxidoreductase 1 (NQO1) to benzene toxicity. JBC. 1998;263(27):13572–8.

15. Rubio V, Zhang J, Valverde M, Rojas E, Shi Z. Essential role of Nrf2 in protection against hydroquinone- and benzoquinone-induced cytotoxicity. Toxicol In Vitro. 2011;25(2):521–9.

16. Tahmasebi Mirgani M, Isacchi B, Sadeghizadeh M, Marra F, Bilia AR, Mowla SJ, et al. Dendrosomal curcumin nanoformulation downregulates pluripotency genes via miR-145 activation in U87MG glioblastoma cells. Int J Nanomedicine. 2014;9:403–17.

17. Balogun E, Hoque M, Gong P, Killeen E, Green CJ, Foresti R, et al. Curcumin activates the haem oxygenase-1 gene via regulation of Nrf2 and the antioxidant-responsive element. BJ. 2003;371(Pt 3):887–95.

18. Garg R, Gupta S, Maru G. Dietary curcumin modulates transcriptional regulators of phase I and phase II enzymes in benzo[a]pyrene-treated mice: mechanism of its anti-initiating action. J Carcinog. 2008;29(5):1022–32.

19. González-Reyes S, Guzmán-Beltrán S, Medina-Campos ON, Pedraza-Chaverri J. Curcumin Pretreatment Induces Nrf2 and an Antioxidant Response and Prevents Hemin-Induced Toxicity in Primary Cultures of Cerebellar Granule Neurons of Rats. Oxid Med Cell Longev. 2013;2013(2013):1–19.

20. Aneck-Hahn N, Bornman M, Jager CD. A relevant battery of screening assays to determine estrogenic and androgenic activity in environmental samples for South Africa, WISA, Biennial 19 Conference and Exhibition Durban International Convention Centre, Durban, South Africa. 2006.

18

Comparison of the effects of Crataegus oxyacantha extract, aerobic exercise and their combination on the serum levels of ICAM-1 and E-Selectin in patients with stable angina pectoris

Leila Jalaly[1*], Gholamreza Sharifi[1], Mohammad Faramarzi[2], Alireza Nematollahi[3], Mahmoud Rafieian-kopaei[4], Masoud Amiri[5] and Fariborz Moattar[6]

Abstract

Background: Adhesion molecules play an important role in the development and progression of coronary atherosclerosis. The aim of this study was comparing the effect of Cratagol herbal tablet, aerobic exercise and their combination on the serum levels of Intercellular adhesion molecule (ICAM)-1 and E-Selectin in patients with stable angina pectoris.

Methods: Eighty stable angina pectoris patients aged between 45 and 65 years, were randomly divided into four groups including three experimental groups and one control group: aerobic exercise (E), Crataegus oxyacantha extract (S), aerobic exercise and Crataegus oxyacantha extract (S+E), and control (C). Blood sampling was taken 24 h before and after 12 weeks of aerobic exercise and Crataegus oxyacantha extract consumption. The results of serum levels of ICAM-1 and E-selectin were compared.

Results: Intergroup comparison of the data revealed a significant reduction ($P < 0.01$) in serum levels of ICAM-1 and E-selectin in experimental groups. Analysis of data showed that the serum levels of ICAM-1 had significant difference when group S+E was compared with groups S and C, but not group E ($P = 0.021$, $P = 0.000$ and $P = 0.068$, respectively). Also the difference between the levels of E-selectin was significant comparing S+E and S but not E with group C ($P = 0.021$, $P = 0.000$ and $P = 0.052$, respectively).

Conclusions: Twelve weeks effects of aerobic exercise and Crataegus oxyacantha extract consuming is an effective complementary strategy to significantly lower the risk of atherosclerosis and heart problems.

Keywords: Aerobic exercise, Cratagol, ICM-1, E-selectin, Stable angina pectoris

Background

Stable angina pectoris is a type of ischemic heart disease described by the discomfort (pain rarely called) in the depth of the chest which has no specific location [1]. The heart coronary inflammation and atherosclerosis are the main causes of chest angina [2, 3]. As mediating agents during different stages of the atherosclerosis, adhesion molecules play important roles in leukocyte recruitment to the surface of vascular endothelium especially in the earlier stages of atherosclerosis. In addition, in atherosclerosis region the leukocyte recruitment on the endothelial cell surface is performed by Cell adhesion molecules (CAMs). As a result, inflammatory agents and adhesion molecules can cause insufficient blood circulation in myocardial tissue and the lack of oxygen leads to the disintegration of these tissues resulting in unstable improper performance of biochemical, mechanical and electrical activities of myocardium. Thus

* Correspondence: Leila_jalaly@yahoo.com
[1]Department of Exercise Physiology, Isfahan (Khorasgan) Branch, Islamic Azad University, Isfahan, Iran
Full list of author information is available at the end of the article

eliminating or reducing of these agents can increase the availability of oxygen to tissues and may help to reduce the heart problems. Among the adhesion cells that have been proved their role in cardiovascular disease especially in atherosclerosis, are Intercellular adhesion molecule (ICAM)-1, Vascular cell adhesion molecule (VCAM)-1 and E-selectin [4, 5]. Intercellular adhesion molecules (ICAMs) are cell surface glycoproteins that in inflammatory condition expressed on a wide variety of cell types including leukocytes, epithelial cells, endothelial cells and fibroblasts while, they are low-expressed in the normal conditions in the vascular endothelial cells, lymphocytes, and monocyte [6].

The demonstration of soluble E-selectin in blood can thus be considered as conclusive evidence of endothelial activation. E-selectin facilitates the earlier stages of polymorphonuclear adhesion to the endothelial cell, constituting an early serum marker of the inflammatory response and promoting cellular damage by ischemia [7]. In the prevention and treatment decade, more attention has been focused on the role of inflammatory factors in the development of atherosclerosis [8]. Therefore the chemical drugs such as non-steroidal anti-inflammatory drugs (NSAIDs) have been used frequently for management of this condition. The meta-analysis of these non-steroidal anti-inflammatory drugs has showed their strong relation with the risk of myocardial infarction, shock and heart stroke [9]. Among the common anti-inflammatory drugs herbal medicines are well known. Several botanicals including Crataegus oxyacantha extract has been shown to play a role in the improve of cardiovascular diseases such as hypertension, hyperlipidemia, and in particular, congestive heart failure [10–13]. In this regard, it was found that these effects may in part be due to the presence of antioxidant flavonoid components [1, 12]. According to conducted researches in attempt to discover new ways to reduce these diseases, it seems that Crataegus oxyacantha extract can be effective to reduce inflammatory adhesion molecules such as ICAM-1 and E-selectin that are new indicators in the development and progression of cardiovascular disease.

Aerobic training can caused reduction in serum levels of ICAM-1 and E-selectin, too [14]. However, the changes in serum levels of CAM-1 and E-selectin in response to aerobic exercise reported conflictingly in various research findings [15–18]. Nevertheless, as far as we know, there is no report on the effect of Crataegus on plasma inflammatory factor and adhesion molecule levels. Walker et al. and Yuen et al. [19, 20] studied the effect of aerobic exercise in interaction with plant Crataegus, but in these studies only the favorable effects on blood pressure, asthma, and enhanced exercise capacity after consumption of herbal Crataegus were reported.

The probable effect of herbal remedy in combination with physical activity is the method, which can be considered to be special. Because of the importance of this issue, this study was aimed to focus on anti-inflammatory effects of Crataegus oxyacantha extract and aerobic training in patients with stable angina to determine how efficient are these methods, and to focus on the effect of Crataegus oxyacantha extract for the first time in combination with aerobic exercise on serum ICAM-1 and E-selectin.

Methods

Crataegus oxyacantha extract

Patients were given the Crataegus oxyacantha extract in Cratagol tablets form. Cratagol was produced at Goldaru pharmaceutical company (Isfahan, Iran) as a Coated tablets in packs of 30 tablets containing 240 mg of dried extract of Crataegus (Hawthorn) leaves and flowers that had been standardized as 4–6 mg Vitexin-2- ramnozide per each tablet. Crataegus oxyacantha extract in Cratagol tablets was produced at EPO Istituto Farmochimico Fltoterapico S.r.l. company (20141 Milano, Italy) (Additional file 1: Appendix A. Supplementary Information). Also Cratagol tablets containing adjuvants Avicel, corn starch, talc, magnesium stearate and Arvzyl. In addition, the researchers had no organizational or financial dependence to the company manufacturing crataegus extract.

Placebo tablets

Placebo tablets were prepared from Goldaru pharmaceutical company (Isfahan, Iran). The placebo was prepared from granulated of inert powder of lactose and the core of pressed tablets was coated similar to that of Cratagol and the produced tablets were entirely similar to the original product in terms of color, size and appearance. The tablets were encoded and they were used in clinical studies through the Double Blind Method. Original and placebo tablets were previously coded and after the required experiments the type of drugs based on their codes in studied subjects were determined, then statistical analysis were performed.

Expriments

Subjects were included patients with stable angina who were under treatment at the Imam Ali cardioligy subspecialty polyclinic of Shahrekord, Iran. The diagnosis of stable angina pectoris in the patients was performed by Professor of Cardiology with coronary angiography test. Patients whose angiography test history was carried out between 1 and 12 months ago and there were no new symptoms of pain or discomfort during this period and also their coronary atherosclerosis was less than 50 %, with clear treatment history within past 3 months, aged between 45 and 65 years were selected for this study. 1500 potential cases of stable angina patients who were under treatment at the Imam Ali cardioligy sub-specialty polyclinic of Shahrekord, Iran were investigated. Most of these patients were out of our entrance requirements, also unwillingness to participate the study, severe heart failure, lack of accessibility, pharmacological interventions and death were of the criteria for which the participants were eliminated and also patients with severe heart failure and/or treated with digoxin, cisapride, anticoagulant, anti-arrhythmic drugs were excluded. Finally, 80 patients (44 male and 36 female) suffering from ischemic heart disease of stable angina were recruited and randomly assigned into four groups (20 patients (11 male and 9 female)): three experimental groups including aerobic exercise and placebo (E), Crataegus oxyacantha extract (S), aerobic exercise and Crataegus oxyacantha extract (S + E) and one control group (C) and were followed for 12 weeks. Patients in each group were homogenate with regards to age, sex, weight, and Body Mass Index (BMI). Because of the relationship between individual characteristics such as sex, age, BMI, and weight and inflammatory markers measured in this study, we attract the reviewer's attention to the fact that the researchers tried to reduce bias in the results by choosing four homogenated groups. In particular, in order to excluding the effect of sex on the results, the number of males and females were equal in both groups, however, the distribution of men and women based on their number was accidental. Random number tables were used where each value was randomly selected with an equal chance of choosing any integer among 1–44 (men) and 45–80 (women) by QuickCalcs online calculator (http://www.graphpad.com/quickcalcs/randomn2.cfm) (Additional file 2: Table S1 and S2), which allocated the numbers randomly to control and experimental groups. Also, the amount of physical activity, nutrition, diet, smoking, alcohol, symptoms and duration of angina were accurately determined through medical record questionnaires and reports contained in patient records. As well as, we had no crossover or contamination between groups and the current study was carried out as multiple parallel groups until the end of experiments. The patients in all 4 groups were administered with Methoral (50 mg/day), Aspirin (80 mg/day), and sublingual Nitroglycerin in case of discomfort. Crataegus oxyacantha extract were additionally taken by patients in the experimental groups (S) and (S+E), twice a day, and each time one tablet along with chemical medication with a little water before meals. The control group (C) did not take any Crataegus oxyacantha extract. The control group in this study was not influenced by any intervention and also did not receive the placebo tablets, but during the experimental period, the weekly report of their nutritional status and physical activity were recorded and were under control. This project was approved by the ethics committee of the Medical University of Shahrekord, Iran and was recorded in the clinical trial center with registration number IRCT201303098435N1. The participants had sufficient information and awareness to participate in the study and the process by which they filled out the consent form was controlled and documented (Fig. 1).

Exercise program

Aerobic exercise program was performed on a treadmill (after one week pre-adaptation) with an intensity of 40–60 % of heart rate reserve (HRR) and a rating of perceived exertion (RPE) of 11–13 (on 6–20 Borg scale), twice a week, each time 20–30 min, for 3 month (12 week) [21]. Meanwhile, The patient's conditions and emotions, intensity and duration of exercise, blood pressure, resting and exercise heart rate were controlled at the beginning, during, and after exercise by digital stethoscope (Geratherm Medical AG, German) and recorded. The exercise was stopped in case of discomfort in the chest, asthma, dizziness, fatigue and loss of systolic blood pressure more than 10 mm Hg and the exercises were continued, modified or interrupted under the opinion of psychiatrists. The data obtained from exercise and blood tests were collectively recorded in separate sheets for final analysis. Training exercise was carried out by specialized expert, under the direction of Professor of Cardiology in the Imam Ali sub-specialty polyclinic of Shahrekord, Iran.

Blood tests

Fasting blood test was performed 24 h before study and also after 12 weeks. Blood tests were performed in specialized laboratories from 5 ml blood sample of arm vein of each patient. After 5 min of coagulation time, the samples were centrifuged at 3000 rpm for 10 min. Immediately blood tests were performed to determine the levels of ICAM-1 and E-Selectin in serum using a detection kit in specialized laboratories.

Measurements

Serum concentrations of ICAM-1, and E-selectin were carried out using standard ELISA Kit (Boster, USA), with a sensitivity of 10 pg/ml and 4 pg/ml respectively. An ELISA reader (Ststfax 2100, USA) was also used.

Statistical analysis

Data were analyzed using SPSS 17 and the results presented as mean ± standard deviation. Comparisons between groups were made using the Kolmogorov-Smirnov test as well as ANOVA followed by Least significant difference (LSD) test. A two-sided P-value of 0.05 was considered as statistically significant.

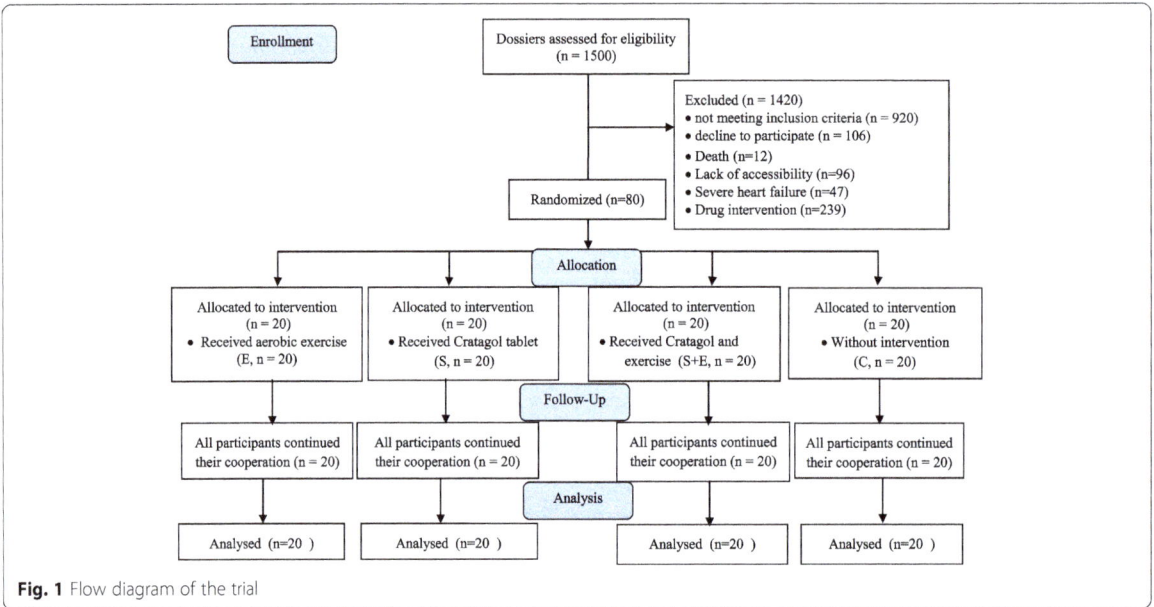

Fig. 1 Flow diagram of the trial

Results

The data were classified according to average and standard deviation in intervention and control groups. The Kolmogorov-Smirnov test showed normal distribution of data in all stages of pre-test and post-test. Statical analysis showed that there were not any significant baseline difference in serum levels of ICAM-1 between groups ($F = 0.28$, $P = 0.834$). Also, there were not any significant baseline difference in the levels of E-selectin between groups ($F = 0.97$, $P = 0.411$).

The result of descriptive data for inflammatory factors mean difference in each group, as well as the result of t-test related to control and experimental groups between pre-test and post-test are presented in Table 1. A significant decline ($p < 0.01$) was observed in the

mean difference between pre-test and post-test in all three experimental groups including aerobic exercise (E), Crataegus oxyacantha extract (S), combination of aerobic exercise and consumption of Crataegus oxyacantha extract (S+E) in the levels of ICAM-1 and E-selectin, while in the control group the decrease due to intake of chemical drugs did not show any significant difference (ICAM-1, $P = 0.412$, E-selectin, $P = 0.313$) (Table 1).

Statical Analysis of data showed a significant difference in serum levels of ICAM-1 in experimental groups ($F = 5.91$, $P = 0.002$). Post hoc test showed that the serum levels of ICAM-1 had significant difference when group S + E was compared with groups S and C, but not group E ($P = 0.021$, $P = 0.000$ and $P = 0.068$, respectively). Also, significant differences in the levels of E-selectin was observed among experimental groups ($F = 3.34$, $P = 0.023$). Post hoc test showed that the difference between the levels of E-selectin was significant comparing S+E and S but not E with group C ($P = 0.021$, $P = 0.000$ and $P = 0.052$, respectively).

According to the weekly reports of patients' condition during the study (12 weeks) there was not seen any side effects and evaluation of this case is out of our duty.

Discussion

The purpose of this study was comparing the effect of Crataegus oxyacantha extract consumption, aerobic exercise or their combination on the serum levels of ICAM-1 and E-Selectin in patients with stable angina pectoris.

One of the important finding of the present study was the reduction in serum levels of ICAM-1 and E-Selectin due to aerobic exercise. The changes in serum levels of

Table 1 Descriptive data t-test between pre-test and post-tes

Variables	Group($n = 20$)	Means ± SD		P
		Pre-test	Post-test	
ICAM-1(ng/ml)	E	65.5 ± 39.7	20.8 ± 2.7	0.001
	S	61.3 ± 38.1	23.1 ± 3.7	0.001
	S+E	90 ± 53.5	21.9 ± 3.9	0.001
	C	56.1 ± 36	42.1 ± 33.1	0.412
E-selectin(ng/ml)	E	3.2 ± 1.5	1.8 ± 1	0.001
	S	3.4 ± 1.9	2.2 ± 1.3	0.003
	S+E	3.5 ± 1.3	1.8 ± 0.7	0.001
	C	2.7 ± 1.3	2.4 ± 1.2	0.313

Aerobic exercise ((E), $n = 20$, 11 males, 9 female), Crataegus oxyacantha extract ((S), $n = 20$, 11 males, 9 female), Aerobic exercise and Crataegus oxyacantha extract supplements ((S + E), $n = 20$, 11 males, 9 female), Control ((C), $n = 20$, 11 males, 9 female), significant ($P < 0.05$) in all groups except control (C)

ICAM-1 and E-selectin in response to aerobic exercise reported conflictingly in various research findings but Studies have shown that ICAM-1 and E-selectin have a similar relationship [15–17, 22–24]. Much evidence suggests that inflammation plays important role in the process of atherosclerosis [16]. During inflammation process, cytokines such as TNF-a, IL-1B, IL-6, IL-10, IL-1ra, sTNF-R are produced and activated at the site of inflammation [8]. In the adhesion step, when leukocytes are approaching the side of endothelial cells, molecules such as VCAM- and ICAM-1 [25] and E-selectin [26] accumulated. Changes in adhesion molecules such as ICAM-1 and E-Selectin are closely related to leukocyte accumulation and inflammatory factors C-reactive protein (CRP), Interleukin (IL)-6, Tumor necrosis factor (TNF)-a, and Creatine kinase (CK). So the activity of endothelial injuring markers is influenced by inflammatory factors [15]. The increased expression of ICAM-1 is dependent on nuclear factor-kappa B (NF-KB) And the increased level of cytokines particularly Interleukin-1 beta (IL-1B), is responsible for the production of E-selectin [6, 7, 27]. Studies showed that physical activity can reduce the resting levels of these cytokines by reducing obesity, leptin and increasing the adiponectin and insulin sensitivity [16, 28–30]. Exercise training can effect on adhesion molecules and endothelial injuring markers by decreasing of inflammatory factors particularly NF-KB and IL-1B [22, 31].

One of the most important finding of this study was the reduction in the serum levels of ICAM-1 and E-selectin after taking Crataegus oxyacantha extract. Crataegus extract via its protective effect against oxidative stress caused by released free radicals, which in turn it can improve cardiac function and reduce infarct size in a rat model of prolonged coronary ischemia and reperfusion [10]. Chen et al. [32] stated that Crataegus improved endothelial function so exposed anti hypertension properties. Crataegus stabilizes collagen function trough prevention of its degradation by secreted enzymes from leukocytes during inflammation, so the adverse effect of atherosclerotic plaques and produced endothelial injury markers on vessels can be prevented. it also inhibit the action of free radicals so improves coronary artery dilation and blood supply to the heart muscle via prevention the activity of phosphodiesterase-Cyclic adenosine mono-phosphate enzyme resulting in increase of cyclic Adenosine monophosphate (AMP) in myocardium and increase of its contractile strength. It increases the time of excitability of heart muscle by blocking potassium channels, which ultimately will lead to improved arrhythmia [33, 34].

Of the other important finding in this study was the reduction in serum levels of ICAM-1 and E-Selectin due to aerobic exercise along with Crataegus oxyacantha extract consumption. Walker et al. [19] were examined the promising hypotensive effect of Crataegus extracts. In this study, the blood pressure values at rest, after exercise and after a stress test were evaluated which both of systolic and diastolic blood pressure decreased in all experimental groups. In addition, the desire to reduce anxiety in those who had received Crataegus was seen compared to the other groups [19]. Crataegus extract in comparison with placebo increased the exercise tolerance in the congestive heart failure. Since the patients during the treatment period were not exposed to any other cardio-active drug, it was proved that advancing in exercise tolerance was due to the action of the Crataegus extract [20]. Exercise program improves environmental inflammatory markers associated with endothelial dysfunction such as soluble intercellular adhesion molecules and vascular, colony factor stimulating of granulocyte and macrophage and chemo attractant protein 1 by increasing of available nitro oxide [16, 27, 35]. Because of its anti-hypertension property, Crataegus can help to improve endothelial function and to reduce the production of inflammatory markers and adhesion molecules through inducing endothelium-dependent no-mediated vasorelaxation by eNOS phosphorylation [12, 32, 36]. Physical activity decreased the oxidative stress by modifying the anti-oxidative defenses in serum [37–39]. In addition, the prescription of Crataegus extract through its protective effect against oxidative stress can result in improvement of cardiac function [10, 40, 41]. Endurance activities and reduction in carbohydrate storage of the body increase the epinephrine, norepinephrine, the growth hormone, and cortisol by the endocrine system, resulting in increase of lipid oxidation [42], While the other part of the beneficial effects of Crataegus can be considered for reduction of lipid peroxidation and oxidative stress in vascular tissue [10, 40, 43]. Since adipose tissue is one of the main locations of secretion the inflammatory markers and cytokines, endurance exercise in combination with Crataegus consumption increases lipolysis rate and decreases the body fat, so it can be considered as an effective strategy to reduce inflammatory mediators and cell adhesion molecules [11, 44]. This may explain the observed stronger effect in the combination group (S+E). Therefore in this study, the exercise along with consumption of Crataegus oxyacantha extract resulted in double reducing of plasma ICAM-1 and E-selectin. While we could not fully control diet, rest, exercise and mental stress outside the clinic environment.

Conclusion

Our findings suggest that aerobic exercise and Crataegus oxyacantha extract over a period of 12 weeks significantly reducing of plasma Cell adhesion molecules in patients with stable angina pectoris. However, since aerobic exercise and herbal drug induces many physiological processes in the body, evaluation of the interaction between aerobic exercise and herbal drug effects in patients with heart disease needs further study.

Additional files

Additional file 1: Appendix A. (DOCX 6257 kb)

Additional file 2: Appendix B. Table S1. Random numbers between 1 and 44 (males). **Table S2.** Random numbers between 45 and 80 (female). (DOCX 23 kb)

Competing interest
The authors declare that they have no competing interest.

Authors' contribution
LJ designed the study, conducted the research, participated in the sequence alignment and drafted the manuscript. GS participated in the sequence alignment. MF participated in the sequence alignment and participated in the design of the study. AN and MR conceived of the study, and participated in its design and coordination and helped to draft the manuscript. MA performed the statistical analysis. FM participated in the sequence alignment. All authors read and approved the final manuscript.

Acknowledgements
We thank the pharmaceutical company Goldaru (Isfahan, Iran) for providing the Cratagol herbal heart tablet, and also president and personnel of medical plants research center university of medical siences and Imam Ali subspecialty polyclinic (shahrekord, Iran) for the corporation in project.
Authors: All research done by the authors.
Financial support: yes.

Author details
[1]Department of Exercise Physiology, Isfahan (Khorasgan) Branch, Islamic Azad University, Isfahan, Iran. [2]Associate Professor in Exercise Physiology, Shahrekord University, Shahrekord, Iran. [3]Subspecialist of Cardiology and Assistant Professor, Shahrekord Univercity of Medical Sciences, Shahrekord, Iran. [4]Medical Plants Research Center, Shahrekord Univercity of Medical Sciences, Shahrekord, Iran. [5]Health Research Center, Shahrekord Univercity of Medical Sciences, Shahrekord, Iran. [6]School of Pharmacy and Pharmaceutical Sciences, Isfahan University of Medical Sciences and Health Services, Isfahan, Iran.

References
1. Braunwald E. Heart disease: a textbook of cardiovascular medicine. 5th ed. Philadelphia: WB Saunders Co; 2001. p. 1210–15.
2. Khastkhodaei S, Sharifi G, Salahi R, Rahnamaeian M, Moattar F. Clinical efficacy of Stragol herbal heart drop in ischemic heart failure of stable chest angina. Eur J Intern Med. 2011;104:7.
3. Roitman J, Lafontaine T. The exercise professionals guide to optimizing health: strategies for preventing and reducing chronic disease. Philadelphia: Lippincott William & Wilkins; 2011. p. 288.
4. Mogharnasi M, Gaeini AA, Sheikholeslami Vatani D. Effect of sprint training and detraining period on cellular adhesion molecule (sICAM-1) in wistar rats. Olympic. 2008;16:19–30 (Persian).
5. O'Brien KA, Ling S, Abbas E, Dai A, Zhang J, Wang WC, et al. A chinese herbal preparation containing radix Salviae Miltiorrhizae, radix Notoginseng and Borneolum Syntheticum reduces circulating adhesion molecules. Evid Based Complement Alternat Med. 2011;2011(Article ID 790784):6.
6. Xu Y, Li S. Blockade of ICAM-1: a novel way of vasculitis treatment. Biochem Biophys Res Commun. 2009;381:459–61.
7. Macias C, Villaescusa R, Valle LD, Boffil V, Cordero G, Hernández A, et al. Endothelial adhesion molecules ICAM-1, VCAM-1 and E-selectin in patients with acute coronary syndrome. Rev Esp Cardiol. 2003;56(2):137–44.
8. Pedersen BK. The anti-inflammatory effect of exercise: its role in diabetes and cardiovascular disease control. Biochem Soc. 2006;42:105–17.
9. Trelle S, Rechenbach S, Wandel S, Hildebrand P, Tschannen B, Villiger PM, et al. Cardiovascular safety of non-steroidal anti-inflammatory drugs: network metaanalysis. BMJ. 2011;342:c7086.
10. Veveris M, Koch E, Chatterjee SS. Crataegus special extract WS 1442 improves cardiac function and reduces infarct size in a rat model of prolonged coronary ischemia and reperfusion. Life Sci. 2004;74(15):1945–55.
11. Li HB, Fang KY, Lü CT, Li XE. Study on lipidregulating function for the extracts and their prescriptions from Semen Cassiae and fructus crataegi. Zhong Yao Cai. 2007;30(5):573–5.
12. Chang WT, Dao J, Shao ZH. Hawthorn: potential roles in cardiovascular disease. Am J Chin Med. 2005;33(1):1–10.
13. Walker AF, Marakis G, Simpson E, Hope JL, Robinson PA, Hassanein M, et al. Hypotensive effects of hawthorn for patients with diabetes taking prescription drugs: a randomised controlled trial. Br J Gen Pract. 2006; 56(527):437–43.
14. Saetre T, Enoksen E, Lyberg T, Stranden E, Jorgensen JJ, Sundhagen JO, et al. Supervised exercise training reduces plasma levels of the endothelial inflammatory markers E-selectin and ICAM-I in patients with peripheral arterial disease. Angioligy. 2011;62(4):301–5.
15. Jee H, Jin Y. Effects of prolonged endurance exercise on vascular endothelial and inflammation markers. J Sports Sci Med. 2012;11:719–26.
16. Kasapis C, Thompson PD. The effects of physical activity on serum C-Reactive Protein and inflammatory markers. J Am Coll Cardiol. 2005;45:1563–9.
17. Hatunic M, Finucane F, Burns N, Gasparro D, Nolan JJ. Vascular inflammatory markers in early-onset obese and type 2 diabetes subjects before and after three months' aerobic exercise training. Diab Vasc Dis Res. 2007;4:231–4.
18. Niebauer J, Clark AL, Webb-Peploe KM, Coats AJS. Exercise training in chronic heart failure: effects on pro-inflammatory markers. Eur J Heart Fail. 2005;7:189–93.
19. Walker AF, Marakis G, Morris AP, Robinson PA. Promising hypotensive effect of hawthorn extract: a randomized double-bind pilot study of mild, essential hypertension. Phytother Res. 2002;16:48–54.
20. Yuen YP, Lai CK, Poon WT, Ng SW, Chan AYW, Mak TWL. Adulteration of over-the-counter slimming products with pharmaceutical analogue–an emerging threat. Hong Kong Med J. 2007;13(3):216–20.
21. Ehrman JK, Gordon PM, Visich PS. Visich, Keteyian SJ. Clinical exercise physiology. USA(Champaign): Human Kinetics 2013;776.
22. Hejazi SM, Abrishami LH, Mohammad Khani J, Boghrabadi V. The effects of 8-week aerobic exercises on serum levels of cell adhesion molecules among middle-aged women. Adv Stud Biol. 2013;5(6):279–89.
23. Reihmane D, Tretjakovs P, Kaupe J, Sars M, Valante R, Jurka A. Systemic pro-inflammatory molecule response to acute submaximal exercise in moderately and highly trained athletes. Environ Exper Biol. 2012;10:107–12.
24. Nassis GP, Papantakou K, Skenderi K, Triandafillopoulou M, Karouras SA, Yannakoulia M, et al. Aerobic exercise training improves insulin sensitivity without changes in body weight, body fat, adiponectin and inflammatory markers in over weight and obese girls. Metabolism. 2005;54(11):1472–9.
25. Muller WA. Mechanisms of transendothelial migration of leukocytes. Circ Res. 2006;105:223–30.
26. van Buul JD, Hordijk PL. Endothelial adapter proteins in leukocyte transmigration. Thromb Haemost. 2009;101:649–55.
27. Niebauer J. Effects of exercise training on inflammatory markers in patients with heart failure. Heart Fail Rev. 2008;13:39–49.
28. Golbid S, Badran M, Laher I. Antioxidant and anti-inflammatory effects of exercise in diabetic patients. Exp Diabetes Res. 2012;Article ID 941868:1–16.
29. Ploeger HE, Takken T, de Greef MHG, Timmons BW. The effects of acute and chronic exercise on inflammatory markers in children and adults with a chronic inflammatory disease: a systematic review. Exerc Immunol Rev. 2009;15:6–41.
30. Sixt S, Beer S, Bluher M, Korff N, Peschel T, Sonnabend M, et al. Long-but not short-term multifactorial intervention with focus on exercise training improves coronary endothelial dysfunction in diabetes mellitus type 2 and coronary artery disease. Eur Heart J. 2010;31:112–9.
31. Blake GJ, Ridker PM. Novel clinical marker of vascular wall inflammation. Circ Res. 2001;89(9):763–71.
32. Chen ZY, Peng C, Jiao R, Wong YM, Yang N, Huang Y. Anti-hypertensive nutraceuticals and functional foods. J Agric Food Chem. 2009;57:4485–99.
33. Chevallier A. Herbal remedies. USA (New York): Dorling Kindersley, 2008;288.

34. Al Makdessi S, Sweidan H, Mullner S, Jacob R. Myocardial protection by pretreatment with Crataegus oxyacantha. Arzneimittelforschung. 1996;46(1):25–7.
35. Giannuzzi P, Temporelli PL, Corra' U, Tavazzi L. Antiremodeling effect of long-term exercise training in patients with stable chronic heart failure: results of the exercise in left ventricular dysfunction and chronic heart failure (ELVD-CHF) trial. Circulation. 2003;108:554–9.
36. Mori S, Takemoto M, Yokote K, Asaumi S, Saito Y. Hyperglycemia-induced alteration of vascular smooth muscle phenotype. J Diabet Complicat. 2002;16(1):65–8.
37. Sun L, Shen W, Liu Z, Guan S, Liu J, Ding S. Endurance exercise causes mitochondrial and oxidative stress in rat liver: effects of a combination of mitochondrial targeting nutrients. Life Sci. 2010;86:39–44.
38. Hovanloo F, Hedayati M, Ebrahimi M, Abednazari H. Effect of various time courses of endurance training on alterations of antioxidant enzymes activity in rat liver tissue. Pejouhesh. 2011;35(1):14–9.
39. Stanković M, Radovanović D. Oxidative stress and physical activity. SportLogia. 2012;8(1):1–11.
40. Peschel W, Bohr C, Plescher A. Variability of total flavonoids in Crataegus - factor evaluation for the monitored production of industrial starting material. Fitoterapia. 2008;79(1):6–20.
41. Machha A, Achike FI, Mustafa AM, Mustafa MR. Quercetin, a flavonoid antioxidant, modulates endothelium-derived nitric oxide bioavailability in diabetic rat aortas. Nitric Oxide. 2007;16(4):442–7.
42. Wegge JK, Roberts CK, Ngo TH, Bamard RJ. Effect of diet and exercise intervention on inflammatory and adhesion molecules in postmenopausal women on hormone replacement therapy and at risk for coronary artery disease. Metabolism. 2004;53:377–81.
43. Vessal M, Hemmati M, Vasei M. Antidiabetic effects of quercetin in streptozocin-induced diabetic rats. Comp Biochem Physiol C Toxicol Pharmacol. 2003;135c(3):357–64.
44. Zoppini G, Targher G, Zamboni C, Venturi C, Cacciatori V, Moghetti P, et al. Effects of moderate-intensity exercise training on plasma biomarkers of inflammation and endothelial dysfunction in order patients with type 2 diabetes. Nutr Metab Cardiovasc Dis. 2006;16(8):543–9.

19

Nanoparticles as potential new generation broad spectrum antimicrobial agents

Clarence S. Yah[1,2*] and Geoffrey S. Simate[3]

Abstract

The rapid emergence of antimicrobial resistant strains to conventional antimicrobial agents has complicated and prolonged infection treatment and increased mortality risk globally. Furthermore, some of the conventional antimicrobial agents are unable to cross certain cell membranes thus, restricting treatment of intracellular pathogens. Therefore, the disease-causing-organisms tend to persist in these cells. However, the emergence of nanoparticle (NP) technology has come with the promising broad spectrum NP-antimicrobial agents due to their vast physiochemical and functionalization properties. In fact, NP-antimicrobial agents are able to unlock the restrictions experienced by conventional antimicrobial agents. This review discusses the status quo of NP-antimicrobial agents as potent broad spectrum antimicrobial agents, sterilization and wound healing agents, and sustained inhibitors of intracellular pathogens. Indeed, the perspective of developing potent NP-antimicrobial agents that carry multiple-functionality will revolutionize clinical medicine and play a significant role in alleviating disease burden.

Introduction

In recent past, microbial infections have become a global health burden due to emerging and resistant strains of viruses [1], bacteria [2], pathogenic fungi [3] and protozoa [4] defying clinical treatment. Consequently, this has culminated into prolonged treatment, higher health expenditure, mortality risk, and low life expectancy [2]. In view of ineffective antimicrobial agents, there is need to seek new alternative and safer antimicrobial agents against these "super bugs" of viruses, bacteria, fungi and protozoa. With the development of biomedical nanomaterials, new antimicrobial agents have begun to emerge either as novel and/or augmenting the activities of the current conventional antimicrobials. This is motivated by the vast physiochemical and functionalization (ligand attachment) properties of nanoparticles (NPs) [5–7]. The NPs physiochemical properties are highly diverse in nature and are highly applicable in biomedical field including antimicrobial and drug delivery [6, 8, 9]. Some examples of these biomedical NPs include silver nanoparticles (AgNPs) [10], carbon nanotubes (CNTs) [11], gold NPs (AuNPs) [12], zinc oxide NPs (ZnO-NPs) [13], and iron oxide NPs (FeO-NPs) [14].

The antimicrobial actions of NPs include cidal destruction of cell membranes, blockage of enzyme pathways, alterations of microbial cell wall, and nucleic materials pathway [1]. However, the antimicrobial mechanisms of the actions are yet to be fully elucidated since some of the NPs drugs are still at their infancy. The high potency of NPs antiviral, antibacterial, antifungal and antiprotozoal activities may revolutionize and bring another turning point in pharmacological therapy. In that regard, this review looks at the status quo of nanomaterials as alternative antimicrobial agents in terms of their broad spectrum ability, the crossing of difficult membrane barriers, delivery and sustained inhibition of intracellular pathogens and sterilization abilities as shown in Fig. 1. This perspective status quo of NP antimicrobial agents with multiple functions will play a significant impact on the treatment of diseases.

Broad spectrum nanoparticle-antimicrobial agents

The global emergence of multidrug-resistant microorganisms (viruses, bacteria, fungi and protozoa) has made conventional treatment of infectious diseases difficult. Therefore, the discovery of alternative new classes of antiviral [15], antibiotics [16], antifungal [17], and

* Correspondence: cyah@nmmu.ac.za
[1]Department of Biochemistry and Microbiology, Nelson Mandela Metropolitan University, Port Elizabeth, South Africa
[2]Department of Epidemiology, Johns Hopkins Bloomberg School of Public Health, E7146, 615 N. Wolfe Street, Baltimore 21205, MD, USA
Full list of author information is available at the end of the article

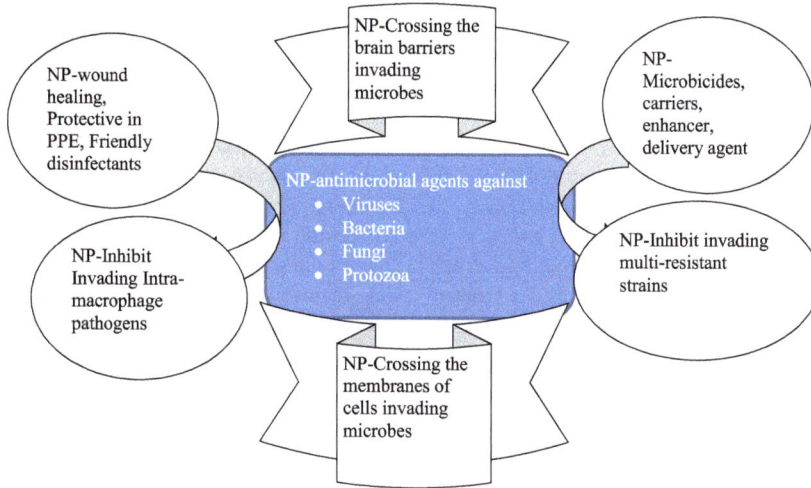

Fig. 1 Multiple functionality and broad spectrum activities of nanoparticles antimicrobial agents. The diverse vast antimicrobial uses of nanoparticle bioconjugates. Used for wound healing, use as anticancers, anti multi-resistant pathogens, aid drugs to cross the blood brain barriers, help in the inhibition of microbes that hide in macrophages. NP = acronyms for Nanoparticles. PPE = Personal Protective equipment incorporated with nanoparticles capable of destroying microbes

antiprotozoal [18] agents that can treat resistant strains is paramount. Research has shown that these emerging broad-spectrum antimicrobial nanomaterial can knock-out diverse pathogenic organisms of different phyla, across diverse and/or within species of viruses, bacteria and fungi [19–22]. For example, Fig. 2 shows the broad spectrum NP-antimicrobial effect of AgNPs. The AgNP

antimicrobial agent has multi-functionality of antibacterial [22], antifungal [22], antiviral [23], anti-parasitic [4], and anti-inflammatory properties [14, 24].

One of the mechanisms of NP-antimicrobial actions is cell wall lysis. For example, a study by Addae et al. [12] in an attempt to produce a transducer agent for photothermal therapy (PTT) found the destruction of *Bacillus*

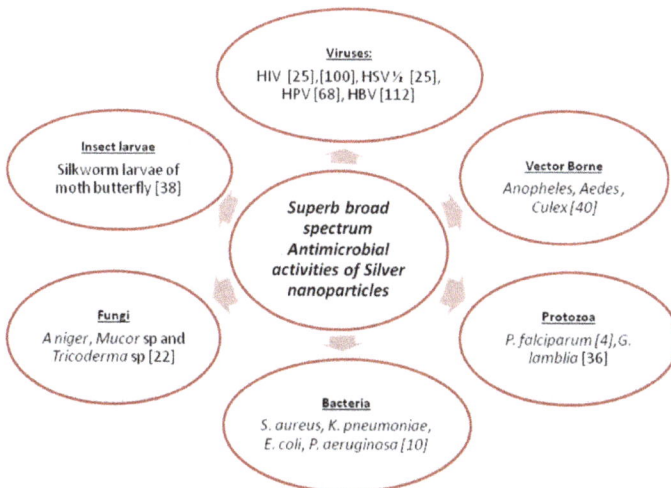

Fig. 2 Broad spectrum NP-antimicrobial activities of silver nanoparticles. The Figure describes the antimicrobial spectrum of silver bio-conjugate nanoparticles against diverse genera of microorganisms. HIV = Human immunodeficiency virus, HSV = Herpes Simplex Virus 1, HPV = Human papillomavirus, HBV = Hepatitis B virus, *P. falciparum* = *Plasmodium falciparum*, *G. lamblia* = *Gardia lamblia*, *S. aureus* = *Staphylococcus aureus*, *E. coli* = *Escherichia coli*, *P. aeruginosa* = *Pseudomonas aeruginosa*, sp = species

species cell membranes when treated with Au/CuS NPs. The destruction of *Bacillus* species in this study proved that Au/CuS NPs are potent NP-antimicrobial agents.

The NPs are potential broad spectrum antibiotics because they can inhibit wide range of multidrug-resistant strains of bacteria that have defied most antibiotic treatment. For example, in the study by Adeli et al. [10] it was found that AgNPs were able to inhibit pan-multidrug resistant strains of *S. aureus, K. pneumoniae, E. coli,* and *P. aeruginosa* that were resistant to all the antibiotic drugs including imipenem. Another similar study by Kathiravan et al. [22] showed that AgNPs can inhibit both bacteria (*S. aureus, E coli, B subtilis*) and fungi species (*A niger, Mucor* sp and *Tricoderma* sp). In addition, earlier findings by Fayaz et al. [25] showed that the AgNPs-coated condom have antiviral (against HIV-1 and HSV-1/2), antibacterial (against *E. coli, S. aureus, M. luteus, K. pneumonia*) and anti-fungi (against *Candida* spp.) properties. This suggests that AgNPs can be used to treat all multi-drug resistant pathogens from diverse phyla from all clinical sources.

The broad spectrum antimicrobial activities have also been demonstrated by CNTs. For example, a study by Tank et al. [26] showed that silica coated silicon nanotubes (SCSNTs) exhibit enhanced antimicrobial activities when compared to other non-silica coated silicon nano-particles. Other studies also found that CNTs containing lysine such as multiwalled CNT (MWCNT)-epilsonpolylysine [27], and SWCNT-poly(L-lysine) (PLL), and poly(L-glutamic acid) [28] exhibit very strong broad antimicrobial activities against a wide range of bacteria. A study by Amiri et al. [29] showed MWCNT-lysine exhibiting very strong broad antimicrobial activity against *S. aureus, S. agalactiae, S. dysgalactiae, E.coli, K. pneumonia* and *Salmonella typhimurium.*

In addition to antimicrobial activities, hybrids of nanomaterials such as cholesterol-containing liposomes phytonanosilver and CNTs have been found to exhibit high antioxidant activity as well as antimicrobial activities against *E. coli, Staphylococcus aureus* and *Enterococcus faecalis* [30]. This shows that when two or more NPs are combined, they tend to enhance the broad spectrum activity of the nano-antimicrobial agents. The hybrid behaviour was equally found when CNTs and AgNP-based nanomaterials were combined and the resulting hybrid biocomposite was found to exhibit stronger and excellent antimicrobial properties [27]. Similarly, chitosan-CNT hybrid showed excellent antimicrobial activities against bacteria and fungi [9]. Other CNTs antimicrobial hybrids include ZnO coated MWCNTs (ZnO/MWCNTs) [13], Triad CNT-NPs/Polymer nanocomposites [11], functionalized MWCNTs-CdS and functionalized-MWCNTs-Ag2S [31], and CdTe QDs/single-walled aluminosilicate nanotubes [32]. Furthermore, Cefalexin-immobilized

multi-walled CNTs have been found to broadly enhance the antimicrobial activities against a wide range of pathogens including *E. coli, P. aeruginosa, S. aureus* and *Bacillus subtilis* [8] as shown in Table 1. The combination of AgNPs and CNTs including MWCNT-AgNPs [33] on fiber membrane has also been found to enhance the filtration and antimicrobial potentials against all types of bacteria. In addition, Poly(N-vinylcarbazole) (PVK)-SWCNT nanocomposite coated membrane for water purification were found to destroy all bacterial species including spore forming organisms such as *Bacillus subtilis* [34]. Apart from filtration and demonstration of antimicrobial activities the MWCNT-AgNPs hybrid composite membrane has been found to significantly reduce biofilm formation which can easily be extended to other types of support membranes [33]. Table 1 summaries the types of NPs and their susceptibility to various organisms.

Nanoparticle anti-parasitic effect

Despite the efforts made in the treatment of parasitic infections, infections by parasites particularly those of giardiasis, schistosomiasis, trypanosomiasis, malaria, leishmaniasis, dengue fevers, Japanese encephalitis, and filariasis continue to increase particularly in tropical and low income countries [24, 35, 36]. The problems associated with parasitic infections include drug toxicity, ineffectiveness, and developments of resistance to conventional anti-parasitic drugs. Furthermore, treatment costs are high, thus limiting supply of drugs in low income countries [37]. As a results of the limitation in anti-parasitic drugs, newer approaches such as nano-biotechnology have shown significant improvement in the treatment of parasitic infections [24]. This is based on the unique properties of NPs including those of AgNPs, AuNPs, chitosan, selenium oxide, and other metallic oxide based NPs that have shown excellent inhibitory effects against parasitic infections including insect larvae [24, 35–38].

Parasites such as *Leishmania* can reside and survive inside macrophages without being exposed to cell damage by reactive oxygen species (ROS) and anti-parasitic drugs [37]. However, AgNPs, because of their trans-membrane mechanisms and sustained anti-parasitic delivery, can inhibit intracellular *Leishmania* and enhance their destruction via ROS [37].

Other NPs including the combination of silver, chitosan, and curcumin nanoparticles have been used in the treatment of *Giardia lamblia* as demonstrated in experimental animals [36]. The findings also showed that *Giardia lamblia* can be successfully eradicated from stool and intestine [36]. The potential of NPs if fully optimized may lead to the development of newer synergic antimicrobials where two or more nano-antimicrobials are combined to generate an effective efficacy in the

Table 1 Summary of the types of nanoparticles susceptibility to organisms

Type of NP	Method of NPs characterization	Size of NP	Types organisms inhibited	Outcome	Toxicity	Author
Fe-Oxide NP & AgNP	UV–vis spectroscopy, Fourier Transform Infrared Spectroscopy (FTIR), Transmission Electron Microscopy (TEM)	Fe-oxide NP 20–40 nm, AgNP 10–20 nm	Bacillus, E. coli and Staphylococcus species	Fe-Oxide NPs were sensitive against Bacillus, E. coli and Staphylococcus species.	The very smaller size AgNP were toxic against the pathogens	[14]
Ag NPs.	TEM, Field Emission Transmission Electron Microscopy (FESEM), FTIR, UV–Vis spectra, Raman spectroscopy, X-ray Difraction (XRD)	Average 18–20 nm	Escherichia coli, Pseudomonas spp. Bacillus species, Staphylococcus species, Aspergillus niger, Aspergillus flavus, Penicillium	Inhibited the growth and multiplication of E. coli, Pseudomonas species, Bacillus spp. and Staphylococcus species, A. niger, A. flavus, Penicillium spp	ND	[98]
Silver, chitosan, and curcumin nanoparticles	NA	-	Giardia lamblia	The highest effect was achieved by combining the three nanoforms. The parasite was found to be eradicated from stool and intestine.	None of the nanoparticle exhibited toxic effect	[36]
AgNPs	UV spectra, TEM	2–30 nm; averagely 20 nm	S. aureus, Klebsiella pneumoniae, Escherichia coli, and Pseudomonas aeruginosa	The AgNPs produced had strong antibacterial effect against all the pathogenic bacteria	ND	[10]
polyvinylpyrrolidone (PVP)-coated silver nanoparticles	-	1–10 nm	HIV-1	PVP-coated AgNP exhibit potent cyto-protective and post-infected anti-HIV-1 activities toward Hut/CCR5 cells.	ND	[99]
PVP-coated silver nanoparticles	-	30–50 nm	HIV-1	PVP-coated AgNPs Inhibited cell-associated HIV-1 and cell-free HIV-1 transmission.	PVP-coated AgNPs were non toxic to cells explant	[100]
mercaptoethane sulfonate (MES)-coated silver and gold nanoparticles	-	4 nm	Herpes simplex virus type 1 (HSV-1)	The MES-coated silver and gold nanoparticles inhibited HSV-1 infection in cell culture	The MES-coated silver and gold were non toxic to host cells	[101]
PVP-coated silver nanoparticles	-	69 nm +/– 3 nm	Respiratory syncytial virus (RSV)	Inhibited RSV infection	showed low toxicity to cells	[102]
AgNP and polysaccharide-coated AgNP	-	10–80 nm	Monkey pox virus (MPV)	The AgNPs of approximately 10 nm inhibit MPV infection in vitro, as an anti-viral	Non of te GgNPs were cytotoxic (Vero cell monolayer sloughing)	[103]
AgNPs	-	10–50 nm	Hepatitis B virus (HBV)	AgNPs inhibited in vitro HBV RNA and extracellular virions	ND	[104]
AgNPs and polysaccharide-coated AgNP	-	10 nm	Tacaribe virus (TCRV)	AgNPs inhibited the TCRV infection in vitro	ND	[105]
Ag-NPs-coated PUC	High resolution Scanning Electron Microscopy (HrSEM), UV Spectra	30–60 nm	E. coli, S. aureus, M. luteus, K. pneumoniae, and Candida tropicalis, Candida krusei, Candida glabrata, and Candida albicans and HIV-1	Ag-NPs-coated PUC with HIV-1 and HSV-1/2 was able to inactivate their infectiousness as well as bacterial and fungal species	ND	[25]

Table 1 Summary of the types of nanoparticles susceptibility to organisms *(Continued)*

Nanoparticle	Characterization	Size	Organism	Activity	Cytotoxicity	Ref
Mycosynthesized silver nanoparticles	UV spectra, TEM, Nanosight-LM 20;	4–46 nm	HSV 1 and 2 and with human parainfluenza virus type 3.	Smaller-sized AgNPs were able to inhibit the infectivity of the viruses	ND	[23]
AgNPs	UV–vis spectroscopy, SEM, TEM, FTIR and XRD.	18 to 45 nm with an average size of 32 nm	Anopheles stephensi, Aedes aegypti, and Culex quinquefasciatus	AgNPs showed biolarvicidal effect to A. stephensi, A. aegypti, and C. quinquefasciatus.	ND	[39]
AgNPs	UV–vis spectroscopy, SEM, FTIR and XRD.	41–60 nm.	Anopheles stephensi, Aedes aegypti, and Culex quinquefasciatus	The AgNPs were effective in destroying the vectors of mosquito vector blood born parasites	ND	[40]
AgNPs	Atomic force microscopy (AFM), UV-vis spectroscopy, FTIR	60–95 nm	3 instar larvae of Culex quinquefasciatus	AgNPs exhibited high mortality against larvae of Culex quinquefasciatus	ND	[78]
AgNPs	UV–vis spectroscopy, SEM, energy-dispersive X-ray (EDX) spectroscopy.	43.52 to 142.97 nm	Aedes aegypti	The Bt-AgNPs showed larvicide effect against mosquito larva A. aegypti	ND	[106]
Polyvinyl-N-carbazole (PVK) and single-walled carbon nanotubes (SWNTs) (PVKSWNT)	UV vis spectra, FTIR, SEM	NA	E. coli MG 1655 and B. subtilis-102	The nano-composite showed antimicrobial activity against both Gram-positive and negative bacterial isolates.	The PVK-SWNT were non toxic to fibroblast cells	[34]
MWCNT-lysine functionalized	FTIR, Thermal gravimetric analysis (TGA), Raman spectra and TEM	N/A	S. aureus, Streptococcus agalactiae, S. dysgalactiae, E. coli, K. pneumonia, S. typhimurium	The functionalized MWCNT with lysine expressed high antimicrobial effect against all bacterial cells	ND	[29]
MWCNT-AgNPs	Inductively coupled plasma atomic emission spectroscopy (ICP-AES), XRD, FTIR	3 to 30 nm	Escherichia coli	MWCNT-AgNPs exhibited strong antimicrobial activities and reduce biofilm formation.	ND	[33]
Silicon nanotubes (SNTs), silicon nanoparticles (SNPs)	SEM–EDX, TEM, Brunauer-Emmett-Teller (BET), STM, Raman spectroscopy.	average diameter of 14	Multidrug-resistant Staphylococcus aureus	SCSNTs were effective in limiting the growth of multidrug-resistant S aureus	ND	[26]
Ag-Fe/SWCNTs	TEM, SEM, XRD, Raman spectra	1–10 nm Ag-Fe NP dispersed and tightly attached to the outer surfaces of SWCNTs	Escherichia coli.	Purified Ag-Fe/SWCNT hybrid nanoparticles were effective against E. coli.	ND	[104]
SWCNTs combine with H_2O_2 or NaOCl	TEM, SEM-EDX	SWCNTs 1–1.5 nm	Bacillus anthracis Spores	The combined effect of SWCNTs and H_2O_2 or NaOCl exhibited sporicidal effect on B. anthracis spores	ND	[87]
SWNT/PLL/PGA	Uv spectra, TEM, SEM, Quartz crystal microgravimetry	SWNT is 0.8–1.2 nm	E. coli and S. epidermidis	SWNT/PLL/PGA highly inactivated E. coli and S. epidermidis	ND	[28]
Zirconia (ZrO2) nanoparticles	SEM, EDX, AFM, U vis spectra, FTIR	50e100 nm, average size 50 nm	Staphylococcus aureus, Escherichia coli, Candida albicans, Aspergillus niger	Zirconia (ZrO2) nanoparticles exhibited antifungal and antibacterial against the test organisms.	ND	[111]

Table 1 Summary of the types of nanoparticles susceptibility to organisms *(Continued)*

Nanoparticle	Characterization	Size	Organism	Effect	Toxicity	Ref
Au/CuS core/shell nanoparticles (NPs)	HRTEM, SEM, energy dispersive X-ray spectroscopy (EDS)	2–5 nm.	*B. anthracis* spores and cells	The Au/CuS NPs were highly efficient in inactivating *B. anthracis* cells, but not effective to the spores.	ND	[12]
Sialic-acid functionalized gold nanoparticles	TEM	2 nm and 14 nm	Influenza virus	The NPs inhibition influenza virus infection	The functionalized AuNPs were nontoxic to the cells	[107]
Titanium dioxide nanoparticles (TiO2 NPs)	XRD, FTIR, SEM, EDX, AFM.	Average size of 70 nm.	*Pediculus humanus capitis* De Geer (Phthiraptera: Pediculidae); larvae of cattle tick *Hyalomma anatolicum* (a.) *anatolicum* Koch (Acari: Ixodidae), and fourth instar larvae of malaria vector *Anopheles subpictus* Grassi (Diptera: Culicidae).	The TiO2 NPs showed significant mortality against the vectors borne organisms	ND	
Chrysosporium tropicum mediated silver and gold nanoparticles	Microscan reader, XRD, TEM, SEM	AuNPs: 2–15 nm and AgNP: 20–50 nm	*Aedes aegypti* larvae.	The AuNPs used as an efficacy enhancer shown mortality 3 times higher *Aedes aegypti* larvae.	ND	[41]
Zinc oxide nanoparticles (ZnO NPs)	UV–visible spectroscopy, XRD, FTIR, SEM	60–120 nm.	larvae of cattle tick *Rhipicephalus (Boophilus) microplus*, Canestrini (Acari: Ixodidae); head louse *Pediculus humanus capitis*, De Geer (Phthiraptera: Pediculidae); larvae of malaria vector, *Anopheles subpictus*, Grassi; and filariasis vector, *Culex quinquefasciatus*, Say (Diptera: Culicidae). R. microplus larvae	The ZnO NPs had significant inhibitory effect on the parasites	ND	[110]
Cobalt nanoparticles (CoNPs)	XRD, FTIR FESEM with energy dispersive X-ray spectroscopy, and TEM	average size of 84.81 nm.	malaria vector *Anopheles subpictus* and dengue vector *Aedes aegypti (Diptera: Culicidae).*	The larvicidal effect was observed in the cobalt acetate solution and against the *A. subpictus* and *A. aegypti*	ND	[108]
Copper(II) nanohybrid solids, LCu(CH3COO)2 and LCuCl2	TEM, dynamic light scattering, and IR spectroscopy	5–10 and 60–70 nm of LCu(CH3COO)2 and LCuCl2	*Plasmodium falciparum* (MRC 2).	The two compounds showed significant antimalarial activities against the parasites	The copper(II) nanohybrid solids were nontoxic to human hepatocellular carcinoma cells	[109]

eradication and probably the elimination of parasitic infections. Some studies have shown that modified *Plasmodium berghei* sporozoite (Tg-Pb/PfCSP) and self-assembling protein NP (SAPN) vaccine presenting *Plasmodium falciparum* circumsporozoite protein epitopes (PfCSP-SAPN) can stimulate humoral and cellular responses against *Plasmodium falciparum* using the complement classical pathway cascade [4]. The results indicates the potential application of the circumsporozoite protein epitopes (PfCSP-SAPN) in the development of protective effector memory CD8+ T-cells [4] capable of generating strong long-lived IgG.

Nanoparticle anti-vector borne diseases
As a result of the increase in the prevalence of vector borne diseases, the production of environmentally friendly and safe NP insecticides synthesized from plants are currently available. These include those of AgNPs synthesized from the leaf extracts of *Heliotropium indicum* [39], and *Azadirachta indica* [40]. These insecticides have shown maximum efficacy against blood feeding mosquitoes of *Anopheles stephensi, Aedes aegypti,* and *Culex quinquefasciatus* [39, 40]. This shows that eco-friendly NPs have the potential of controlling vector transmitted infections that have significantly contributed to disease burden, social debility, poverty and death in mostly low income countries [39, 40]. However, due to NPs non-specific actions to environmental organisms, this may deter their usefulness as vector control agents [40–42].

Wound healing and nanoparticles
Wound dressing and wound healing are very important components of reducing morbidity and mortality of wound related burden. A wound is a debilitated tissue that results from a breakdown in the skin giving rise to a physiological condition for microbial manifestation including opportunistic pathogens [43, 44] affecting wound healing [45]. Depending on the degree of wound, whether acute or chronic, wound care is necessary to reduce infection or abnormal bacterial presence that may cause stress and other health consequences [44, 46]. Over the years, wound dressing and healing have been problematic to clinicians [46]. Because there is no single appropriate wound dressing material that can act as a potent sterile antimicrobial agent capable of absorbing excess exudate, preserving the wound from external sources of infection, preventing excess heat at the wound, impermeable to gases, and a dressing that is easy to remove without further trauma to the wound [47] has complicated wound healing. Wound dressing materials such as gauze are associated with painful removal and may cause trauma and associated stress [48].

Nevertheless, the research on NPs in wound dressing materials has come at an opportune time. The NP

wound dressing materials provide biocompatible antimicrobial agents that are inexpensive, soft, and flexible, and conform to the contours of the body [49, 50]. For example, AgNPs wound dressing antimicrobial nanomaterials have been introduced to supplement traditional wound dressing because the slow release of the AgNPs allow the dressing to be changed less frequently, but is highly effective and efficient in wound healing with less antimicrobial resistance [49]. Furthermore, a study by Guidelli et al. [51] showed that natural latex rubber blended with AgNPs gradually released the AgNPs, but was useful in promoting and facilitating wound healing as well as the reduction in scar formation [49]. The AgNPs may also mediate wound healing via reduced mitochondria activity that does not affect the host cell viability with rapid re-establishment of the body integrity [52]. According to a study by Tian et al. [53] AgNPs exert positive broad spectrum antimicrobial properties by reducing wound inflammation, and modulation of fibrogenic cytokines.

Similarly, other findings by John and Moro [54] showed that NPs hydrogel wound dressing consist of methacrylate backbone and terminal hydroxyl group capable of providing versatile and excellent wound healing. This is because the NPs hydrogel dressing powders have thermal insulators capable of absorbing some of the blood or wound exudate, thus providing an impermeable potent antimicrobial environment to wound pathogens as well as protecting the wound from external contamination [50, 54]. The NPs hydrogel are cost effective, user friendly, easy to apply, do not adhere to the wound and have minimal need for secondary dressing [54].

Apart from AgNPs, other NPs equally used in wound healings include those of gold [55], curcumin-encapsulated NPs [56], chitin/nanosilver composite with good blood clotting ability [57], conjugated iron oxide NPs [58], and nitric oxide releasing NPs [59]. However, the significant acceleration of wound healing by nanomaterials still remains a mystery and the mechanisms of action are still to be fully elucidated and unfold.

Nanoparticles microbicides activities
With the increase in sexually transmitted infections (STI) fuelling the HIV burden and other health problems, microbicides may be considered as alternative preventive methods of STI and HIV [60, 61]. Microbicides are antimicrobial agents that are self-applied on the vagina or rectum to protect against STIs [19, 62, 63]. Hence they act as chemical, biological and/or physical barriers that prevent transmission of pathogens during sexual intercourse [62, 64, 65]. They may be in gel, creams, rings, or films form and can be used with condoms, thus offering additional protection or used alone especially by those who do not appreciate the use of

condoms [19]. The microbicides may be used by both HIV positive and heathy individuals to prevent transmission of the virus. Studies have shown that microbicides may provide prevention against HIV and STI infections for those practicing receptive anal and/or vaginal intercourse [63]. In addition, microbicides can provide individuals with protection especially those who are unaware of their partner HIV status including those on antiretroviral therapies (ART) and undetectable HIV viral load [63].

Research studies have shown that NPs-microbicides including those of dendrimer-nanoscale-microbicides hold potential safety efficacy against viruses [19, 66–68]. For example, the VivaGel™ (SPL7013Gel) dendrimer is carefully formulated against HIV and HSV and does not interfere with vaginal or rectal physiological pH [19, 69]. The dendrimer VivaGel™ microbicide is meant to disrupt and block viral attachment and/or prevent the viral adsorption from targeting cells of the rectum or vagina. In the case of HIV the gp120 of the virus are blocked from attaching to the CD4 receptors of human white blood cells [19]. In a study by Chonco et al. [60], it was found that carbosilane dendrimer microbicide are capable of exhibiting HIV thus blocking potential in epithelial monolayer in vitro model cells. Other dendrimers such as heparan sulfate-binding peptide were found to inhibit human papillomaviruses [68] thus, acting as promising antiviral microbicides.

Nanoparticles inhibition of intra-macrophage pathogens

Pathogenic organisms that traverse cell membranes or reside in nerve cells cause persistence infections and, thus are difficult to treat [70]. Bacteria such as *Brucella*, *Mycobacterium*, *Listeria* species and viruses including HIV, and herpes simplex are intracellular pathogens that invade treatment and persistently exhibit latent infections [70–72]. Therefore, some drugs find it difficult to reach such cells, thus complicating the elimination and eradication of such microbial pathogens [73]. Some of the pathogens may invade cells and exist as intra-macrophage pathogens and central nervous infections escaping drugs action as well as immunological responses [71, 73]. Health care workers (HCWs) find it very difficult and frustrating when providing treatment to such intravascular disease causing pathogens due to failure of conventional antimicrobial drugs to destroy such organisms. Drugs for treating such diseases including HIV, encephalopathy and cerebrovascular infections may not lack potency, but due to shortcomings of poor or inefficient intracellular penetration and sustained drugs concentration, may limit treatment efficiency and efficacy [73]. The problems associated with such drugs may include lack of solubility and bio-distribution to

reach target areas, thus do not have sufficient drug delivery profile.

Nano-drugs such as polymeric NPs, dendrimers, polymer micelles, and solid lipid NPs have been shown to exhibit excellent antimicrobial profiles and have potent ligand conjugates that improve the pharmacological and therapeutic profile of such drugs to cross such cell membranes, internalize and render efficient antimicrobial potentials [70, 71, 73]. The delivery process provide NP-drugs with multiple functions of carrier, delivery, and antimicrobial capabilities [71, 73, 74]. These attributes are due to the small size (1–100 nm), vast NPs-functionalization ability, and the robust physiochemical properties, even if biodegradability and the toxicological challenges may be hindering beneficial health outcomes [75, 76].

As mentioned earlier, organisms such *Brucella* species, *Mycobacterium tuberculosis* exist as intra-macrophage pathogen rendering standard treatment very difficult [71, 72]. For example, *Brucella* species usually invade, reside and survive within phagocytic, dendritic and trophoblast cells, thus making treatment potential very difficult to clinicians [71]. Similarly, *Mycobacterium tuberculosis* bacteria responsible for tuberculosis reside inside macrophage resulting into persistent tuberculosis [77]. The same effect has been demonstrated by herpes simplex virus that hides and resides in nerve cells causing latent herpes zosters infections [78]. The use of NPs could be beneficial for such treatments because of the NPs antimicrobials potentials, ease membrane crossing ability and delivery potentials of materials into such cells. They play the role of carrier, delivery and sustain antimicrobials effect in such cells. For example, AgNPs have huge biocidal effect and have been shown to cross the macrophage cell wall and inhibit intra-macrophage *Bacillus abortus*; a maternal bacterium that tend to resist treatment and causes perinatal morbidity during pregnancy [79].

Furthermore, some pathogens are highly resistant to extreme temperatures and difficult to be eliminated by antibiotics or other chemicals. Nanomaterials and other emerging materials have been reported to be potent antimicrobial agents capable of destroying such pathogens that are tolerant to extreme temperatures and resistant to treat with conventional antibiotics [80]. For example, SWCNTs coupled within 20 minutes near infrared (NIR) treatment significantly increases the potential effect of antimicrobials against *Bacillus anthracis* spores when compared to non NIR treated SWCNTs [67]. In addition, a study by Martínez-Gutierrez et al. [81] found that 24 nm AgNPs were not only potent antibacterial agents against resistant strains of bacteria, but also had anti-coagulation activities as well as inflammatory response in macrophages. This indicates that nanomaterials can easily be modified as efficient intravascular agent for the destruction of intravascular pathogens as well as delivery agents since they are capable of crossing membrane cell walls without any cell damage or harm [82]. However, the mechanisms of cell membrane or pathways used by the NPs antimicrobial agents in crossing/cell uptake are still to be fully explained [82].

Nanoparticles penetration of the brain barriers and difficult to reach tissues or cells

Infections of the brain are often very difficult to treat because of the difficulty of most antimicrobial agents to cross the blood brain barrier and inhibit microbial agents [84]. This is due to the fact that the brain is made up of complex cell networks that filter foreign materials, protect and prevent the brain from injuries and diseases [83]. However, some small microbes such as viruses as well as some bacteria are still capable of bypassing and crossing the blood brain barrier [83, 84]. Substances entering the brain are mediated through a tight regulated systematic process of membrane transporters [82–84]. This tight regulatory system prevents most pharmacological antimicrobial agents from crossing the blood brain barrier and exercising their pharmacological activities [82–84]. In this regard nanotechnological antimicrobial agents could bring a novel dimensional approach that is capable of overcoming and bypassing the complex brain cell network, and inhibiting the brain pathogens, thus reducing the burden of microbial brain infections [85]. The NPs can potentially carry and potentially deliver antimicrobial across the blood brain barrier. In fact, it is known that NPs have very small nanosizes that exhibit vast physiochemical multifunctional properties that play a significant role of crossing the blood brain barrier with ease. These features of being able to transiting difficult biological system with ease without disrupting or damaging the cell membranes and sustaining the antimicrobials have made NPs and/or nanomaterials (nano-functionalized-ligands) very attractive for biomedical applications [5, 86]. For example, a single oral administration of poly-lactide-co-glycolide NP-encapsulated antituberculosis drugs consisting of rifampicin + isoniazid + pyrazinamide + ethambutol conjugate in murine mice was found to cross the blood brain barrier and sustained for 9 days in the brain [86]. Furthermore, based on colony forming unit enumerations and pathological examinations, the study showed that 5 oral doses administered every 10th day improved the pharmacologic activities of the polymer NP-antituberculosis drugs resulting in an undetectable level of *Mycobacterium tuberculosis* in the mice meninges [86].

The mechanisms of action of how the polymer- antituberculosis nanomaterials bypassed the complex cell network of blood brain barriers are yet to be uncovered. It is envisaged that the development of emerging novel NP-antimicrobial agents will soon revolutionize clinical

medicine [86]. It is anticipated that the crossing of the blood brain barrier by NP-antimicrobial agents including other classes of drugs would reduce the burden of infections including meningitis caused by vast majority of pathogens.

Nanoparticles enhancement of antimicrobial activities of other agents

The NPs play a significant role in enhancing the activities of other agents leading to effective and efficient treatment action. For example, the combination of SWCNTs and hydrogen peroxide (H_2O_2) or NaOCl increases the sporicidal effect on the spores of organisms such as *Bacillus* species when compared to treatment with H_2O_2 or NaOCl alone at the same concentrations [87]. In such treatments, synergistic mechanisms of efficacy are established due to contribution of multiple antimicrobial effects. Further analysis shows that SWCNTs do not only play the role of antimicrobial effect, but also increases permeability/susceptibility of the *Bacillus* species pathogen to H_2O_2 or NaOCl, thus significantly developing high effective sporicidal effect [87]. Furthermore, findings by Gilbertson et al. [6] found that oxygen functional groups when functionalized on MWCNTs, enhances several MWCNT properties such as redox activity, electrochemical and antimicrobial activities. The redox activities include the ability to enhance the oxidation of glutathione, and the reduction of surface carboxyl groups that promote the functional performance of MWCNTs antimicrobial activities for biomedical application [6]. This synergetic effect has equally been shown by AgNPs which enhanced the angiogenic properties of natural latex rubber for cell growth and wound healing [51].

Nanoparticles disinfectants

The inventive approach of nanomaterials as disinfectant relate to their stability, homogeneity, high efficiency and efficacy of broad biocide spectrum of virucidal, bactericidal, fungicidal, antiparasitic and sporicidal as well as mycobactericidal and mycoplasmicidal potentials [88–90]. These excellent disinfectant properties as well as the additional ability of NPs surface functionalization and the dispersion on the NPs surfaces have been exhibited by a wide range of NPs [5–7]. Such functional groups provide very potent additional antimicrobial properties and include ligands such as hydroxyl, carboxyl, amine, and other chemical radicals [5]. The NPs including those of silver, copper and gold [91] have excellent cleaning and disinfecting properties. Some of these NPs are now being used as cleaning disinfectants in hospitals. In such instances, the surfaces may be coated with potent nanomaterials against nosocomial pathogens including the stubborn multi-drug resistant pathogens of Methicillin-resistant *Staphylococcus aureus*

(MRSA) that are responsible for most nosocomial infections [88, 92]. For example, silicone polymers of AuNPs have shown to actively reduce the microbial load on clinical surfaces, particularly, when the surfaces are activated with white light [93].

To minimize the risk of microbial and other contamination of hospital HCW during various clinical procedures and examination procedures, hospital protective equipment are re-enforced with nanomaterials-antimicrobial agents that have been developed. Some of the HCW antimicrobial protective materials include surgical mask, gloves and many other latex personal protective equipment (PPE). For example, mixtures of silver nitrate and titanium dioxide NP coated on hospital facemask used during very delicate clinical procedures have shown to have significant protection against infectious agents [91, 93, 94]. The use of NPs-antiseptics has also led to an increase in surface area to volume ratio, thus improving the lethal action of NPs-antiseptics against pathogens [91, 93].

As a result of the biocidal action and non-toxic nature of some NPs such as AgNPs, they are widely coated on medical devices to reduce infections [95]. In addition, nanomaterials of silver are being used in pet-animal shampoos as disinfection, cleaning and softening agents [96]. The AgNPs can also be coated on filters used for the purification of water. In some studies, PVK and SWNTs were found to destroy bacterial cell membranes [34].

Furthermore, NPs are currently being used as preservatives in packages to prevent food spoilage. For example, allyl isothiocyanate (AIT) and CNTs can be incorporated into packaging materials so as to prevent the contamination of food by *Salmonella choleraesuis* [97]. The allyl isothiocyanate (AIT) and CNTs work by providing an antimicrobial film that reduces the microbial contamination, control oxidation and reduces the colour changes for up to 40 days [97].

Nanoparticles antimicrobial mechanisms of action
Traditionally, most antimicrobial agents inhibit microbial growth through several mechanisms such as cell wall inhibition and lysis, inhibition of protein synthesis, alteration of cell membranes, inhibition of nucleic acid (NA) synthesis and antimetabolite activity [113]. The NP-antimicrobials, on the other hand, may encompass and differ slightly due to their vast physiochemical properties with respect to size, shape, surface area, surface energy, charge, crystallinity, agglomeration, aggregation and chemical composition [114–116]. Although most NP-antimicrobial mechanisms of action are still unknown and are currently under investigations [117], studies show that NPs can mediate bacterial cell membranes degradation [118–120]. For example, Li et al. [120] found the degradation of *S. aureus* by Catechin-Cu NPs. The Catechin-Cu NPs was also found to exert

different mechanisms of action during *E. coli* cell wall degradation, which is an indication of different impacts on the Gram negative and Gram positive bacteria [120]. The multiple effects have also been observed in CuNP-antimicrobial actions which include the generation of reactive oxygen species and lipid peroxidation [118]. Other CuNP-antibacterial actions include protein oxidation and DNA degradation in *E. coli* cells [118]. Another study by Xie et al. [121] showed that zinc oxide (ZnO) NPs exerted bactericidal effect by disruption of the cell membrane and oxidative stress in *Campylobacter jejuni*. The NP-antimicrobials such as AgNP have also been shown to bind to lippopolysaccharides, surface proteins or porin, collapsing the microbial cell wall and limiting the membrane potential [122]. Similarly, AgNP have been found to induce efflux of phosphate, reduction of cellular ATP level, interacting with sulphahydryl (or thiol) group and altering cytoplasmic components as well as inhibiting the respiratory enzymes and blocking of DNA replication in both Gram negative and Gram positive bacterial pathogens [122]. These studies show that different NPs have very different physiochemical properties and thus exhibit different antimicrobial mechanisms of action.

Nanoparticles toxicity
The NPs antimicrobial agents have excellent potent and low tendency of inducing resistance when compared to non-NPs-antimicrobial agents [123]. However, the NP-antimicrobial agents' pharmacological properties may be hampered by potential toxicity [123, 124]. As stated in previous sections of this review paper, NPs facilitate the penetration and delivery of antimicrobial agents into biological membranes including microbial cells, thereby enhancing and increasing biological activities [76, 113]. This means that the toxicity of different NP-antimicrobial polymers needs a time-dependent understanding and characterization [125]. Generally, antimicrobial agents' biocompatibility inhibition cannot occur without producing some undesirable health effects, either local or systemic. In fact, the most deterring effect of most drugs is their potential toxicity to organisms of which NPs-antimicrobials agents are not an exception. Therefore, effective NP-antimicrobial agents' dose-related response is an important factor in relation to human exposure and other organisms. Few studies have described the toxicity of NP-antimicrobials (Table 1) with controversies. For example, a study by Cooper and Spitzer [126] shows that AgNPs antimicrobials at sub-lethal dose disrupt cytoskeleton and neurite dynamics when cultured in adult neural stem cells. For example, at sub-lethal dose of 1.0 μg/mL, AgNP cultured in neural stem cells induced the formation of f-actin inclusions, indicating a disruption of actin function [126]. Similar findings were reported by

Baram-Pinto [101] that AgNPs capped with Mercap-toethane Sulfonate showed some serious effects in mammalian cells. Some results showed that PVK-SWCNT-antimicrobial agents were nontoxic to fibroblast cells as opposed to pure SWCNTs [34]. Multivalent Sialic acid functionalized AuNPs-antimicrobials agents have also been shown to demonstrate no toxic effect on Madin-Darby canine kidney cells [107]. Similarly, copper (II) nanohybrid solids-antimicrobial have shown no toxic effect on human hepatocellular carcinoma cells [109]. In another study, no cytotoxicity was reported when rats were treated with antibacterial AgNP-loaded titanium nanotube [127]. The rat cells expressed no toxicity thus demonstrating the competence of NPs-antimicrobials as future antimicrobial agents. However, despite several studies, the current available information is insufficient to ascertain the adverse effects of NP-antimicrobials on human health. Therefore, it is imperative that further research is carried out to mitigate any toxicological problems that may arise.

Summary and future perspectives

Research has shown that the functionalization-immobilization and/or hybridization of NPs can enhance and improve the antimicrobial activities of the nanomaterials against a wide range of multi-resistant strains of pathogenic microorganisms. For example, a single type of NP-antimicrobial agent could show multiple antimicrobial properties against many pathogens. However, these characteristics may also alter the microbial flora of the body since their antimicrobial action is non-specific. Most of the studies reviewed showed that AgNPs were the widely used and have several antibacterial, antiviral, antifungal, anti-parasite, anti-insect and anti-vector borne properties. Generally, most NP-antimicrobial drugs were able to target and transit difficult membrane barriers, deliver and sustain the NP-antimicrobial doses resulting in disease clearance which is a difficult phenomenon for conventional antimicrobials. However, more information on the toxicological effects of NP-antimicrobial agents is needed so as to enhance and broaden their biomedical application [76]. In some instances, depending on the size of the NP, the particle tended to be toxic rather than demonstrating antimicrobial effect of inhibiting pathogens. For example, very small AgNPs were found to cover the pathogen, inhibiting oxygen supply to the pathogen thus reducing respiration and toxically killing the pathogen rather than inhibiting the microbial growth [14]. However, very small NPs may also be toxic to human pathogens. For example, AgNPs ranging from 10–20 nm were found to be toxic to *Bacillus* species, *E. coli* and *Staphylococcus* species. [14]. Therefore, it is imperative that further research is carried out to mitigate such problems.

Competing interest
The authors declare that they have no competing interests.

Authors' contributions
CSY conceived, CSY and GSS collected and CSY drafted the manuscript. CSY and GSS analysed the data and additional information. Both authors have read and approved the final manuscript.

Acknowledgements
We acknowledge the Social Aspects for HIV/AIDS Research Alliance (SAHARA) unit of the HIV/AIDS, STIs and TB (HAST) at the Human Sciences Research Council (HSRC) of South Africa for providing conducive infrastructural environment during the course of the sourcing and writing of the manuscript.

Disclaimer
The contents of this paper reflect authors views who are responsible for the accuracy of the information presented herein. This paper does not constitute a standard, specification, nor is it intended for design, construction, bidding, or permit purposes.

Author details
[1]Department of Biochemistry and Microbiology, Nelson Mandela Metropolitan University, Port Elizabeth, South Africa. [2]Department of Epidemiology, Johns Hopkins Bloomberg School of Public Health, E7146, 615 N. Wolfe Street, Baltimore 21205, MD, USA. [3]School of Chemical and Metallurgical Engineering, University of the Witwatersrand, P/Bag 3, Wits 2050, Johannesburg, South Africa.

References
1. Galdiero S, Falanga A, Vitiello M, Cantisani M, Marra V, Galdiero M. Silver nanoparticles as potential antiviral agents. Molecules. 2011;16:8894–918.
2. Tanwar J, Das S, Fatima Z, Hameed S. Multidrug resistance: an emerging crisis. Interdiscip Perspect Infect Dis. 2014;2014:541340. 7 pages.
3. Sharma RK, Ghose R. Synthesis of zinc oxide nanoparticles by homogeneous precipitation method and its application in antifungal activity against *Candida albicans*. Ceram Int. 2015;41:967–75.
4. McCoy ME, Golden HE, Doll TA, Yang Y, Kaba SA, Zou X, et al. Mechanisms of protective immune responses induced by the *Plasmodium falciparum* circumsporozoite protein-based, self-assembling protein nanoparticle vaccine. Malar J. 2013;22:2–136.
5. Ngoy JM, Iyuke SE, Neuse WE, Yah CS. Covalent functionalization for multi-walled carbon nanotube (*f-MWCNT*) -folic acid bound bioconjugate. J Appl Sci. 2011;11(15):2700–11.
6. Gilbertson LM, Goodwin DG, Taylor AD, Pfefferle L, Zimmerman JB. Toward tailored functional design of Multi-Walled Carbon Nanotubes (MWNTs): electrochemical and antimicrobial activity enhancement via oxidation and selective reduction. Environ Sci Technol. 2014;48:5938–45.
7. Parise A, Thakor H, Zhang X. Activity inhibition on municipal activated sludge by single-walled carbon nanotubes. J Nanoparticle Res. 2014;16:2159.
8. Qi X, Gunawan P, Xu R, Chang MW. Cefalexin-immobilized multi-walled carbon nanotubes show strong antimicrobial and anti-adhesion properties. Chem Eng Sci. 2015;84:552–6.
9. Venkatesan J, Jayakumar R, Mohandas A, Bhatnagar I, Kim SK. Antimicrobial activity of chitosan-carbon nanotube hydrogels. Materials. 2014;7:3946–55.
10. Adeli M, Hosainzadegan H, Pakzad I, Zabihi F, Alizadeh M, Karimi F. Preparation of the silver nanoparticle containing starch foods and evaluation of antimicrobial activity. Jundishapur J Microbiol. 2013;6(4):e5075.
11. Subbiah R, Veerapandian M, Sadhasivam S, Yun K. Triad CNT-NPs/Polymer nanocomposites: fabrication, characterization, and preliminary antimicrobial study. Synth React Inorg Met-Org Nano-Met Chem. 2011;41:345–55.
12. Addae E, Dong X, McCoy E, Yang C, Chen W, Yang L. Investigation of antimicrobial activity of photothermal therapeutic gold/copper sulphide core/shell nanoparticles to bacterial spores and cells. J Biol Eng. 2014;8:11.
13. Sui M, Zhang L, Sheng L, Huang S, She L. Synthesis of ZnO coated multi-walled carbon nanotubes and their antibacterial activities. Sci Total Environ. 2013;452–453:148–54.

14. Sunitha A, Rimal IRS, Sweetly G, Sornalekshmi S, Arsula R, Praseetha PK. Evaluation of antimicrobial activity of biosynthesized iron and silver Nanoparticles using the fungi *Fusarium oxysporum* and *Actinomycetes sp.* on human pathogens. Nano Biomed Eng. 2013;5(1):39–45.

15. Hoffmann H-H, Kunz A, Simon VA, Palese P, Shawa ML. Broad-spectrum antiviral that interferes with de novo pyrimidine biosynthesis. Proc Natl Acad Sci U S A. 2011;108(14):5777–82.

16. Kollef MH. Broad-spectrum antimicrobials and the treatment of serious bacterial infections: Getting It Right Up Front. Clin Infect Dis. 2008;47(Supplement 1):S3–13.

17. Kwon DS, Mylonakis E. Posaconazole: a new broad-spectrum antifungal agent. Expert Opin Pharmacother. 2007;8(8):1167–78.

18. Navarrete-Vazquez G, Chávez-Silva F, Argotte-Ramos R, Rodríguez-Gutiérrez Mdel C, Chan-Bacab MJ, Cedillo-Rivera R, et al. Synthesis of benzologues of Nitazoxanide and Tizoxanide: a comparative study of their in vitro broad-spectrum antiprotozoal activity. Bioorg Med Chem Lett. 2011;21(10):3168–71.

19. Rupp R, Rosenthal SL, Stanberry LR. VivaGel™ (SPL7013 Gel): A candidate dendrimer –microbicide for the prevention of HIV and HSV infection. Int J Nanomedicine. 2007;2(4):561–6.

20. Marambio-Jones C, Hoek EMV. A review of the antibacterial effects of silver nanomaterials and potential implications for human health and the environment. J Nanoparticle Res. 2010;12:1531–51.

21. San CY, Don MM. Biosynthesis of silver nanoparticles from *Schizophyllum Commune* and *in-vitro* antibacterial and antifungal activity studies. J Phys Sci. 2013;24(2):83–96.

22. Kathiravan V, Ravi S, Ashokkumar S, Velmurugan S, Elumalai K, Khatiwada CP. Green synthesis of silver nanoparticles using Croton sparsiflorus morong leaf extract and their antibacterial and antifungal activities. Spectrochim Acta A Mol Biomol Spectrosc. 2015;139:200–5.

23. Gaikwad S, Ingle A, Gade N, Rai M, Falanga A, Incoronato N, et al. Antiviral activity of mycosynthesized silver nanoparticles against herpes simplex virus and human parainfluenza virus type 3. Int J Nanomedicine. 2013;8:4303–14.

24. Elmi T, Gholami S, Fakhar M, Azizi F. A review on the use of nanoparticles in the treatment of parasitic infections. J Mazand Uni Med Sci. 2013;23:127–34.

25. Fayaz AM, Ao Z, Girilal M, Chen L, Xiao X, Kalaichelvan P, et al. Inactivation of microbial infectiousness by silver nanoparticles-coated condom: a new approach to inhibit HIV- and HSV-transmitted infection. Int J Nanomedicine. 2012;7:5007–18.

26. Tank C, Raman S, Karan S, Gosavi S, Lalla NP, Sathe V, et al. Antimicrobial activity of silica coated silicon nano-tubes (SCSNT) and silica coated silicon nano-particles (SCSNP) synthesized by gas phase condensation. J Mater Sci Mater Med. 2013;24(6):1483–90.

27. Zhou J, Qi X. Multi-walled carbon nanotubes/epilson-polylysine nanocomposite with enhanced antibacterial activity. Lett Appl Microbiol. 2010;52:76–83.

28. Aslan S, Deneufchatel M, Hashmi S, Li N, Pfefferle LD, Elimelech M, et al. Carbon nanotube-based antimicrobial biomaterials formed via layer-by-layer assembly with polypeptides. J Colloid Interface Sci. 2012;388(1):268–73.

29. Amiri A, Zardini HZ, Shanbedi M, Maghrebi M, Baniadam M, Tolueinia BB. Efficient method for functionalization of carbon nanotubes by lysine and improved antimicrobial activity and water-dispersion. Mater Lett. 2012;72:153–6.

30. Barbinta-Patrascu ME, Ungureanu C, Iordache SM, Iordache AM, Bunghez IR, Ghiurea M, et al. Eco-designed biohybrids based on liposomes, mint-nanosilver and carbon nanotubes for antioxidant and antimicrobial coating. Mater Sci Eng C Mater Biol Appl. 2014;39:177–85.

31. Neelgund GM, Oki A, Luo Z. Antimicrobial activity of CdS and Ag2S quantum dots immobilized on poly(amidoamine) grafted carbon nanotubes. Colloids Surf B Biointerfaces. 2012;100:215–21.

32. Geraldo DA, Arancibia-Miranda N, Villagra NA, Mora GC, Arratia-Perez R. Synthesis of CdTe QDs/single-walled aluminosilicate nanotubes hybrid compound and their antimicrobial activity on bacteria. J Nanoparticle Res. 2012;14:1286.

33. Booshehri AY, Wang R, Xu R. The effect of re-generable silver nanoparticles/multi-walled carbon nanotubes coating on the antibacterial performance of hollow fibermembrane. Chem Eng J. 2013;230:251–9.

34. Ahmed F, Santos CM, Mangadlao J, Advincula R, Rodrigues DF. Antimicrobial PVK:SWNT nanocomposite coated membrane for water purification: Performance and toxicity testing. Water Res. 2013;47:3966–75.

35. Santos-Magalhães NS, Mosqueira VC. Nanotechnology applied to the treatment of malaria. Adv Drug Deliv Rev. 2010;62(4–5):560–75.

36. Said DE, ElSamad LM, Gohar YM. Validity of silver, chitosan, and curcumin nanoparticles as anti-Giardia agents. Parasitol Res. 2012;111(2):545–54.

37. Allahverdiyev AM, Abamor ES, Bagirova M, Ustundag CB, Kaya C, Kaya F, et al. Antileishmanial effect of silver nanoparticles and their enhanced antiparasitic activity under ultraviolet light. Int J Nanomedicine. 2011;6:2705–14.

38. Das S, Bhattacharya A, Debnath N, Datta A, Goswami A. Nanoparticle-induced morphological transition of Bombyx mori nucleopolyhedrovirus: a novel method to treat silkworm grasserie disease. Appl Microbiol Biotechnol. 2013;97(13):6019–30.

39. Veerakumar K, Govindarajan M, Hoti SL. Evaluation of plant-mediated synthesized silver nanoparticles against vector mosquitoes. Parasitol Res. 2014;113:4567–77.

40. Poopathi S, De Britto LJ, Praba VL, Mani C, Praveen M. Synthesis of silver nanoparticles from Azadirachta indica—a most effective method for mosquito control. Environ Sci Pollut Res. 2015;22:2956–63.

41. Soni N, Prakash S. Efficacy of fungus mediated silver and gold nanoparticles against Aedes aegypti larvae. Parasitol Res. 2012;110:175–84.

42. Kramer MF, Cook WJ, Roth FP, Zhu J, Holman H, Knipe DM, et al. Latent herpes simplex virus infection of sensory neurons alters neuronal gene expression. J Virol. 2003;77(17):9533–41.

43. Sharman D. Moist wound healing: a review of evidence, application and outcome – Review. Diabet Foot J. 2003;6(3):112–20.

44. Yah SC, Enabulelel O, Eghafona NO, Udemezue OO. Prevalence of *Pseudomonas* in burn wounds at the University of Benin teaching Hospital. Benin City, Nigeria. J Exp Clin Anat (JECA). 2004;3(1):12–5.

45. Hiro ME, Pierpont YN, Ko F, Wright TE, Robson MC, Payne WG. Comparative evaluation of silver containing antimicrobial dressing on the In-vitro and In vivo processing of wound healing. ePlasty. 2012;12:409–19.

46. Yah SC, Yusuf EO, Haruna T. Patterns of antibiotics susceptibility of isolates and plasmid analysis of *Staphylococcus aureus* from Postoperative Wound Infections. Int J Biol Chem Sci. 2009;3(4):810–8.

47. Jones V, Grey JE, Harding KG. Wound dressings. BMJ. 2006;332:777–80.

48. Stashak TS, Farstvedt E, Othica A. Update on wound dressings: Indications and best use. Clin Tech Equine Pract. 2004;3:148–63.

49. Kwan KH, Liu X, Yeung KW. Silver nanoparticles improve wound healing. Nanomedicine. 2011;6(4):595–6.

50. Caló E, Khutoryanskiy VV. Biomedical applications of hydrogels: a review of patents and commercial products. Eur Polym J. 2015;65:252–67.

51. Guidelli EJ, Kinoshita A, Ramos AP, Baffa O. Silver nanoparticles delivery system based on natural rubber latex membranes. J Nanoparticle Res. 2013;15:1536.

52. Rigo C, Ferroni L, Tocco L, Roman M, Munivrana I, Gardin C, et al. Carlo Barbante 4 and Barbara ZavanActive silver nanoparticles for wound healing. Int J Mol Sci. 2013;14:4817–40.

53. Tian J, Wong KK, Ho CM, Lok CN, Yu WY, Che CM, et al. Topical delivery of silver nanoparticles promotes wound healing. Chem Med Chem. 2007;2:129–36.

54. John JS, Moro DG. Hydrogel wound dressing and biomaterials formed in situ and their uses. Patent US7910135 B2. 2011.

55. Leu JG, Chen SA, Chen HM, Wu WM, Hung CF, Yao YD, et al. The effects of gold nanoparticles in wound healing with antioxidant epigallocatechin gallate and α-lipoic acid. Nanomedicine. 2012;8(5):767–75.

56. Krausz AE, Adler BL, Cabral V, Navati M, Doerner J, Charafeddine RA, et al. Curcumin-encapsulated nanoparticles as innovative antimicrobial and wound healing agent. Nanomedicine. 2015;11(1):195–206.

57. Madhumathi K, Kumar PTS, Abhilash S, Sreeja V, Tamura H, Manzoor K, et al. Development of novel chitin/nanosilver composite scaffolds for wound dressing applications. J Mater Sci Mater Med. 2010;21920:807–13.

58. Ziv-Polat O, Topaz M, Brosh T, Margel S. Enhancement of incisional wound healing by thrombin conjugated iron oxide nanoparticles. Biomaterials. 2010;31(4):741–7.

59. Mihu MR, Sandkovsky U, Han G, Friedman JM, Nosanchuk JD, Martinez LR. The use of nitric oxide releasing nanoparticles as a treatment against *Acinetobacter baumannii* in wound infections. Virulence. 2010;1(2):62–7.

60. Chonco L, Pion M, Vacas E, Rasines B, Maly M, Serramía MJ, et al. Carbosilane dendrimer nanotechnology outlines of the broad HIV blocker profile. J Control Release. 2012;161(3):949–58.

61. Fields S, Song B, Rasoul B, Fong J, Works MG, Shew K, et al. New candidate biomarkers in the female genital tract to evaluate microbicide toxicity. PLoS ONE. 2014;9(10):e110980.

62.   Gary AB, Nuttall J, Romano J. The future of HIV microbicides: challenges and opportunities. Antivir Chem Chemother. 2009;19:143–50.

63.   Galea JT. Preparing for rectal microbicides: sociocultural factors affecting product uptake among potential South American users. Am J Public Health. 2014;104(6):e113–20.

64.   Morris GC, Wiggins RC, Woodhall SC, Bland JM, Taylor CR , Jespers V, et al. MABGEL 1: first phase 1 trial of the anti-HIV-1 monoclonal antibodies 2F5, 4E10 and 2G12 as a vaginal microbicide. PLoS ONE. 2014;9(12):e116153.

65.   Harper CC, Holt K, Nhemachena T, Chipato T, Ramjee G, Stratton L, et al. Willingness of clinicians to integrate microbicides into HIV prevention practices in southern Africa. AIDS Behav. 2012;16(7):1821–9.

66.   McCarthy TD, Karellas P, Henderson SA, Giannis M, O'Keefe D F, Heery G, et al. Dendrimers as drugs: discovery and preclinical and clinical development of dendrimer-based microbicides for HIV and STI prevention. Mol Pharm. 2005;2:312–8.

67.   Gong E, Matthews B, McCarthy T, Chu J, Holan G, Raff J, et al. Evaluation of dendrimer SPL7013, a lead microbicide candidate against herpes simplex viruses. Antivir Res. 2005;68:139–46.

68.   Donalisio M, Rusnati M, Cagno V, Civra A, Bugatti A, Giuliani A, et al. Inhibition of human respiratory syncytial virus infectivity by a dendrimeric heparan sulfate-binding peptide. Antimicrob Agents Chemother. 2012;56(10):5278–88.

69.   Price CF, Tyssen D, Sonza S, Davie A, Evans S, Lewis G R, et al. SPL7013 Gel (VivaGel®) retains potent HIV-1 and HSV-2 inhibitory activity following vaginal administration in humans. PLoS ONE. 2011;6(9):e24095.

70.   Imbuluzqueta E, Gamazo C, Ariza I, Blanco-Prieto MJ. Drug delivery systems for potential treatment of intracellular bacterial infections. Front Biosci (Landmark Ed). 2010;15:397–417.

71.   Alizadeh H, Salouti M, Shapouri M. Bactericidal effect of silver nanoparticles on intramacrophage brucella abortus 544. Jundishapur J Microbiol. 2014;7:e9039.

72.   Xie S, Tao Y, Pan Y, Qu W, Cheng G, Huang L, et al. Biodegradable nanoparticles for intracellular delivery of antimicrobial agents. J Control Release. 2014;187:101–17.

73.   Upadhyay RK. Drug delivery systems, CNS protection, and the blood brain barrier. Biomed Res Int. 2014;2014:869269. 37 pages.

74.   Zhang L, Pornpattananangkul D, Hu CMJ, Huang CM. Development of nanoparticles for antimicrobial drug delivery. Curr Med Chem. 2010;17:585–94.

75.   Yah CS, Iyuke SE, Simate GS. Nanoparticles toxicity and their routes of exposures. Pak J Pham Sci. 2012;25(2):477–91.

76.   Simate GS, Yah CS. The use of carbon nanotubes in medical applications - is it a success story? Occup Med Health Aff. 2014;2(1):147.

77.   Welin A. Survival strategies of Mycobacterium tuberculosis inside the human macrophage. Linköping University Medical Dissertations. Sweden Linköping University: Division of Medical Microbiology Department of Clinical and Experimental Medicine , Faculty of Health Sciences Linköping University SE-58185 Linköping; 2011.

78.   Kumar KR, Nattuthurai N, Gopinath P, Mariappan T. Synthesis of eco-friendly silver nanoparticles from Morinda tinctoria leaf extract and its larvicidal activity against Culex quinquefasciatus. Parasitol Res. 2015;114:411–7.

79.   Malone FD, Athanassiou A, Nores LA, Dalton ME. Poor perinatal outcome associated with maternal Brucella abortus infection. Obstet Gynecol. 1997;90(4 Pt 2):674–6.

80.   Dong X, Tang Y, Wu M, Vlahovic B, Yang L. Dual effects of single-walled carbon nanotubes coupled with near-infrared radiation on Bacillus anthracis spores: inactivates spores and stimulates the germination of surviving spores. J Biol Eng. 2013;7:19.

81.   Martinez-Gutierrez F, Thi EP, Silverman JM, de Oliveira CC, Svensson SL, Vanden Hoek A, et al. Antibacterial activity, inflammatory response, coagulation and cytotoxicity effects of silver nanoparticles. Nanomedicine. 2012;8(3):328–36.

82.   Briones E, Colino CI, Lanao IM. Delivery systems to increase the selectivity of antibiotics in phagocytic cells. J Control Release. 2008;125:210–27.

83.   Masserini M. Nanoparticles for brain drug delivery. ISRN Biochemistry. 2013;2013:238428. 18 pages.

84.   Gandhi M, Bohra H, Daniel V, Gupta A. Nanotechnology in blood brain barrier. Int J Pharm Biol Arch. 2010;1(1):37–43.

85.   Haque S, Md S, Alam MI, Sahni JK, AliN J, Baboota S. Nanostructure-based drug delivery systems for brain targeting. Drug Dev Ind Pharm. 2012;38(4):387–411.

86.   Khuller GK, Pandey R. Oral nanoparticle-based antituberculosis drug delivery to the brain in an experimental model. J Antimicrob Chem. 2006;57:1146–52.

87.   Lilly M, Dong X, McCoy E, Yang L. Inactivation of Bacillus anthracis spores by single-walled carbon nanotubes coupled with oxidizing antimicrobial chemicals. Environ Sci Technol. 2012;46(24):13417–24.

88.   McDonnell G, Russell AD. Antiseptics and disinfectants: activity, action, and resistance. Clin Microbiol Rev. 1999;12(1):147–79.

89.   Gutiérrez LG. Nanoparticulate titanium dioxide nanomaterial modified with functional groups and with citric extracts adsorbed on the surface, for the removal of a wide range of microorganisms. Patent. WO/2014/204290. 2010.

90.   Vetten MV, Yah CS, Singh T, Gullumian M. Challenges facing sterilization and depyrogenation of nanoparticles: effects on structural stability and biomedical applications. Nanomedicine. 2014;10(7):1391–9.

91.   Bouchard M, Bouchard J-M. Disinfectant cleaner. Patent no. US20110195131A1. 2011.

92.   Turos E, Shim JY, Wang Y, Greenhalgh K, Reddy GS, Dickey S, et al. Antibiotic-conjugated polyacrylate nanoparticles: new opportunities for development of anti-MRSA agents. Bioorg Med Chem Lett. 2007;17(1):53–6.

93.   Ismail S, Perni S, Pratten J, Parkin I, Wilson M. Efficacy of a novel light-activated antimicrobial coating for disinfecting hospital surfaces. Infect Control Hosp Epidemiol. 2011;32(11):1130–2.

94.   Li Y, Leungb P, Yaoa L, Songa QW, Newtona E. Antimicrobial effect of surgical masks coated with nanoparticles. J Hosp Infect. 2006;62(1):58–63.

95.   Reiche T, Lisby G, Jorgensen S, Christensen A B, Nordling J. A prospective, controlled, randomized study of the effect of a slow-release silver device on the frequency of urinary tract infection in newly catheterized patients. BJU Int. 2000;85:54–9.

96.   Troncarelli MZ, Brandão HM, Gern JC, Guimarães AS, Langoni H. Nanotechnology and antimicrobials in veterinary medicine. Badajoz, Spain: FORMATEX; 2013.

97.   Dias MV, Soares Nde F, Borges SV, de Sousa MM, Nunes CA, de Oliveira IR, et al. Use of allyl isothiocyanate and carbon nanotubes in an antimicrobial film to package shredded, cooked chicken meat. Food Chem. 2013;141(3):3160–6.

98.   Ajitha B, Reddy YAK, Reddy PS. Biosynthesis of silver nanoparticles using Plectranthus amboinicus leaf extract and its antimicrobial activity. Spectrochim Acta A Mol Biomol Spectrosc. 2014;128:257–62.

99.   Sun RW, Chen R, Chung NP, Ho CM, Lin CL, Che CM. Silver nanoparticles fabricated in Hepes buffer exhibit cytoprotective activities toward HIV-1 infected cells. Chem Commun (Camb). 2005;40:5059–61.

100. Lara HH, Nilda V, Ayala-Nuñez NV, Ixtepan-Turrent L, Rodriguez-Padilla C. Mode of antiviral action of silver nanoparticles against HIV-1. J Nanobiotechnol. 2010;8:1.

101. Baram-Pinto D, Shukla S, Perkas N, Gedanken A, Sarid R. Inhibition of herpes simplex virus type 1 infection by silver nanoparticles capped with mercaptoethane sulfonate. Bioconjug Chem. 2009;20:1497–502.

102. Sun L, Singh AK, Vig K, Pillai S, Shreekumar R, Singh SR. Silver nanoparticles inhibit replication of respiratory sincitial virus. J Biomed Biotechnol. 2008;4:149–58.

103. Rogers JV, Parkinson CV, Choi YW, Speshock JL, Hussain SM. A preliminary assessment of silver nanoparticles inhibition of monkeypox virus plaque formation. Nanoscale Res Lett. 2008;3:129–33.

104. Liu X, Yu L, Liu F, Sheng L, An K, Chen H, et al. Preparation of Ag–Fe-decorated single-walled carbon nanotubes by arc discharge and their antibacterial effect. J Mater Sci. 2012;47:6086–94.

105. Speshock JL, Murdock RC, Braydich-Stolle LK, Schrand AM, Hussain SM. Interaction of silver nanoparticles with Tacaribe virus. J Nanobiotechnol. 2010;8:19–27.

106. Banu AN, Balasubramanian C, Vinayaga MP. Biosynthesis of silver nanoparticles using Bacillus thuringiensis against dengue vector, Aedes aegypti (Diptera: Culicidae). Parasitol Res. 2014;113:311–6.

107. Papp I, Sieben C, Ludwig K, Roskamp M, Böttcher C, Schlecht S, et al. Inhibition of influenza virus infection by multivalent sialic-acid-functionalized gold nanoparticles. Small. 2010;6:2900–6.

108. Marimuthu S, Rahuman AA, Kirthi AV, Santhoshkumar T, Jayaseelan C, Rajakumar G. Eco-friendly microbial route to synthesize cobalt nanoparticles using Bacillus thuringiensis against malaria and dengue vectors. Parasitol Res. 2013;112(12):4105–12.

109. Mohapatra SC, Tiwari HK, Singla M, Rathi B, Sharma A, Mahiya K, et al. Antimalarial evaluation of copper(II) nanohybrid solids: inhibition of plasmepsin II, a hemoglobin-degrading malarial aspartic protease from Plasmodium falciparum. J Biol Inorg Chem. 2010;15(3):373–85.

110. Kirthi AV, Rahuman A, Rajakumar G, Marimuthu S, Santhoshkumar T, Jayaseelan C, et al. Acaricidal, pediculocidal and larvicidal activity of

synthesized ZnO nanoparticles using wet chemical route against blood feeding parasites. Parasitol Res. 2011;109:461–72.

111. Gowri S, Gandhi RR, Sundrarajan M. Structural, optical, antibacterial and antifungal properties of zirconia nanoparticles by biobased protocol. J Mater Sci Technol. 2014;30(8):782e790.

112. Lu L, Sun RW, Chen R, Hui CK, Ho CM, Luk JM, et al. Silver nanoparticles inhibit hepatitis B virus replication. Antivir Ther. 2008;13:253–62.

113. Pelczar M, Reid R, Chan ECS. Microbiologia. São Paulo: McGraw-Hill; 1980. p. 2008.

114. Senior K, Müller S, Schacht VJ, Bunge M. Antimicrobial precious-metal nanoparticles and their use in novel materials. Recent Pat Food Nutr Agric. 2012;4(3):200–9.

115. Yah CS. The toxicity of gold nanoparticles in relation to their physiochemical properties. Biomed Res. 2013;24(3):400–13.

116. Gatoo MA, Naseem S, Arfat MY, Dar AM, Qasim K, Zubair S. Physicochemical properties of nanomaterials: implication in associated toxic manifestations. Biomed Res Int. 2014;2014:498420.

117. Dorotkiewicz-Jach A, Augustyniak D, Olszak T, Drulis-Kawa Z. Modern therapeutic approaches against pseudomonas aeruginosa infections. Curr Med Chem. 2015;22(14):1642–64.

118. Chatterjee AK, Chakraborty R, Basu T. Mechanism of antibacterial activity of copper nanoparticles. Nanotechnology. 2014;25(13):135101.

119. Dong Q, Dong A, Morigen. Evaluation of novel antibacterial N-halamine nanoparticles prodrugs towards susceptibility of escherichia coli induced by DksA protein. Molecules. 2015;20(4):7292–308.

120. Li H, Chen Q, Zhao J, Urmila K. Enhancing the antimicrobial activity of natural extraction using the synthetic ultrasmall metal nanoparticles. Sci Rep. 2015;5:11033.

121. Xie Y, He Y, Irwin PL, Jin T, Shi X. Antibacterial activity and mechanism of action of zinc oxide nanoparticles against Campylobacter jejuni. Appl Environ Microbiol. 2011;77(7):2325–31.

122. Bawskar M, Deshmukh S, Bansod S, Gade A, Rai M. Comparative analysis of biosynthesised and chemosynthesised silver nanoparticles with special reference to their antibacterial activity against pathogens. IET Nanobiotechnol. 2015;9(3):107–13.

123. Piras AM, Maisetta G, Sandreschi S, Gazzarri M, Bartoli C, Grassi L, et al. Chitosan nanoparticles loaded with the antimicrobial peptide temporin B exert a long-term antibacterial activity in vitro against clinical isolates of Staphylococcus epidermidis. Front Microbiol. 2015;6:372.

124. Mogharabi M, Abdolahi M, Faramarzi MM. Toxicity of nanomaterials. Daru. 2014;22:9.

125. Nuñez-Anita RE, Acosta-Torres LS, Vilar-Pineda J, Martínez-Espinosa JC, de la Fuente-Hernández J, Castaño VM. Toxicology of antimicrobial nanoparticles for prosthetic devices. Int J Nanomedicine. 2014;9:3999–4006.

126. Cooper RJ, Spitzer N. Silver nanoparticles at sublethal concentrations disrupt cytoskeleton and neurite dynamics in cultured adult neural stem cells. Neurotoxicology. 2015;48:231–8.

127. Uhm SH, Lee SB, Song DH, Kwon JS, Han JG, Kim KN. Fabrication of bioactive, antibacterial TiO2 nanotube surfaces, coated with magnetron sputtered Ag nanostructures for dental applications. J Nanosci Nanotechnol. 2014;14(10):7847–54.

20

Immunomodulatory effect of hypertonic saline in hemorrhagic shock

Javad Motaharinia[1], Farhad Etezadi[2], Azadeh Moghaddas[1] and Mojtaba Mojtahedzadeh[1*]

Abstract

Multiple organ dysfunction syndrome (MODS) and nosocomial infection following trauma-hemorrhage are among the most important causes of mortality in hemorrhagic shock patients. Dysregulation of the immune system plays a central role in MODS and a fluid having an immunomodulatory effect could be advantageous in hemorrhagic shock resuscitation. Hypertonic saline (HS) is widely used as a resuscitation fluid in trauma-hemorrhagic patients. Besides having beneficial effects on the hemodynamic parameters, HS has modulatory effects on various functions of immune cells such as degranulation, adhesion molecules and cytokines expression, as well as reactive oxygen species production. This article reviews clinical evidence for decreased organ failure and mortality in hemorrhagic shock patients resuscitated with HS. Despite promising results in animal models, results from pre-hospital and emergency department administration in human studies did not show improvement in survival, organ failure, or a reduction in nosocomial infection by HS resuscitation. Further post hoc analysis showed some benefit from HS resuscitation for severely-injured patients, those who received more than ten units of blood by transfusion, patients who underwent surgery, and victims of traumatic brain injury. Several reasons are suggested to explain the differences between clinical and animal models.

Keywords: Hypertonic saline, Hemorrhagic shock, Trauma, Anti-inflammatory, Multiple organ failure, Acute lung injury

Introduction

Multiple organ dysfunction syndrome (MODS) and nosocomial infection following trauma-hemorrhage are the most common causes of mortality in hemorrhagic shock patients [1]. The most important pathogenic mechanism underlying MODS is disproportionate excitation and dysregulation of systemic inflammatory response triggered by injury and microbial invasion. Although fluid resuscitation is the mainstay of therapy in hemorrhagic shock, reperfusion of ischemic tissues produces additional injury known as ischemia reperfusion injury (IRI) [2].

Hypertonic saline (HS) now is widely used as a resuscitation fluid during critical illness because of its beneficial hemodynamic properties, such as rapid expansion of intravascular volume, reduction of endothelial and tissue edema that improves microcirculation, improvement of blood viscosity caused by hemodilution, and increased myocardial contractility [3, 4].

Besides the improvement in hemodynamic parameters, studies on hemorrhagic shock models have shown that HS can reduce organ failure [5–8]. Recently, new findings have suggested that HS modulates local and systemic inflammatory response [9–16]. It is demonstrated that an increase of 10 to 20 mOsm/kg in plasma osmolality caused by HS can affect some functions of immune cells such as degranulation [10, 14], reactive oxygen species (ROS) production [10, 14, 17], adhesion molecules expression [15], cytokine production [18, 19], and phagocytic ability [12]. However, recent studies showed that some immunomodulatory effects of HS such as inhibition of b2 integrin expression on neutrophil surface and alteration in inflammatory cytokine production mediated via sodium- or chloride-dependent events rather than by its osmolality [16, 20].

Activation of the innate immune system and inflammatory responses are associated with IRI [2, 21]. The beneficial effects of HS can be partly explained by its ability to suppress the various functions of neutrophil including adhesion molecule expression, release of proteolytic enzymes, and production of ROS [10, 13]. Endothelial

* Correspondence: mojtahed@tums.ac.ir
[1]Department of Pharmacotherapy, Faculty of Pharmacy, Tehran University of Medical Sciences, 16 Azar Ave, Enghelab Sq, Tehran, Iran
Full list of author information is available at the end of the article

cells (ECs) activation increases the adherence of neutrophils promoting capillary congestion and the no-reflow phenomenon [22]. By inhibiting the Intercellular adhesion molecule-1 and b2 integrin upregulation, HS decreases neutrophil rolling and adherence to ECs, thereby improving microcirculation and vascular permeability [23–25]. Reactive oxygen species production during reperfusion of ischemic tissues is thought to be the main reason for uncontrolled oxidative stress [21]. Several models of hemorrhagic shock and IRI demonstrated that HS attenuates oxidative stress by decreasing inducible nitric oxide synthase expression and increasing heme oxygenase −1 expression [26–28].

Although the beneficial effects of HS and its immunomodulatory mechanisms have been demonstrated in experimental studies of hemorrhagic shock, resuscitation with HS has failed to improve patient outcomes in human studies. Several meta-analyses and review articles have concluded that there is insufficient evidence for improved survival of hemorrhagic shock patients resuscitated using HS; however, these are dated [29–31]. More recent and larger clinical studies have been performed and, as for the earlier clinical studies, these trials have provided conflicting results.

This article reviews clinical evidence for decreased organ failure and mortality in hemorrhagic shock patients resuscitated with HS, and proposes reasons for the discrepancy between results of experimental studies and clinical trials.

Methods

Materials for this review were obtained by searching PubMed, CINAHL, Scopus, Cochrane Central Register of Controlled Trials, and Cochrane Database of Systematic Reviews. Keywords used as search terms were hypertonic saline, hypertonic solution, hypertonic NaCl, hemorrhagic shock, trauma, inflammation, anti-inflammatory, multiple organ failure syndrome, lung injury, and mortality. The search was limited to publications from 1990 to the present.

Randomized controlled trials that compared HS with or without dextran to isotonic crystalloid solutions were assessed for the study endpoints of patient survival and organ failure. Papers that assessed HS resuscitation for concomitant hemorrhagic shock and traumatic brain injury (TBI) were excluded. Only English language articles were assessed in this review.

HS resuscitation in clinical studies of hemorrhagic shock

To date, several randomized clinical trials (RCT) have been conducted on hemorrhagic shock. Only 11 RCTs met the criteria mentioned in the method [32–42]. In most, trauma patients with hypotension were included and randomly allocated for treatment with hypertonic

solutions (7.5 % HS (HS7.5 %) and dextran 70 (HSD) or isotonic crystalloid solutions in pre-hospital settings or in emergency departments. All trials were prospective and double-blind and subjects received the same 250 ml dose of either HS or isotonic crystalloid solution. Resuscitation was continued by isotonic crystalloid solutions when needed.

Four of the 11 trials were designed for emergency departments [33, 34, 37, 40], the others for pre-hospital settings. In six trials only HSD was used as the HS [32, 33, 35, 36, 40, 41]; in the others, both HS and HSD were applied [34, 37–39, 42]. Unfortunately, most of these studies were conducted prior to 2000; hence, authors assessed only early mortality and hemodynamic variables as end points and did not report secondary endpoints such as the development of acute respiratory distress syndrome (ARDS) or MODS. These studies also did not report the pretreatment acid–base status of the patients. Early and late mortality as primary outcomes and MODS and infection as secondary outcomes were reported in only four studies [35, 40–42].

Table 1 shows that, in the 11 trials assessing more than 2530 cases, results showed that a small volume of HSD or HS improved hemodynamic variables such as blood pressure and cardiac output. Importantly, nearly all confirmed that the use of HSD or HS was safe and effective for trauma patients.

Results from evaluating trials were not able to show any survival improvement; only Younes et al. demonstrated in 1997 that HSD treatment significantly improved survival after 24 h of resuscitation [40]. In other studies, *post hoc* sub-group analysis suggests that certain populations could be more likely to benefit from HS; these included patients with TBI, with low mean arterial pressure (MAP), who required massive transfusions, or underwent surgery.

Younes et al. studied 212 hypovolemic shock patients in an emergency department. Patients were randomly assigned for treatment with a 250 ml bolus of 7.5 % HS + 6 % dextran (HSD, $n = 101$) or 0.9 % normal saline (NS, $n = 111$) and resuscitation was followed using a standard algorithm [40]. The groups were assessed at 24 h and 30 days of survival and prognostic factors such as sex, age, cause of hypovolemia induction, revised trauma score, Glasgow index, and MAP on admission were evaluated. The results showed that the 24 h survival rate was significantly higher for the HSD group (87 %) than the NS group (72 %) ($p \le 0.007$). Multivariate analysis showed that RTS and MAP were independent predictors for 24 h survival for the HSD group. HSD improved the long-term survival rate significantly only in the patients with MAP values of <70 mmHg ($p < .01$). The overall rate of complications (renal failure, ARDS, heart failure, infections, and neurological complications) were similar for both groups (24 %). The authors concluded that the administration of HS as

Table 1 Prospective double-blinded randomized clinical trials on HS or HSD resuscitation in hemorrhagic shock patients

Study	Population	Resuscitation fluid	End point	Results
[32]	20 pre-hospital trauma patients with SBP ≤ 100 mmHg	HSD or LR	Survival to hospital discharge and hemodynamic variables	Improved SBP and overall survival rate.
[33]	32 trauma patients with a SBP < 80 mm Hg admitted to ED	HSD or LR	Survival to hospital discharge and hemodynamic variables	There were no differences in survival rate.
[34]	106 trauma patients with SBP <80 mm Hg for 6 % HSD or < 90 mmHg for HS and were 18 years or older admitted to ED	HS or HSD or LR	Survival to hospital discharge and hemodynamic variables	There were no differences in overall survival between any of the groups.
[35]	422 pre-hospital trauma patients ≥ 16 years with SBP ≤ 90 mmHg 72 % of participants had sustained penetrating trauma	HSD or LR	Primary end points included: survival at 24 h and 30 days (if possible). Secondary end points included: complications and safety of HSD	In the HSD 6 % group which requiring surgery: there was a significant treatment effect in favor of HSD 6 % ($p = 0.02$). This effect was significant in those patients sustaining penetrating trauma ($p = 0.01$), but not in those with blunt trauma.
[36]	166 pre-hospital trauma patients with SBP ≤ 90 mmHg	HSD or LR	Survival to hospital discharge and hemodynamic variables	There was no difference in overall survival and there is a trend to improve survival in patients with severe head injuries.
[37]	105 trauma patients ≥ 18 years with SBP < 80 mm Hg admitted to ED	HSD or HS or NS	Survival to hospital discharge, hemodynamic variables	There were no significant differences in overall complication and mortality rates in the three groups.
[38]	194 pre-hospital trauma patients with SBP < 90 mm	HSD or HS or LR	Survival to hospital discharge, hemodynamics variables, MTOS and neurological outcome scores	Overall survival in the four treatment groups was not statistically significant. Survival in the hypertonic group, however, was significantly higher than that predicted by the MTOS norms. The survival rate in the HS group was higher than that in the LR group for the cohort with baseline Glasgow Coma Scale scores of 8 or less ($P < .05$ by logistic regression and $P < .01$ by Cox proportional-hazards analysis)
[39]	258 pre-hospital trauma patients with SBP < 90 mm Hg.	HSD or HS or NS	Survival to hospital discharge, hemodynamics variables, MTOS and neurological outcome scores	There were no differences in overall survival. Improved survival vs. predicted MTOS in high-risk HS & HSD 6 % patients, HS patient with GCS 8 or less and HSD 6 % patients with unobtainable BP at the time of randomization.
[40]	212 hypovolemic shock patients admitted to ED	HSD or NS	Survival at 24 h and 30 days and complications	The 24 h survival rate was significantly higher in HSD 6 % (87 %) compared with NS (72 %) ($P < .007$). HSD 6 % improved long term survival rate significantly only in the patients with MAP < 70 mmHg ($p < .01$).
[41]	209 pre-hospital blunt trauma patients with SBP ≤90 mm Hg "The study was stopped for futility after the second interim analyses."	HSD or LR	Primary outcome was 28 day ARDS-free survival. Secondary outcome; nosocomial infection, multiple organ failure syndrome	There was no significant difference in ARDS-free survival. There was an improved in ARDS-free survival in the patients (19 % of the population) requiring 10 U or more of packed RBC in the first 24 h. (HR, 2.18; 95 % CI, 1.09–4.36).
[42] RCT, multi center	853 pre-hospital hypovolemic shock patients with SBP ≤ 70 mm Hg or SBP ≈ 71–90 mm Hg with HR equal or higher than 108 beats per minute. (62 % of patients were with blunt trauma.) . "The study was stopped early (23 % of proposed sample size) for futility and potential safety concern."	HSD or HS or NS	Primary outcome was 28 day survival. Secondary outcomes included: fluid and blood requirements in the first 24 h, physiologic parameters of organ dysfunction, 28 day ARDS–free survival, multiple organ dysfunction score and nosocomial infections	There was no significant difference in 28 day survival between treatment groups. There was a higher mortality for the post-randomization subgroup of patients who did not receive blood transfusions in the first 24 h, who received hypertonic fluids compared to NS ($P < 0.01$). There were no differences between groups in organ failure or nosocomial infections.

HSD dextran 70 in HS. *HS* hypertonic saline 7.5 %. *NS* 0.9 % saline. *LR* ringer's lactate. *SBP* systolic blood pressure. *MAP* mean arterial pressure. *MTOS* major trauma outcome study. *BP* blood pressure. *RTS* revised trauma score. *ARDS* acute respiratory distress syndrome. *CI* confidence interval. *HR* hazard ratio. *RBC* red blood cells. *HR* heart rate. *RCT* randomized clinical study. *ED* emergency department an initial treatment of hypovolemic patients admitted through the emergency department is safe and associated with a beneficial outcomes. Further study is needed to identify the survival benefits in patients treated with HS in a pre-hospital setting.

Vassar et al. could not prove differences in survival between differently resuscitated patients in a pre-hospital setting [38]. They resuscitated injured patients with a systolic blood pressure (SBP) of <90 mmHg using four solutions ($n = 150$ in each group) containing 250 ml of lactated Ringer's (LR), 7.5 % HS, 7.5 % sodium chloride + 6 % dextran 70, or 7.5 % sodium chloride + 12 % dextran 70 followed by conventional isotonic solutions as needed. There was no overall difference in survival between groups, but actual survival in the hypertonic group was significantly higher than that predicted by Major trauma outcome study (MTOS) norms. The survival rate in the HS group was higher than that in the LR group for patients with baseline Glasgow Coma Scale scores of ≤ 8 ($p < 0.05$ by logistic regression; $p < 0.01$ by Cox proportional hazards analysis). The authors concluded that infusion of a small volume of 7.5 % HS early in resuscitation was safe and improved the survival rates of severely-injured patients when compared with MTOS norms. The addition of dextran to hypertonic solution showed no benefits.

Prior this study, in 1991, Vassar et al. published the results of 166 pre-hospital trauma patients recording SBP ≤ 90 mmHg [36]. They resuscitated patients with 250 ml of either 7.5 % HSD ($n = 83$) or LR solution ($n = 83$). Although the results of this study showed no difference in overall survival between HSD and LR patients, it did show a trend of improved survival in patients with severe head injuries. Administration of small volumes of HSD before hospitalization increased the blood pressure of severely injured patients more effectively than did LR solution and tended to improve survival in patients with severe head injuries.

Mattox et al. randomly assigned hypovolemic shock patients to be administered with HSD or isotonic crystalloid solution (LR, NS, plasmalyte) [35]. Survival at 24 h and 30 days (if possible) were primary end points and improvement in 24 h physiological status, reduction in post-injury complications, and safety of HSD solutions (in the volume given) with regard to seizures, anaphylactoid reactions, and coagulopathies were secondary end points. The authors estimated that 700 patients would be required to show a difference in survival, but only 422 patients were enrolled. Seventy-two percent of participants had sustained penetrating trauma. HSD has improved survival significantly in the subpopulation of patients requiring surgery ($p = 0.02$). This effect was significant in those patients sustaining penetrating trauma ($p = 0.01$), but not in those with blunt trauma. Only 22

patients were followed for as long as 30 days. Thus, analysis was not performed.

The HSD group had fewer complications such as ARDS, renal failure, sepsis, pneumonia, and coagulopathy than the standard treatment group (7 versus 24). HSD related coagulopathy, anaphylactoid reactions, and seizures were not reported. The authors concluded that bolus administration of 250 ml of 7.5 % HSD is safe and was as effective as standard resuscitation solutions in the pre-hospital management of traumatic hypotension. HSD may also offer a potential benefit in a subgroup of patients with penetrating injuries, active hemorrhage, or those requiring urgent laparotomy or thoracotomy. Studies with larger sample sizes will be required to establish which subgroups of trauma patients will maximally benefit from pre-hospital use of a small volume of HS [35].

Lack of conclusive evidence led to meta-analysis to reevaluate the effect of HSD on early mortality (24 h survival). The first was performed by Wade et al. in 1997. They included eight RCT of trauma patients treated with HSD until that date and demonstrated that HSD administrated as the initial fluid therapy enhanced survival of patients with hypotension caused by trauma (OR = 1.46; 95 % CL; 1.01–2.12). All included studies in this meta-analysis have been summarized in the present article. Further improvement in survival was found in patients with penetrating trauma requiring surgery (OR = 1.97; 1.07–3.61) or blood transfusion. The authors concluded that initial fluid therapy with HSD was beneficial in patients requiring blood transfusion, surgery, or patients with penetrating injuries who required surgery [29].

The second meta-analysis examined eight double-blind RCTs in which HSD and HS were compared with isotonic solution [32–39] and also compared HS and isotonic solution in two trials for the treatment of hypovolemic trauma patients (These studies was not reviewed in the present article due to unpublished data). Analysis was done on 615 patients who were treated with 6 % HSD and 340 who were treated with HS. The primary end point was 30 day survival after injury or until discharge. Results showed that the survival rate did not differ for HS and isotonic resuscitation ($p = 0.46$; OR = 0.98; 95 % CI; 0.71–1.36). The authors concluded that there is a trend toward superiority of 6 % HSD for improved survival, but it was not significant. The results of the meta-analysis showed that resuscitation with HS alone did not demonstrate efficacy for survival of trauma patients with hypovolemia [30].

Bunn et al. conducted meta-analysis in 2004 to determine whether HS decreases mortality in hypovolemic patients with and without head injury [31]. Most of the 17 trials (869 participants) included in the analysis had small precipitants and only five trials conducted on trauma patients were judged to provide adequate quality [32–39] (Nine of the studies that have been included in this meta-analysis was not reviewed in the present article due to unpublished data and included TBI patients). The authors concluded that there was insufficient data to support efficacy of HS in resuscitation of patients with trauma, burns, or those who underwent surgery. They stated that further large and qualified trials were needed to adequately compare hypertonic and isotonic crystalloid.

Bulgar et al. in 2008 designed a RCT to evaluate effect of HS on late mortality, multiple organ failure, and nosocomial infection in blunt traumatic injury with hypovolemic shock. In this study, 209 patients with SBP of ≤ 90 mmHg were randomized to receive either HSD ($n = 110$) or LR ($n = 99$) in a pre-hospital setting. The primary outcome was 28 day ARDS-free survival and the secondary outcomes were nosocomial infection, MODS, resource utilization, mortality, and noninfectious complications. There was no significant difference in ARDS-free survival (adjusted hazard ratio = 1.01; 95 % confidence interval (CI); 0.63–1.60); however, there was evidence of improvement in ARDS-free survival by patients (19 % of the population) requiring 10 units or more of packed red blood cells in the first 24 h. (Odds ratio (OR) = 2.18; 95 % CI; 1.09–4.36). Further evaluation using Cox proportional hazards methods to assess the effect of treatment by red cells transfused again reached the same hazard ratio for 28 day survival (2.49; 95 % CI; 1.1–5.6). There were no significant differences in the secondary outcome measures. The authors concluded that although there were no significant differences in ARDS-free survival and secondary outcomes, there was a survival benefit in the subgroup of patients at highest risk for ARDS, such as those requiring 10 units or more of packed red blood cells in the first 24 h [41].

Bulger et al. in 2011 conducted a larger trial on traumatic hemorrhagic shock in patients. The resuscitation outcome consortium (ROC) trial was a randomized, double-blind, multicenter study. Two series of patients were included; those who recorded SBP ≤ 70 mmHg and those with heart rates (HR) of ≤ 108 beats per minute and SBP of 71 to 90 mmHg. Patients randomly received a 250 ml bolus of HSD, HS, or NS followed by additional crystalloid as determined by medical requirements in a pre-hospital setting. The primary outcome was 28 day survival and the secondary outcomes were incidence of ARDS, multi-organ failure, infection, number of ventilator days, and physiological and functional outcomes in the first 28 days after intervention. Because only 23 % of the proposed sample size was achieved and because of the increase in mortality among patients receiving no blood transfusions in the first 24 h, the Data Safety Monitoring Board halted the study prematurely. The 28 day mortality rates did not differ between HS, HSD and NS groups (74.5 % HSD (absolute difference in 28 day survival probabilities = 0.1; 95 % CI;–7.5 to 7.8), 73.0 % HS (–1.4; 95 % CI,–8.7 to 6.0), and 74.4 % NS ($p = 0.91$). The rate of organ failure or nosocomial infections in patients treated with NS was higher than those in the HS and HSD groups, but these differences were not statistically significant. The authors concluded that initial resuscitation with hypertonic solution in a pre-hospital setting did not improve 28 day survival. Future studies are warranted to better define the use of these fluids in a pre-hospital setting [42].

The Colloids versus Crystalloids for the Resuscitation of the Critically Ill (CRISTAL) trial enrolled 2857 intensive care unit patients admitted for hypovolemic shock to evaluate a possible decrease in mortality for the use of fluid resuscitation with colloids ($n = 1443$) versus crystalloids (1414). No difference in 28 day mortality was noted, but 90 day mortality improved in those resuscitated with colloids (30.7 % vs. 34.2 %). Patients receiving colloids also recorded more days free of vasopressor therapy and mechanical ventilation at 7 and 28 days, respectively. The incidence of organ failure did not differ between groups; however, the population of this study was heterogeneous (sepsis, trauma, others cases of hypovolemic shock) and differed from the previously discussed trials, which exclusively examined traumatic hemorrhagic shock patients. Patients in the crystalloid and colloid groups mainly received isotonic solutions (96 %) and hydroxylethyl starch (69 %), respectively. Subgroup analysis was not performed to compare hypertonic saline resuscitation versus isotonic crystalloids or colloids [43].

Discussion

Bolus administration of HS is safe and effective and improved hemodynamic states from hemorrhagic hypotensive states [29–31]. In clinical studies, it has been shown that a bolus of 4 ml/kg of 7.5 % HS can enhance plasma sodium and osmolality from 147 to 154 mEq/l and 10 to 20 mOsm/kg, respectively; however, the increase in osmolality is temporary and starts to decline after 30 to 60 min [38–41]. This temporary increase in plasma osmolality can affect some functions of the immune system, which can persist for up to 24 h after HS administration [10, 42].

The immunomodulatory effects of hypertonic saline have clinical significance and include a reduction in the incidence of acute lung injury and infectious complications following hemorrhagic shock. Animal studies have shown that HS decreased acute lung injury and improved survival [5–8]; however, evidence that HS benefits survival in hemorrhagic shock patients is inconclusive.

The timing of HS administration appears to be critical. It has been shown that delayed administration of HS exacerbates the inflammatory response and tissue damage following trauma [44, 45]. A septic shock model study showed that the beneficial effects of HS diminished if it is administered after isotonic resuscitation [46]. The results of experimental and clinical studies indicate that the best time to administer HS to prevent inflammatory side effects is early during resuscitation in a pre-hospital setting. The results of pre-hospital resuscitation in clinical studies showed no significant effect on survival or improvement in outcome.

Several reasons for the disagreement between results from animal studies and clinical settings have been proposed. First, the amount and duration of HS infusion used in clinical studies could have been insufficient to decrease the inflammatory response in humans. Although the experimental studies in human showed anti-inflammatory effects of HS [10, 13], because of low sample size of these studies, it could not be concluded that HS can produce clinically relevant anti-inflammatory effects in every traumatic patient.

Another reason for disagreement may be the difference in model design. Animals were resuscitated using either HS or isotonic crystalloids immediately after blood withdrawal [5–8]. In clinical studies under real conditions, resuscitation may be delayed and isotonic fluid administration continued after hypertonic treatment. Evidence suggests that fluid resuscitation with isotonic solutions potentiate neutrophil activation associated with increased organ damage [11, 47, 48]. It has also been demonstrated that hypervolemia alone or massive resuscitation in trauma patients increases the risk of ARDS and mortality [49, 50]. It appears that isotonic resuscitation following HS administration attenuates the protective effects of HS on tissue injury and subsequent MODS.

Another matter for debate is whether trauma patients included in clinical studies actually had experienced IRI or had severe inflammatory conditions for which HS could be beneficial because HS only benefits a subpopulation who require more blood transfusions, have been severely injured, or require surgery. In these populations, severe inflammatory processes are generated in response to trauma. In these situations, the anti-inflammatory effect of hypertonic saline could be apparent.

Some patients could have existing metabolic acidosis at the time of treatment. Crystalloid fluids containing high chloride ion concentrations cause hyperchloremic metabolic acidosis [51]. Metabolic acidosis caused by lactate accumulation gradually disappears in hemorrhagic shock patients if tissue perfusion is restored, but the effect of HS resuscitation on acid–base status is not easily predictable. Moon et al. [52] showed that HS infusion in hemorrhagic shock models produces immediate and transient metabolic acidosis by increasing the plasma chloride concentration relative to the plasma sodium concentration. Metabolic acidosis affects some aspects of the immune system, increasing neutrophil phagocytosis, intracellular death, cytokines, ROS production, complement activation, and impairing leukocyte chemotaxis [53]. Metabolic acidosis is also associated with gut barrier dysfunction and may increase oxidative stress [54]. It is likely that hyperchloremic acidosis caused by administration of HS increases acidosis in already acidotic patients. Acidic conditions, particularly hyperchloremic acidosis, inhibit or weaken the immunomodulatory effects of HS and must be considered at the time of treatment.

Conclusion

Hypertonic saline is safe when used as a resuscitation fluid in the early phase of trauma/hemorrhagic shock. Animal studies have demonstrated some benefit for survival rates, but clinical trials have failed to support such results in humans. HS has been advantageous for patients experiencing severe injury and requiring massive blood transfusions or surgery and in patients with TBI. Evidence suggests that these patients might experience a significant inflammatory response which can be ameliorated by the anti-inflammatory effects of HS.

The present study suggests that further clinical trials with large sample sizes be undertaken to clarify which subgroup of trauma/shock patents gain the most advantage from HS resuscitation. New clinical trials should be designed to better quantify the clinical benefits of continuing resuscitation after administration of the first HS bolus. It is also necessary to consider the acid–base status of a patient before administration of HS solution because the high chloride content of HS may worsen pre-existing lactic acidosis from superimposed hyperchloremic acidosis.

Abbreviations
HS: Hypertonic saline; HSD: Hypertonic saline-dextran; MODS: Multiple organ dysfunction syndrome; IRI: Ischemia reperfusion injury; ROS: Reactive oxygen species; TBI: Traumatic brain injury; EC: Endothelial cell; MTOS: Major trauma outcome study; MAP: Mean arterial pressure; HR: Heart rate; SBP: Systolic blood pressure; ARDS: Acute respiratory distress syndrome; RCT: Randomized clinical trials; LR: Lactated ringer's; NS: Normal saline; ROC: Resuscitation outcomes consortium; CRISTAL: Colloids versus crystalloids for the resuscitation of the critically ill.

Competing interests
The authors declare that they have no competing interests.

Authors' contributions
MM Designing the review method and Reviewing the final manuscript FE Reviewing the final manuscript. AM Contributing to write the manuscript. JM Reviewing the literature, preparing the manuscript and final revision. All authors read and approved the final manuscript.

Acknowledgment
The authors would like to express their special thanks of gratitude to Professor Mohammad Abdollahi for his comments on this manuscript, although any errors are their own and should not tarnish the reputations of this respected person.

Author details
[1]Department of Pharmacotherapy, Faculty of Pharmacy, Tehran University of Medical Sciences, 16 Azar Ave, Enghelab Sq, Tehran, Iran. [2]Department of

Anesthesiology & Critical Care, Sina Hospital, Tehran University of Medical Sciences, Tehran, Iran.

References

1. Durham RM, Moran JJ, Mazuski JE, Shapiro MJ, Baue AE, Flint LM. Multiple organ failure in trauma patients. J Trauma. 2003;55(4):608–16.
2. Lenz A, Franklin GA, Cheadle WG. Systemic inflammation after trauma. Injury. 2007;38(12):1336–45.
3. Rocha-e-Silva M, de Figueiredo LF P. Small volume hypertonic resuscitation of circulatory shock. Clinics. 2005;60(2):159–72.
4. Strandvik GF. Hypertonic saline in critical care: a review of the literature and guidelines for use in hypotensive states and raised intracranial pressure. Anaesthesia. 2009;64(9):990–1003.
5. Coimbra R, Hoyt DB, Junger WG, Angle N, Wolf P, Loomis W, et al. Hypertonic saline resuscitation decreases susceptibility to sepsis after hemorrhagic shock. J Trauma. 1997;42(4):602–6. discussion 6–7.
6. Angle N, Hoyt DB, Coimbra R, Liu F, Herdon-Remelius C, Loomis W, et al. Hypertonic saline resuscitation diminishes lung injury by suppressing neutrophil activation after hemorrhagic shock. Shock. 1998;9(3):164–70.
7. Shi HP, Deitch EA, Da Xu Z, Lu Q, Hauser CJ. Hypertonic saline improves intestinal mucosa barrier function and lung injury after trauma-hemorrhagic shock. Shock. 2002;17(6):496–501.
8. Vincenzi R, Cepeda LA, Pirani WM, Sannomiya P, Rocha ESM, Cruz Jr RJ. Small volume resuscitation with 3 % hypertonic saline solution decrease inflammatory response and attenuates end organ damage after controlled hemorrhagic shock. Am J Surg. 2009;198(3):407–14.
9. Kolsen-Petersen JA. Immune effect of hypertonic saline: fact or fiction? Acta Anaesthesiol Scand. 2004;48(6):667–78.
10. Junger WG, Rhind SG, Rizoli SB, Cuschieri J, Shiu MY, Baker AJ, et al. Resuscitation of traumatic hemorrhagic shock patients with hypertonic saline-without dextran-inhibits neutrophil and endothelial cell activation. Shock. 2012;38(4):341–50.
11. Alam HB, Stanton K, Koustova E, Burris D, Rich N, Rhee P. Effect of different resuscitation strategies on neutrophil activation in a swine model of hemorrhagic shock. Resuscitation. 2004;60(1):91–9.
12. Shields CJ, O'Sullivan AW, Wang JH, Winter DC, Kirwan WO, Redmond HP. Hypertonic saline enhances host response to bacterial challenge by augmenting receptor-independent neutrophil intracellular superoxide formation. Ann Surg. 2003;238(2):249–57.
13. Rizoli SB, Rhind SG, Shek PN, Inaba K, Filips D, Tien H, et al. The immunomodulatory effects of hypertonic saline resuscitation in patients sustaining traumatic hemorrhagic shock: a randomized, controlled, double-blinded trial. Ann Surg. 2006;243(1):47–57.
14. Junger WG, Hoyt DB, Davis RE, Herdon-Remelius C, Namiki S, Junger H, et al. Hypertonicity regulates the function of human neutrophils by modulating chemoattractant receptor signaling and activating mitogen-activated protein kinase p38. J Clin Invest. 1998;101(12):2768–79.
15. Rizoli SB, Kapus A, Parodo J, Rotstein OD. Hypertonicity prevents lipopolysaccharide-stimulated CD11b/CD18 expression in human neutrophils in vitro: role for p38 inhibition. J Trauma. 1999;46(5):794–8. discussion 8–9.
16. Thiel M, Buessecker F, Eberhardt K, Chouker A, Setzer F, Kreimeier U, et al. Effects of hypertonic saline on expression of human polymorphonuclear leukocyte adhesion molecules. J Leukoc Biol. 2001;70(2):261–73.
17. Mojtahedzadeh M, Ahmadi A, Mahmoodpoor A, Beigmohammadi MT, Abdollahi M, Khazaeipour Z, et al. Hypertonic saline solution reduces the oxidative stress responses in traumatic brain injury patients. J Res Med Sci. 2014;19(9):867–74.
18. Ke QH, Zheng SS, Liang TB, Xie HY, Xia WL. Pretreatment of hypertonic saline can increase endogenous interleukin 10 release to attenuate hepatic ischemia reperfusion injury. Dig Dis Sci. 2006;51(12):2257–63.
19. Powers KA, Woo J, Khadaroo RG, Papia G, Kapus A, Rotstein OD. Hypertonic resuscitation of hemorrhagic shock upregulates the anti-inflammatory response by alveolar macrophages. Surgery. 2003;134(2):312–8.
20. Hatanaka E, Shimomi FM, Curi R, Campa A. Sodium chloride inhibits cytokine production by lipopolysaccharide-stimulated human neutrophils and mononuclear cells. Shock. 2007;27(1):32–5.
21. Angele MK, Schneider CP, Chaudry IH. Bench-to-bedside review: latest results in hemorrhagic shock. Crit Care. 2008;12(4):218.
22. Vrints CJ. Pathophysiology of the no-reflow phenomenon. Acute Card Care. 2009;11(2):69–76.
23. Pascual JL, Khwaja KA, Chaudhury P, Christou NV. Hypertonic saline and the microcirculation. J Trauma. 2003;54(5 Suppl):133–40.
24. Oreopoulos GD, Hamilton J, Rizoli SB, Fan J, Lu Z, Li YH, et al. In vivo and in vitro modulation of intercellular adhesion molecule (ICAM)-1 expression by hypertonicity. Shock. 2000;14(3):409–14. discussion 14–5.
25. Pascual JL, Ferri LE, Seely AJ, Campisi G, Chaudhury P, Giannias B, et al. Hypertonic saline resuscitation of hemorrhagic shock diminishes neutrophil rolling and adherence to endothelium and reduces in vivo vascular leakage. Ann Surg. 2002;236(5):634–42.
26. Attuwaybi B, Kozar RA, Gates KS, Moore-Olufemi S, Sato N, Weisbrodt NW, et al. Hypertonic saline prevents inflammation, injury, and impaired intestinal transit after gut ischemia/reperfusion by inducing heme oxygenase 1 enzyme. J Trauma. 2004;56(4):749–58. discussion 58–9.
27. Ke QH, Zheng SS, Liang TB, Xie HY, Xia WL. Effects of hypertonic saline on expression of heme oxygenase enzyme-1 in hepatic ischemia/reperfusion injury rats. Zhongguo Wei Zhong Bing Ji Jiu Yi Xue. 2006;18(1):5–8.
28. Lu YQ, Gu LH, Jiang JK, Mou HZ. Effect of hypertonic versus isotonic saline resuscitation on heme oxygenase-1 expression in visceral organs following hemorrhagic shock in rats. Biomed Environ Sci. 2013;26(8):684–8.
29. Wade C, Grady J, Kramer G. Efficacy of hypertonic saline dextran (HSD) in patients with traumatic hypotension: meta-analysis of individual patient data. Acta Anaesthesiol Scand Suppl. 1997;110:77–9.
30. Wade CE, Kramer GC, Grady JJ, Fabian TC, Younes RN. Efficacy of hypertonic 7.5 % saline and 6 % dextran-70 in treating trauma: a meta-analysis of controlled clinical studies. Surgery. 1997;122(3):609–16.
31. Bunn F, Roberts I, Tasker R, Akpa E. Hypertonic versus near isotonic crystalloid for fluid resuscitation in critically ill patients. Cochrane Database Syst Rev. 2004;3:002045.
32. Holcroft JW, Vassar MJ, Turner JE, Derlet RW, Kramer GC. 3 % NaCl and 7.5 % NaCl/dextran 70 in the resuscitation of severely injured patients. Ann Surg. 1987;206(3):279–88.
33. Holcroft JW, Vassar MJ, Perry CA, Gannaway WL, Kramer GC. Use of a 7.5 % NaCl/6 % Dextran 70 solution in the resuscitation of injured patients in the emergency room. Prog Clin Biol Res. 1989;299:331–8.
34. Vassar MJ, Perry CA, Holcroft JW. Analysis of potential risks associated with 7.5 % sodium chloride resuscitation of traumatic shock. Arch Surg. 1990;125(10):1309–15.
35. Mattox KL, Maningas PA, Moore EE, Mateer JR, Marx JA, Aprahamian C, et al. Prehospital hypertonic saline/dextran infusion for post-traumatic hypotension. The U.S.A. Multicenter Trial. Ann Surg. 1991;213(5):482–91.
36. Vassar MJ, Perry CA, Gannaway WL, Holcroft JW. 7.5 % sodium chloride/ dextran for resuscitation of trauma patients undergoing helicopter transport. Arch Surg. 1991;126(9):1065–72.
37. Younes RN, Aun F, Accioly CQ, Casale LP, Szajnbok I, Birolini D. Hypertonic solutions in the treatment of hypovolemic shock: a prospective, randomized study in patients admitted to the emergency room. Surgery. 1992;111(4):380–5.
38. Vassar MJ, Fischer RP, O'Brien PE, Bachulis BL, Chambers JA, Hoyt DB, et al. A multicenter trial for resuscitation of injured patients with 7.5 % sodium chloride. The effect of added dextran 70. The Multicenter Group for the Study of Hypertonic Saline in Trauma Patients. Arch Surg. 1993;128(9):1003–11. discussion 11–3.
39. Vassar MJ, Perry CA, Holcroft JW. Prehospital resuscitation of hypotensive trauma patients with 7.5 % NaCl versus 7.5 % NaCl with added dextran: a controlled trial. J Trauma. 1993;34(5):622–32. discussion 32–3.
40. Younes RN, Aun F, Ching CT, Goldenberg DC, Franco MH, Miura FK, et al. Prognostic factors to predict outcome following the administration of hypertonic/hyperoncotic solution in hypovolemic patients. Shock. 1997;7(2):79–83.
41. Bulger EM, Jurkovich GJ, Nathens AB, Copass MK, Hanson S, Cooper C, et al. Hypertonic resuscitation of hypovolemic shock after blunt trauma: a randomized controlled trial. Arch Surg. 2008;143(2):139–48. discussion 49.
42. Bulger EM, May S, Kerby JD, Emerson S, Stiell IG, Schreiber MA, et al. Out-of-hospital hypertonic resuscitation after traumatic hypovolemic shock: a randomized, placebo controlled trial. Ann Surg. 2011;253(3):431–41.
43. Annane D, Siami S, Jaber S, Martin C, Elatrous S, Declere AD, et al. Effects of fluid resuscitation with colloids vs crystalloids on mortality in critically

ill patients presenting with hypovolemic shock: the CRISTAL randomized trial. JAMA. 2013;310(17):1809–17.

44. Partrick DA, Moore EE, Offner PJ, Johnson JL, Tamura DY, Silliman CC. Hypertonic saline activates lipid-primed human neutrophils for enhanced elastase release. J Trauma. 1998;44(4):592–7. discussion 8.

45. Chen Y, Hashiguchi N, Yip L, Junger WG. Hypertonic saline enhances neutrophil elastase release through activation of P2 and A3 receptors. Am J Physiol Cell Physiol. 2006;290(4):C1051–9.

46. Inoue Y, Chen Y, Pauzenberger R, Hirsh MI, Junger WG. Hypertonic saline up-regulates A3 adenosine receptor expression of activated neutrophils and increases acute lung injury after sepsis. Crit Care Med. 2008;36(9):2569–75.

47. Watters JM, Tieu BH, Todd SR, Jackson T, Muller PJ, Malinoski D, et al. Fluid resuscitation increases inflammatory gene transcription after traumatic injury. J Trauma. 2006;61(2):300–8. discussion 8–9.

48. Koustova E, Stanton K, Gushchin V, Alam HB, Stegalkina S, Rhee PM. Effects of lactated Ringer's solutions on human leukocytes. J Trauma. 2002;52(5):872–8.

49. Silva PL, Cruz FF, Fujisaki LC, Oliveira GP, Samary CS, Ornellas DS, et al. Hypervolemia induces and potentiates lung damage after recruitment maneuver in a model of sepsis-induced acute lung injury. Crit Care. 2010;14(3):R114.

50. Ertmer C, Kampmeier T, Rehberg S, Lange M. Fluid resuscitation in multiple trauma patients. Curr Opin Anaesthesiol. 2011;24(2):202–8.

51. Constable PD. Hyperchloremic acidosis: the classic example of strong ion acidosis. Anesth Analg. 2003;96(4):919–22.

52. Moon PF, Kramer GC. Hypertonic saline-dextran resuscitation from hemorrhagic shock induces transient mixed acidosis. Crit Care Med. 1995;23(2):323–31.

53. Lardner A. The effects of extracellular pH on immune function. J Leukoc Biol. 2001;69(4):522–30.

54. Kellum JA, Song M, Li J. Science review: extracellular acidosis and the immune response: clinical and physiologic implications. Critical care. 2004;8(5):331–6.

21

Comparative efficacy of esomeprazole and omeprazole: Racemate to single enantiomer switch

Waheed Asghar, Elliot Pittman and Fakhreddin Jamali[*]

Abstract

Background: Both omeprazole and its S enantiomer (esomeprazole) have been available and used to treat symptoms of gastroesophageal reflux disease (GERD) and conditions associated with excessive stomach acid secretion for more than a decade. Controversy exists over improved efficacy of S enantiomer (esomeprazole) over parent racemate (omeprazole). However, a comparison of the clinical outcomes of these products may reveal the rationale for switching from the racemate to single enantiomer. Since enantiomers of omeprazole are equipotent, we compared the outcomes of equal doses of each product to see if both actually differ in their efficacy's or the reported superiority of S enantiomer is just a dose effect.

Methods: A web search was carried out for randomized controlled trials with head-to-head comparisons of omeprazole and S-omeprazole. The data were abstracted and after calculating theodd ratios (OR) for the outcomes reported in each study, the combined overall odd ratios (OR') were estimated. The random effect inverse variance method with omeprazole as the reference (OR" = 1) was used.

Results: Out of 1171 studies, 14 were deemed eligible. There was no significant difference in the therapeutic success between omeprazole and S-omeprazole as a part of triple therapy for the treatment of H. pylori in both intention-to-treat (OR', 1.06; CI, 0.83, 1.36; $p = 0.63$) as well as per-protocol analysis (OR', 1.07; CI, 0.84, 1.36; $p = 0.57$). For the treatment of gastro-oesophageal reflux disease, S-omeprazole was significantly but marginally superior to the racemate (OR', 1.18; CI, 1.01, 1.38; $p = 0.04$). The two products were equipotent in all metrics used to assess intragastric pH except for the % patients maintaining a 24 h gastric pH above 4 (1.57; CI, 1.04, 2.381; $p = 0.03$).

Conclusion: The therapeutic benefit of chiral switch of omeprazole is questionable considering the substantially greater economic burden involved.

Keywords: Omeprazole, Esomeprazole, Enantiomer, GERD, Acid control, *H. pylori*, Comparative efficacy

Background

Stereochemical aspects of drug actions and drug disposition have become a subject of interest since the early 1980s [1]. Most chiral drugs have been used as racemates while the beneficial effects are often attributed mainly to one of the enantiomers. Hence, it was intuitively believed that a product containing the stereochemically pure enantiomer with the main pharmacological activity would be superior to its racemate counterpart. This overwhelming notion has not been without opposition due to increased toxicity risk in humans [2] or in experimental animal [3–5]. Nevertheless,

many attempts have been made during the past decades to switch from racemate to stereochemically pure drug products. This has resulted in the introduction of a few products in the past decade, e.g., levofloxacin, dexibuprofen and esomeprazole. At the time of their development, reasonable rationales for such a switch had been offered without unequivocal data on the superiority of the single enantiomers. For example, omeprazole and S-omeprazole have been the subject of many randomized controlled trials (RCTs) and , cohort and case-control studies. However, these studies and the subsequent systematic reviews [6–12], typically compared non-comparable doses, i.e., 40 mg S-omeprazole vs 20 mg racemic omeprazole. In addition, recently, Gellad et al., who reviewed 4 RCTs that included non-comparative

* Correspondence: fjamali@ualberta.ca
Faculty of Pharmacy and Pharmaceutical Sciences, University of Alberta, 11361 – 87 Avenue, Edmonton, AB T6G 2E1, Canada

doses, concluded mixed evidence for the superiority of the single S enantiomer over the racemate [13]. Thus, a comparison of the available data on comparative doses is needed. From the pharmacological viewpoints, the drug is not stereoselective since its properties are attributed to both enantiomers [14]. Its pharmacokinetics, on the other hand, are stereoselective with the S enantiomer having a higher bioavailability yielding a greater body exposure than R-omeprazole. A 40 mg dose of S-omeprazole, therefore, yields greater than twice the body exposure than a 20 mg dose of the racemate. Thus, clinical trials that have compared 40 vs 20 mg have not assessed comparative doses. Only, a 2005 meta-analysis that focused on *Helicobacter pylori* (*H. pylori*) eradication had included a comparison of equal doses of the racemate and S-omeprazole [15]. The purpose of this work was to analyse all clinical data on the efficacy of equal mg doses of S-omeprazole versus that of racemic omeprazole reported until April 2015. This is with the realization that a dose of the single S enantiomer will result in a greater body exposure when compared to an equal mg dose of the racemate. We stratified the data based on therapeutic, symptomatic and intragastric pH control outcomes. We also analyzed available data based on the type of analysis used; i.e., intention-to-treat and per-protocol. In addition, we assessed the dose-dependency of omeprazole effects.

Methods

Literature search

A web search was conducted using a set of keywords (Appendix 1), in databases including MEDLINE (Medical Literature Analysis and Retrieval System Online database), EMBASE (Excerpta Medica database), CINHAL (Cumulative Index to Nursing and Allied Health Literature), IPA (International Pharmaceutical Abstracts), PASCAL (Dedicated Database for European Science, Technology and Medicine), Cochrane, EBM (The Evidence-Based Medicine database) and Google Scholar. We looked for studies reporting comparative RCTs published until April 2015. The United States Food and Drug Administration (FDA) and pharmaceutical manufacturer's websites were also searched for any relevant literature. Reference lists from review articles were also checked for any relevant information, if available. Two reviewers (W.A. and E.P) independently reviewed the studies for the inclusion and exclusion criteria and conflicts were resolved by mutual agreement.

Data analysis

The data from eligible studies was abstracted and analysed according to published methods [16] and the odds ratios (ORs) of each study were manually calculated for each outcome including: (i) therapeutic success; i.e., as part of triple therapy for eradication of H. pylori or healing of esophagitis or peptic ulcer; (ii) symptomatic relief of heart burn, (gastro-oesophageal reflux disease, GERD; (iii) % of patient with median 24 h intragastric pH above 4. The calculated OR values from all studies were then merged to create the combined odds ratio (OR') using the Review Manager software recommended by Cochrane, and employing the random effect inverse variance method [17]. For cross-over studies, odd ratios were calculated based on the matched samples case–control approach [18]. We chose omeprazole to be the reference (OR' = 1). For metrics that OR could not be calculated (i.e., median pH in 24 h, mean time pH > 4 and % of 24 h with pH > 4) actual measured values were used to assess the differences.

Selection criteria

Only RCTs carried out in an adult population (>18 years age) having both S-omeprazole and omeprazole, in head to head comparisons, at equivalent oral doses, and published in English were included in our analysis. No outcome restriction was considered at this stage. All formulations (capsule, tablet, and suspension, both immediate and delayed release) with approved doses, regimens, with any salt (magnesium/strontium/sodium), and for any duration of treatment were considered eligible. Both the intention-to-treat (all data included regardless of whether or not they completed or received that treatment) and per-protocol studies were included and analysed separately.

Any study conducted in a paediatric population (age < 18 years), comparing inequivalent doses (40 mg vs. 20 mg), or administering the drug by any route other than per-oral were excluded from our analysis. Additionally, studies reporting the use of more than two acid suppressing agents and/or had drug/brand switching during the trial were also excluded.

Heterogeneity

The variability in outcomes measure (i.e., heterogeneity of analysis) was determined using Cochrane's Q and the I2 statistics [19] as reported here (Table 1). The methodological quality of all eligible studies was assessed using the previously published Newcastle-Ottawa scale with scores >5 deemed as acceptable. All eligible studies scored between 6 and 7 [20].

Strengths and weaknesses

To the best of our knowledge, this systematic review presents the only exhaustive and up-to-date analysis of the efficacy of omeprazole (racemate) and esomeprazole (S enantiomer) at equivalent doses. We have also provided a comprehensive analysis of all outcomes reported in the included trials. The fact that most of the eligible studies were sponsored by the maker of the drugs is the limitation of our study. Availability and analysis of data on the prophylactic potential of these drugs would have been further useful and informative.

Drug Discovery and Development in Pharmaceuticals

Table 1 Characteristics of the studies and odds ratio OR (95 % CI) for studies reporting therapeutic and symptomatic relief outcomes

Reference	Outcome	Dose (mg)	Duration (Days)	Mean Age (Years)	Sex (Male %)	OR (95%CI) Intention-to-treat (ITT)	OR (95%CI) Per-Protocol (PP)	Forest Plot of ITT OR (95%CI)
21	Therapeutic	O: 40	7	59	52	1.00	1.00	
		E: 40	7	57	54	1.703 (0.69 to 4.25)	1.70 (0.68 to 4.25)	
22	Therapeutic	O: 40	7	39	63	1.00	1.00	
		E: 40	7	46	58	2.14 (0.58 to 8.00)	1.97 (0.44 to 8.87)	
23	Therapeutic	O: 40	7	39.7	66	1.00	1.00	
		E: 40	7	41.7	64	0.80 (0.49 to 1.29)	0.88 (0.58 to 1.33)	
24	Therapeutic	O: 40	7	45	60	1.00	1.00	
		E: 40	7	46	64	0.86 (0.49 to 1.50)	1.00 (0.61 to 1.64)	
25	Therapeutic	O: 20	7	54	61	1.00	1.00	
		E: 20	7	54	67	1.22 (0.65 to 2.26)	0.92 (0.45 to 1.85)	
26	Therapeutic	O: 20	7	48.9	51	1.00	1.00	
		E: 20	7	48.4	78	1.19 (0.75 to 1.88)	1.36 (0.82 to 2.28)	
Overall effect of all studies combined Heterogeneity: Tau² = 0.00; Chi² = 4.42, df = 5 (P = 0.49); I² = 0%, Test for overall effect: Z = 0.48 (p = 0.63).		O E				1.00 1.06 [0.83, 1.36] (p = 0.63)	1.00 1.07 [0.84, 1.36] (p = 0.57)	
27†	Symptomatic Relief	O: 20	28	48.3	43.1	1.00	NR	
		E: 20	28	48	43.3	1.10 (0.85 to 1.45)	NR	
27†	Symptomatic Relief	O: 20	28	48.3	43.1	1.00	NR	
		E: 20	28	48	43.3	1.10 (0.81 to 1.50)	NR	
28	Symptomatic Relief	O: 20	56	45.3	63.9	1.00	NR	
		E: 20	56	44.7	63.3	1.28 (0.88 to 1.87)	NR	
29	Symptomatic Relief	O: 20	28	46.5	61.4	1.00	NR	
		E: 20	28	45.3	59.6	1.34 (0.96 to 1.89)	NR	
Overall effect of all studies combined Heterogeneity: Tau² = 0.00; Chi² = 4.42, df = 5 (P = 0.49); I² = 0%, Test for overall effect: Z = 0.48 (p= 0.63).		O E				1.00 1.18 [1.01, 1.38] (p = 0.04)*	NR NR	

E: S-omeprazole , O: Omeprazole, NR: Data not reported; †Reference 27 contains two independent set of data; * Statistical significance (p <0.05)

Results

Our search yielded 2467 studies of which, after review of the title and abstract, 73 were deemed potentially relevant. These studies were retrieved in full text and reviewed (Fig. 1). Of those, only 14 studies were deemed eligible after full review [21–34] (Tables 1, 2, 3).

Our final selection included 6 studies [21–26] (Table 1) reporting the treatment of peptic ulcer secondary to *H. pylori* infection with omeprazole or S-omeprazole as part of a 7-day triple therapy. Four of these studies [21–24] compared 40 mg daily doses while the other two [25, 26] used 20 mg daily doses of the two products. Three studies [27–29] (Table 1) were analysed that included data on the relief from GERD offered by omeprazole versus S-omeprazole. Five studies were included which reported [30–34] 24 h median intragastric pH values after administration of omeprazole and S-omeprazole.

There was no significant difference in the therapeutic success between omeprazole and S-omeprazole as a part of triple therapy for the treatment of *H. pylori* in both intention-to-treat (OR, 1.06; CI, 0.83, 1.36; $p = 0.63$; $n = 6$) as well as per-protocol analysis

(OR, 1.07; CI, 0.84, 1.36; $p = 0.57$; $n = 6$). Data for per-protocol analysis were only available for *H. pylori* treatment.

For the treatment of GERD, however, S-omeprazole was found to be marginally superior to omeprazole (OR, 1.18; CI, 1.01, 1.38; $p = 0.04$; $n = 3$).

Among the metrics used to compare the effectiveness of the two products to control intragastric pH (Table 2), only the percent patients maintaining a 24 h gastric pH above 4 was significantly greater for S-omeprazole as compared with racemic omeprazole (OR': 1.57; CI, 1.04, 2.381; $p = 0.03$; $n = 3$). For other pH metrics [35], we found 5 studies that included outcomes of the median intragastric pH, duration of intragastric pH > 4, and percent of patients having intragastric pH > 4 during the 24 h post dose [30–34].

Discussion

Omeprazole is a racemic drug with both enantiomers entering the parietal cells where, in the presence of acid, they are converted to an achiral sulphenamide that, in turn, inhibits the proton pumps therein [36]. The pharmacological effects of omeprazole are, therefore, not

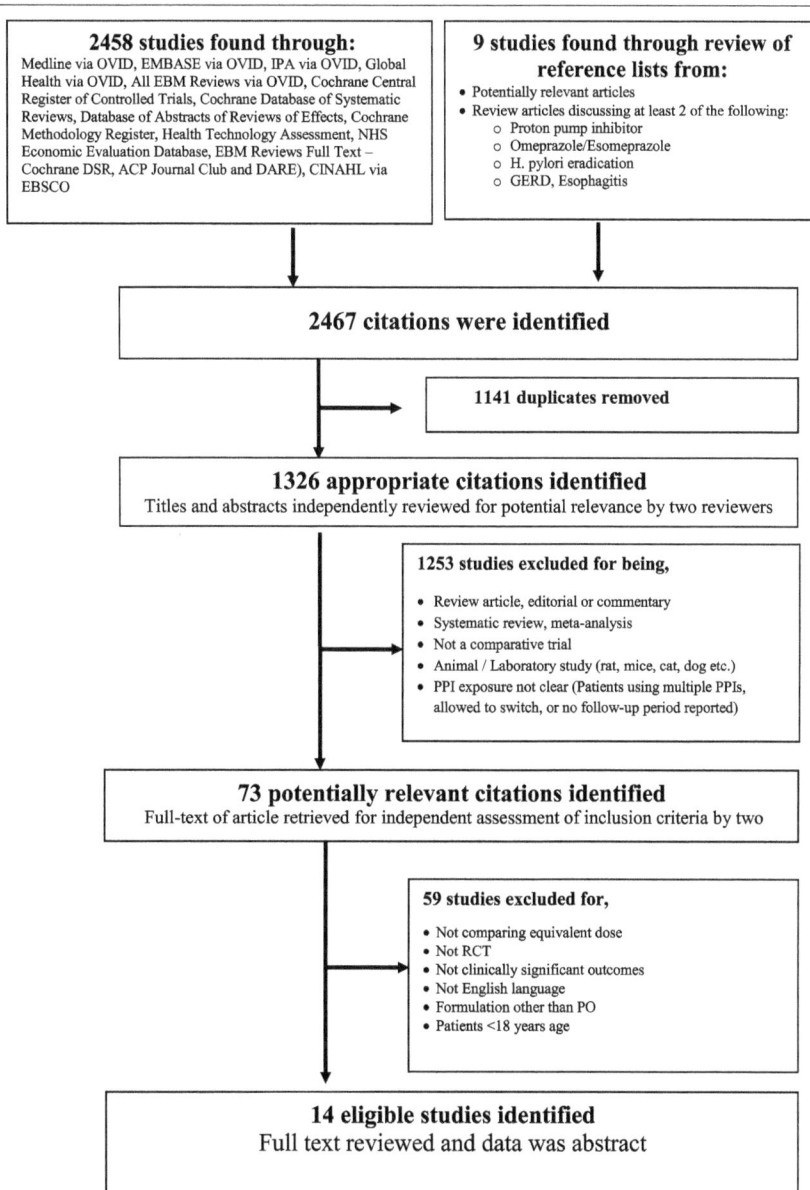

Fig. 1 Flow diagram of the selection process for randomized controlled trials reporting omeprazole vs esomeprazole (Published until April 2015)

stereoselective [14]. Its pharmacokinetics, on the other hand, are stereoselective. Upon its rapid absorption, the drug undergoes a stereoselective first-pass metabolism mediated by CYP2C19 in favour of the R enantiomer. For switching from racemic omeprazole to its S enantiomer, the following rationale were offered [37] (i) omeprazole controls intragastric pH for only 10 h while the S-enantiomer does so for a longer period; (ii) an increase in dose, does not add to the beneficial effects of the racemate but it does so with the S-enantiomer; (iii) there is a less

inter-subject variability in response to S-omeprazole as compared to the racemate.

Our analysis reveals that, indeed, there is no significant difference between the two products in the duration of pH control (Table 2). Indeed, the two products were equally effective in terms of other pH related outcomes except for the effectiveness to maintain the value above 4 for which the OR' was greater for S-omeprazole as compared with the racemate.

Some investigators have compared the therapeutic outcomes of the recommended doses of the two drugs;

Table 2 Characteristics of the studies and odds ratio OR (95%CI) for studies reporting 24 h median intra-gastric pH as outcomes

Reference	Dose (mg)	Duration (Days)	Mean Age (Years)	Sex (Male %)	Outcome measures as reported in the studies included in our analysis			
					Odds of 24 h median intra-gastric pH > 4 OR	Median intra-gastric pH within 24 h post dose (pH)	Mean time pH > 4 within 24 h post dose (h)	% time duration of 24 h with intra-gastric pH > 4 (%)
30	O:40	1	31.7	46	1.00	4.5 (4.36- 4.64)	17.8 (17.4-18.5)	62.0 (59.0-65.0)
	E: 40	1	31.7	46	2.08 (1.10, 3.96)	4.8 (4.64- 4.92)	19.2 (18.6-19.75)	68.4 (65.4-71.4)
31	O:20	1	58	47	NR	6.4 (6.32- 6.42)	NR	NR
	E: 20	1	59	47	NR	6.4 (6.30- 6.52)	NR	NR
32	O:20	5	45	42	1.00	3.6 (3.2- 3.9)	10.5 (8.8-12.2)	43.7 (36.7-50.7)
	E: 20	5	45	42	1.23 (0.63, 2.38)	4.1 (3.8- 4.5)	12.7 (11.0-14.4)	53.0 (46.0-60.0)
33	O:20	7	21.7	75	NR	5.4 (3.5 - 6.8)	22.6 (20.3–24)]	79.2 (40.0-90.2)
	E: 20	7	21.7	75	NR	5.4 (3.5–6.8)	21.1 (17.2–23.8)	81.0 (60.0-90.0)
34	O:20	5	18-6	46	1.00	3.5 (1.6-5.3)	10.4 (3.0–20.2)	44.0 (12.4-83.9)
	E:20	5	18-6	46	1.42 (0.56, 3.63)	3.9 (1.9-5.1)	11.3 (3.7–18.0)	48.0 (15.5-75.3)
Overall effect of all studies combined:	O				1.00	4.39 (3.36, 5.73)	15.24 (12.13, 19.14)	52.01 (39.52, 68.44)
	E				1.57 (1.04, 2.38) ($p = 0.03$)*	4.69 (3.79, 5.81) ($p = 0.67$)	16.43 (13.72, 19.66) ($p = 0.55$)	60.10 (48.58, 74.34) ($p = 0.40$)

* Statistical significance of difference from referance (p < 0.05), NR- Data not reported

i.e., 20 mg omeprazole vs 40 mg S-omeprazole. Thus, since the enantiomers of omeprazole are equipotent, the comparison has been made between 20 and 40 mg of the active compound. In addition, since the R enantiomer undergoes a greater extent of first-pass metabolism, and the S enantiomer has a nonlinear pharmacokinetics, the body exposure of 40 mg S-omeprazole is expected to be even greater than twice that of 20 mg racemic omeprazole. These studies [6–12], with one exception [15], have reported a greater beneficial effect for 40 mg doses of S-omeprazole as compared to 20 mg of the racemic drug. However, our analysed of the available data revealed no differences between 20 and 40 mg of either omeprazole or S-omeprazole with respect to both therapeutic and pH control outcomes (Table 3). This is despite the fact that a 40 mg dose of S-omeprazole is expected to yield a substantially greater drug bioavailability than a 20 mg racemate or single enantiomer [37]. This suggests that the examined dosage range may be at the plateau phase of the dose-effect curve. We were unable to find data comparing the effect of dose elevation on GERD.

Our analysis revealed a marginal but significantly greater effect in the control of GERD for S-omeprazole (OR, 1.18; CI, 1.01, 1.38) as compared to omeprazole (reference, OR 1.0) (Table 1). This difference, although statistically significant, may be of questionable therapeutic value as the OR' is calculated to be very close to unity.

The link between plasma omeprazole concentration and its beneficial effects is complicated and mainly unknown. The drug has an apparent plasma t1/2 of approximately 1 h but a duration of effect of 72 h [38]. Drawing therapeutic inferences based merely on the pharmacokinetics properties alone and in the absence of a clear understanding of the kinetics of pharmacological actions is questionable. It is clear that at the time of drug development, some advantages were speculated, however, due to the emergence of more information over the past decade, a more reliable analysis of the data has become possible. We can now

Table 3 The effect of 20 mg and 40 mg doses of omeprazole and S-omeprazole

Drug and Dosage	Therapeutic outcome	Intra-gastric pH outcome			
	% of patients cured (i.e. treatment of H. pylori) Mean % (SD)	% of patients cured (i.e. 24 h intra-gastric pH >4) Mean % (SD)	Median intra-gastric pH within 24 h post dose Mean pH (SD)	Mean time pH > 4 within 24 h post dose Mean h (SD)	% time duration of 24 h with intra-gastric pH > 4 Mean % (SD)
Omeprazole (O 20)	80.0 (11.3), $n = 2$	37.5 (9.2), $n = 2$	4.7 (1.4), $n = 4$	14.5 (7.0), $n = 3$	55.6 (20.4), $n = 3$
Omeprazole (O 40)	79.8 (7.1), $n = 4$	75.0[a]$n = 1$	4.5[a]$n = 1$	17.8[a]$n = 1$	62.0[a]$n = 1$
S-Omeprazole (E 20)	83.0 (11.3) $n = 2$	49.0 (7.1), $n = 2$	4.9 (1.2), $n = 4$	15.0 (5.3), $n = 3$	60.7 (17.8), $n = 3$
S-Omeprazole (E 40)	84.0 (7.6) $n = 4$	88.0[a]$n = 1$	4.8[a]$n = 1$	19.2[a]$n = 1$	68.4[a]$n = 1$

[a]No variance since $n = 1$; NR- Data not reported

conclude more conclusively that despite the overwhelming economic success of S-omeprazole, the drug offers little or no advantage over its parent racemic product.

Despite the lack of success in therapeutic outcome, the S enantiomer of omeprazole has been mentioned, particularly in public and trade media, as an example of racemic to enantiomer switch success. The market success of the switch cannot be disputed due to the ever-growing market share of the acid-controlling agent (approximately $5 billion in 2013) [39]. This is significant as the monthly cost of S-omeprazole is up to over ten-fold of that of omeprazole.

The advances in stereochemical aspects of drug action and disposition have enhanced our understanding of the mechanisms behind both the beneficial and harmful outcomes of drugs. For example, we have reported that inflammatory disease slows down clearance of racemic verapamil. The extent of this drug-disease interaction is only 3-fold based on achiral analysis but 11-fold when the S enantiomer is considered [40]; pharmacological properties of verapamil are mainly attributed to its S enantiomer. In addition, the well-known enantiomeric bioconversion of some drugs has significantly added to the knowledge of the field [41, 42] so that many pharmaceutical houses were prompted to develop new drugs as stereochemically pure products, or to consider the racemic-enantiomer switch of available drugs, though there have been very few successful results [13]. Based on some data generated using animal models, we have reported that the stereochemically pure enantiomers of the racemic nonsteroidal anti-inflammatory drugs do not provide safer alternatives with regard to the well-known gastrointestinal side effects of these drugs [3–5]. In addition, for ofloxacin to levofloxacin and ibuprofen to dexibuprofen switching, (i.e., another two successful racemic to enantiomer switches) there are no comparative data available to assess the claimed superiority of one over the other. Altogether, it is reasonable to suggest that, despite the earlier intuitive belief, stereochemically pure drugs are not necessarily superior to their corresponding racemates [3]. This by no means implies that the stereochemical aspects of a drug's action and dispositions are not of prime importance in clinical pharmacology or toxicology research.

Conclusion

Overall S-omeprazole appeared to be as effective as omeprazole when used at equivalent doses in treating ulcers as part of triple therapy, and in controlling 24 h intragastric pH. For both omeprazole and S-omeprazole the differences between 20 and 40 mg doses, if any, are marginal.

Appendix 1: List of search terms and key words used

1. exp omeprazole sulfone/or exp omeprazole/or exp omeprazole derivative/or omeprazole.mp.
2. omepr$.mp.
3. (Antra or Aspra or Gastroloc or Losectil or Lozeprel or Mopral or Omepral or Omez or Opal or Ozid or Rome 20 or Prilosec or Losec or Ulcozol or Segazole or Zegacid or Zegerid or Losepine).mp. [mp = title, abstract, subject headings, heading word, drug trade name, original title, device manufacturer, drug manufacturer, device trade name, keyword)
4. (73590-58-6 or 95510-70-6).mp.
5. or/1-4
6. esomeprazole.mp. or exp esomeprazole/ or exp esomeprazole strontium/
7. esome$.mp.
8. (217087-09-7 or 934714-36-0).mp.
9. (Nexium or Essocam or Esomezol or Racipher or Opton or Neptor or Nexemezol).mp. [mp = title, abstract, subject headings, heading word, drug trade name, original title, device manufacturer, drug manufacturer, device trade name, keyword)
10. or/6-9
11. cohort studies.mp. or exp cohort analysis/
12. exp case control study/ or case–control.mp.
13. (randomized controlled trial or random$).mp.
14. 11 or 12 or 13
15. 5 and 10
16. 14 and 15

Competing interest

The authors have no professional affiliation, financial interest or conflict with the subject matter or information discussed here in this manuscript to declare.

Authors' contribution

Web search, article screening, article review, data analysis, manuscript preparation: W. Asghar and E. Pittman. Study design, data review, data analysis, manuscript preparation: F Jamali. All authors read and approved the final manuscript.

Source of funding

University of Alberta Self-Directed Grant (F. Jamali).

References

1. Jamali F, Mehvar R, Pasutto FM. Enantioselective aspects of drug action and disposition: therapeutic pitfalls. J Pharm Sci. 1989;78(9):695–715.
2. Wallin JD, Frishman WH. Dilevalol: a selective beta-2 adrenergic agonist vasodilator with beta adrenergic blocking activity. J Clin Pharmacol. 1989;29(12):1057–68.
3. Valentova J, Hutt AJ. Chiral switch: pure enantiomers of drugs instead of racemic mixtures. Ceska Slov Farm. 2004;53(6):285–93.
4. Davies NM, Wright MR, Russell AS, Jamali F. Effect of the enantiomers of flurbiprofen, ibuprofen, and ketoprofen on intestinal permeability. J Pharm Sci. 1996;85(11):1170–3.
5. Wright MR, Davies NM, Jamali F. Rationale for the development of stereochemically pure enantiomers: are the R enantiomers of chiral nonsteroidal anti-inflammatory drugs inactive? J Pharm Sci. 1994;83(6):911–2.

6.   Edwards SJ, Lind T, Lundell L, Das R. Systematic review: standard- and double-dose proton pump inhibitors for the healing of severe erosive oesophagitis – a mixed treatment comparison of randomized controlled trials. Aliment Pharmacol Ther. 2009;30(6):547–56.

7.   Edwards SJ, Lind T, Lundell L. Systematic review: proton pump inhibitors (PPIs) for the healing of reflux oesophagitis - a comparison of esomeprazole with other PPIs. Aliment Pharmacol Ther. 2006;24(5):743–50.

8.   Gralnek IM, Dulai GS, Fennerty MB, Spiegel BM. Esomeprazole versus other proton pump inhibitors in erosive esophagitis: a meta-analysis of randomized clinical trials. Clin Gastroenterol Hepatol. 2006;4(12):1452–8.

9.   Lucioni C, Mazzi S, Rossi C. Proton pump inhibitors in acute treatment of reflux oesophagitis: a cost-effectiveness analysis. Clin Drug Investig. 2005; 25(5):325–36.

10. Tang HL, Li Y, Hu YF, Xie HG, Zhai SD. Effects of CYP2C19 loss-of-function variants on the eradication of H. pylori infection in patients treated with proton pump inhibitor-based triple therapy regimens: a meta-analysis of randomized clinical trials. PLoS One. 2013;8(4):e62162.

11. Villoria A, Garcia P, Calvet X, Gisbert JP, Vergara M. Meta-analysis: high-dose proton pump inhibitors vs. standard dose in triple therapy for Helicobacter pylori eradication. Aliment Pharmacol Ther. 2008;28(7):868–77.

12. Klok RM, Postma MJ, van Hout BA, Brouwers JR. Meta-analysis: comparing the efficacy of proton pump inhibitors in short-term use. Aliment Pharmacol Ther. 2003;17(10):1237–45.

13. Gellad WF, Choi P, Mizah M, Good CB, Kesselheim AS. Assessing the chiral switch: approval and use of single-enantiomer drugs, 2001 to 2011. Am J Manag Care. 2014;20(3):e90–7.

14. Li XQ, Weidolf L, Simonsson R, Andersson TB. Enantiomer/enantiomer interactions between the S- and R- isomers of omeprazole in human cytochrome P450 enzymes: major role of CYP2C19 and CYP3A4. J Pharmacol Exp Ther. 2005;315(2):777–87.

15. Chiba N. Esomeprazole was not better than omeprazole for resolving heartburn in endoscopy-negative reflux disease. ACP J Club. 2005;142(1):6.

16. Cook DA, West CP. Conducting systematic reviews in medical education: a stepwise approach. Med Educ. 2012;46(10):943–52.

17. Deeks JJ, Higgins J, Altman DG. Analysing Data and Undertaking Meta-Analyses. Cochrane Handbook for Systematic Reviews of Interventions: Cochrane Book Series; 2008. 243-296

18. Hernandez-Diaz S, Hernan MA, Meyer K, Werler MM, Mitchell AA. Case-crossover and case-time-control designs in birth defects epidemiology. Am J Epidemiol. 2003;158(4):385–91.

19. Whitehead A. Meta-analysis of controlled clinical trials (Vol. 7). John Wiley & Sons Ltd; 2002. page 57-97.

20. Hartling L, Milne A, Hamm MP, et al. Testing the Newcastle Ottawa Scale showed low reliability between individual reviewers. J Clin Epidemiol. 2013;66(9):982–93.

21. Anagnostopoulos GK, Tsiakos S, Margantinis G, Kostopoulos P, Arvanitidis D. Esomeprazole versus omeprazole for the eradication of Helicobacter pylori infection: results of a randomized controlled study. J Clin Gastroenterol. 2004;38(6):503–6.

22. Miehlke S, Schneider-Brachert W, Bastlein E, Ebert S, Kirsch C, Haferland C, et al. Esomeprazole-based one-week triple therapy with clarithromycin and metronidazole is effective in eradicating Helicobacter pylori in the absence of antimicrobial resistance. Alimentary pharmacology & therapeutics. 2003; 18(8):799-804.

23. Subei IM, Cardona HJ, Bachelet E, Useche E, Arigbabu A, Hammour AA, et al. One week of esomeprazole triple therapy vs 1 week of omeprazole triple therapy plus 3 weeks of omeprazole for duodenal ulcer healding in Helicobacter pylori-positive patients. Digestive diseases and sciences. 2007; 52(6):1505-12

24. Tulassay Z, Kryszewski A, Dite P, Kleczkowski D, Rudzinski J, Bartuzi Z, et al. One week of treatment with esomeprazole-based triple therapy eradicates Helicobacter pylori and heals patients with duodenal ulcer disease. European journal of gastroenterology & hepatology. 2001;13(12):1457-65.

25. Veldhuyzen Van Zanten S, Lauritsen K, Delchier JC, et al. One-week triple therapy with esomeprazole provides effective eradication of Helicobacter pylori in duodenal ulcer disease. Aliment Pharmacol Ther. 2000;14(12):1605–11.

26. Veldhuyzen Van Zanten S, Machado S, Lee J. One-week triple therapy with esomeprazole, clarithromycin and metronidazole provides effective eradication of Helicobacter pylori infection. Aliment Pharmacol Ther. 2003;17(11):1381–7.

27. Armstrong D, Talley NJ, Lauritsen K, Moum B, Lind T, Tunturi-Hihnala H, et al. The role of acid suppression in patients with endoscopy-negative reflux disease: the effect of treatment with esomeprazole or omeprazole. Alimentary pharmacology & therapeutics. 2004;20(4):413-21.

28. Lightdale CJ, Schmitt C, Hwang C, Hamelin B. A multicenter, randomized, double-blind, 8-week comparative trial of low-dose esomeprazole (20 mg) and standard-dose omeprazole (20 mg) in patients with erosive esophagitis. Dig Dis Sci. 2006;51(5):852–7.

29. Kahrilas PJ, Falk GW, Johnson DA, Schmitt C, Collins DW, Whipple J, et al. Esomeprazole improves healing and symptom resolution as compared with omeprazole in reflux oesophagitis patients: a randomized controlled trial. The Esomeprazole Study Investigators. Alimentary pharmacology & therapeutics. 2000;14(10):1249-58.

30. Rohss K, Hasselgren G, Hedenstrom H. Effect of esomeprazole 40 mg vs omeprazole 40 mg on 24-hour intragastric pH in patients with symptoms of gastroesophageal reflux disease. Dig Dis Sci. 2002;47(5):954–8.

31. Gursoy O, Memis D, Sut N. Effect of proton pump inhibitors on gastric juice volume, gastric pH and gastric intramucosal pH in critically ill patients: a randomized, double-blind, placebo-controlled study. Clin Drug Investig. 2008;28(12):777–82.

32. Lind T, Rydberg L, Kyleback A, et al. Esomeprazole provides improved acid control vs. omeprazole In patients with symptoms of gastro-oesophageal reflux disease. Aliment Pharmacol Ther. 2000;14(7):861–7.

33. Sahara S, Sugimoto M, Uotani T, Ichikawa H, Yamade M, Iwaizumi M, et al. Twice-daily dosing of esomeprazole effectively inhibits acid secretion in CYP2C19 rapid metabolisers compared with twice-daily omeprazole, rabeprazole or lansoprazole. Alimentary pharmacology & therapeutics. 2013; 38(9):1129-37.

34. Miehlke S, Lobe S, Madisch A, Kuhlisch E, Laass M, Grossmann D, et al. Intragastric acidity during administration of generic omeprazole or esomeprazole - a randomised, two-way crossover study including CYP2C19 genotyping. Alimentary pharmacology & therapeutics. 2011;33(4):471-6.

35. Armstrong D. Review article: gastric pH – the most relevant predictor of benefit in reflux disease? Aliment Pharmacol Ther. 2004;20 Suppl 5:19–26. discussion 38–9.

36. Olbe L, Carlsson E, Lindberg P. A proton-pump inhibitor expedition: the case histories of omeprazole and esomeprazole. Nat Rev Drug Discov. 2003;2(2):132–9.

37. Edsbacker S, Andersson T. Pharmacokinetics of budesonide (Entocort EC) capsules for Crohn's disease. Clin Pharmacokinet. 2004;43(12):803–21.

38. Lind T, Cederberg C, Ekenved G, Haglund U, Olbe L. Effect of omeprazole–a gastric proton pump inhibitor–on pentagastrin stimulated acid secretion in man. Gut. 1983;24(4):270–6.

39. Statista. AstraZeneca's top products based on revenue 2010–2013. Pharmaceutical Products & Market [cited 2015 20 Jan]; Available from: http://www.statista.com/statistics/311976/proton-pump-inhibitors-by-us-revenues/

40. Sanaee F, Clements JD, Waugh AW, Fedorak RN, Lewanczuk R, Jamali F. Drug-disease interaction: Crohn's disease elevates verapamil plasma concentrations but reduces response to the drug proportional to disease activity. Br J Clin Pharmacol. 2011;72(5):787–97.

41. Berry BW, Jamali F. Presystemic and systemic chiral inversion of R-(–)-fenoprofen in the rat. J Pharmacol Exp Ther. 1991;258(2):695–701.

42. Caldwell J, Hutt AJ, Fournel-Gigleux S. The metabolic chiral inversion and dispositional enantioselectivity of the 2-arylpropionic acids and their biological consequences. Biochem Pharmacol. 1988;37(1):105–14.

22

The impact of polymer coatings on magnetite nanoparticles performance as MRI contrast agents

Maryam Khalkhali[1], Kobra Rostamizadeh[2,3]*, Somayeh Sadighian[2,4], Farhad Khoeini[1], Mehran Naghibi[5] and Mehrdad Hamidi[2]

Abstract

Background: Superparamagnetic iron oxide nanoparticles (SPIONs) are the most commonly used negative MRI contrast agent which affect the transverse (T_2) relaxation time. The aim of the present study was to investigate the impact of various polymeric coatings on the performance of magnetite nanoparticles as MRI contrast agents.

Methods: Ferrofluids based on magnetite (Fe_3O_4) nanoparticles (SPIONs) were synthesized via chemical co-precipitation method and coated with different biocompatible polymer coatings including mPEG-PCL, chitosan and dextran.

Results: The bonding status of different polymers on the surface of the magnetite nanoparticles was confirmed by the Fourier transform infrared spectroscopy (FT-IR) and thermogravimetric analysis (TGA). The vibrating sample magnetometer (VSM) analysis confirmed the superparamagnetic behavior of all synthesized nanoparticles. The field–emission scanning electron microscopy (FE-SEM) indicated the formation of quasi-spherical nanostructures with the final average particle size of 12–55 nm depending on the type of polymer coating, and X-ray diffraction (XRD) determined inverse spinel structure of magnetite nanoparticles. The ferrofluids demonstrated sufficient colloidal stability in deionized water with the zeta potentials of −24.2, −16.9, +31.6 and −21 mV for the naked SPIONs, and for dextran, chitosan and mPEG-PCL coated SPIONs, respectively. Finally, the magnetic relaxivities of water based ferrofluids were measured on a 1.5T clinical MRI instrument. The r_2/r_1 value was calculated to be 17.21, 19.42 and 20.71 for the dextran, chitosan and mPEG-PCL coated SPIONs, respectively.

Conclusions: The findings demonstrated that the value of r_2/r_1 ratio of mPEG-PCL modified SPIONs is higher than that of some commercial contrast agents. Therefore, it can be considered as a promising candidate for T_2 MRI contrast agent.

Introduction

Magnetic resonance imaging (MRI) is one of the noninvasive powerful imaging techniques with very high spatial resolution that allows precise determination of the 3D shape for differentiate soft body tissue. In order to make an accurate diagnosis and improve the intrinsic contrast between normal tissues and lesions, there is a need to use exogenous contrast agents. Contrast agents in clinic are classified into two categories [1]. The most commonly used MRI contrast agents are those that reduce the longitudinal (T_1) relaxation time and cause positive contrast enhancement based on the paramagnetic ions including chelate complexes of gadolinium (Gd^{3+}) or manganese (Mn^{2+}). Due to some toxicity issues related to gadolinium [2], nowadays, there is a growing interest in negative contrast agents based on magnetic iron oxide nanoparticles (SPIONs) affect the transverse (T_2) relaxation time and cause darker state in the T_2-weighted image wherever accumulate in tissue [3]. As compared to gadolinium compounds, superparamagnetic iron oxide nanoparticles show the advantages of tunable size and shape, as well as possibility of surface modification and more effectiveness at lower concentrations because of their superparamagnetic property [4].

* Correspondence: rostaimzadeh@gmail.com
[2]Zanjan Pharmaceutical Nanotechnology Research Center, Zanjan University of Medical Sciences, Zanjan, Iran
[3]Department of Medicinal Chemistry, School of Pharmacy, Zanjan University of Medical Sciences, Postal Code 45139-56184 Zanjan, Iran
Full list of author information is available at the end of the article

The effectiveness of SPIONs can be limited by their high surface area to volume ratio which leads to an increase in surface energy and tendency to agglomeration. This phenomena consequently makes them recognized by the macrophage system and reduce their circulation time. To overcome this shortcoming, one approach is to modify nanoparticles surface with various surface stabilizing agents that ensure their stability, biodegradability, nontoxicity as well as prolonging their circulation time in vivo. Although surface modification is successful in prolonging the SPIONs circulation time in vivo, according to the Koening – Kellar model, they could also influence the longitudinal (r_1) and transverse (r_2) relaxivities characteristics of SPIONs as a result of change in size, composition, accumulation situation in the biological environment, magnetization, hydrophilicity and surface properties [5–7].

Recently, Xie et al. [8] have prepared superparamagnetic iron oxide nanoparticles (SPIONs) coated with polyethylene glycol (PEG), PEG/PEI (poly ethyleneimine) and PEG/PEI/Tween 80 by the thermal decomposition of Fe(acac)$_3$ and investigated their in vivo MRI contrast effects in the mouse brains. The results showed different vascular imaging effects after 24 h intravenous injection of the synthesized ferrofluids. Ma et al. [9] explored SPION-based MRI contrast agents by a polyol method. SPIONs entrapped into albumin nanospheres and then folic acid as targeting agent was conjugated onto the surface of nanoparticles. The r_2/r_1 value of resultant ferrofluids was around 40 indicating a strong T_2 shortening effect. Ahmad et al. [10] reported synthesis of chitosan-coated nickel-ferrite (NiFe$_2$O$_4$) nanoparticles by a chemical coprecipitation method. The coated nanoparticles were cylindrical in shape and were studied as both T_1 and T_2 contrast agents in MRI. The T_1 and T_2 relaxivities were 0.858 ± 0.04 and 1.71 ± 0.03 mM^{-1} s^{-1}, respectively. In animal study, both a 25 % signal enhancement in the T_1-weighted image and a 71 % signal loss in the T_2-weighted image were observed. This result demonstrated chitosan-coated nickel-ferrite nanoparticles potential as both T_1 and T_2 contrast agents in MRI.

According to the literature [5], it is clear that by careful selection of different coatings on SPIONs, it is possible to provide significant improvement in magnetic resonance activity. The aim of this contribution was to prepare the ferrofluids based on Fe$_3$O$_4$ magnetic nanoparticles (SPIONs) stabilized with various biocompatible polymer coatings such as dextran, chitosan and mPEG-PCL in order to elucidate the influence of the polymer type on the corresponding longitudinal (r_1) and transverse (r_2) relaxivities. SPIONs were characterized by the Fourier transform infrared spectroscopy (FT-IR), Dynamic Light Scattering (DLS) technique, field–emission

scanning electron microscopy (FE-SEM), vibrating sample magnetometer (VSM) analysis, and X-ray diffraction (XRD). Finally T_1 and T_2 weighted phantom MRI images were obtained at a series of colloidal suspension of nanoparticles with different iron concentrations using 1.5 T MRI.

Experimental
Materials and method
Ferrous chloride tetrahydrate (FeCl$_2 \cdot$4H$_2$O), ferric chloride hexahydrate (FeCl$_3$.6H$_2$O), ammonium hydroxide, acetic acid, dextran (M$_w \approx$ 13–23 kDa), poly vinylalcohol (M$_w \approx$ 13–23 kDa) and dichloromethane all were purchased from Merck (Germany). Chitosan of molecular weight in the range of 10^5–3×10^5 g/mol and degree of deacetylation ≥ 75 %, poly (ethylene glycol) monomethyl ether (mPEG, 5000 g/mol), ε-caprolactone and stannous octoate were purchased from Sigma. Ethanol (96 %) and oleic acid were provided by Kimia alcohol (Iran) and Fluka (Switzerland), respectively. All chemicals used as received without further purification. mPEG-PCL copolymer with the average molecular weight of 13 kDa was synthesized and characterized. The detailed procedures of the synthesis of mPEG-PCL copolymer and its corresponding characterization have been described in our previous paper [11].

Synthesis of naked superparamagnetic iron oxide nanoparticles (SPIONs)
Naked magnetite nanoparticles (SPIONs) were synthesized via alkaline coprecipitation of Fe^{2+} and Fe^{3+} ions in aqueous solution [12]. Briefly, a mixture of iron (II) chloride and iron (III) chloride (1:2, molar ratio) dissolved in 45 mL deionized water and put into a three-neck flask and mechanically stirred at 80 °C. Then, 4 mL NH$_4$OH (25 wt %) was added dropwise to the solution under nitrogen protection and the mixture was continuously stirred for another 30 min to complete the reaction. The resultant SPIONs were collected by a 1.4 T magnet, and washed several times with ethanol and deionized water to eliminate excess ammonia and finally dried at 60 °C under vacuum for one day. The yield of reaction was 80 %.

Synthesis of chitosan coated magnetite nanoparticles
Chitosan coated magnetite nanoparticles were synthesized according to the previous published method [13]. Briefly, 0.2 g of the naked magnetite nanoparticles prepared in the previous step were dispersed in 0.5 % chitosan solution (0.5 g chitosan dissolved in 100 mL acetic acid buffer with pH = 4.8) using an ultrasonic bath for 30 min at 60 °C and the mixture stirred mechanically at room temperature for 12 h and a black homogeneous suspension was obtained. During this process surface of

nanoparticles were coated by chitosan and the resulting black precipitate was separated by a permanent magnet and washed five times with deionized water and dried at vacuum conditions.

Synthesis of dextran coated magnetite nanoparticles

Synthesis of dextran coated SPIONs were adapted from the literature [14]. In a typical procedure, $FeCl_3 \cdot 6H_2O$ (12 mmol), $FeCl_2 \cdot 4H_2O$ (6 mmol), and 1.45 g dextran were dissolved in 150 mL deionized water. The mixture was ultrasonicated for 10 min at room temperature whilst pure nitrogen was bubbled into, then, followed by the addition of 4 M potassium hydroxide. After ultrasonication of mixture at 60 °C under nitrogen atmosphere for 60 min, the dark suspension was obtained. The black product was separated by centrifugation for 10 min at 14000 rpm and washed five times with absolute ethanol and deionized water. The final product was dried at room temperature.

Synthesis of mPEG-PCL coated SPIONs (Magnetic micelles)

The synthesis followed the procedure performed by Meerod et al. [15]. In essence, a mixture of iron(II) chloride and iron(III) chloride (1:2, molar ratio) were dissolved in 45 mL deionized water. Then, 4 mL aqueous ammonia (25 %) and 250 μL oleic acid was added to the solution and stirred for 30 min under the N_2 flow. The dark precipitant was isolated by a magnet and thoroughly were washed with ethanol to remove excess oleic acid and dried at 60 °C under vacuum for 24 h. Afterwards, 10 mg of mPEG-PCL and 2 mg of the oleic acid coated magnetite nanoparticles were dispersed in 2 ml dichloromethane, then the mixture was emulsified in 10 mL of 0.5 % (w/v) PVA aqueous solution. Dichloromethane was evaporated slowly by stirring overnight at room temperature and the magnetic micelles were formed.

Characterization of nanoparticles

Fourier transform infrared (FT-IR) spectra for pure polymers and the naked and coated magnetite nanoparticles were recorded using Matson1000 FT-IR spectrometer (Unican, United States) with KBr pellets in the range of 400–4000 cm^{-1}. Crystal structure and the phase analysis of SPIONs were studied by Bruker D8 X-ray diffractometer (Germany) with Cu K_α radiation ($\lambda = 0.1540$ nm) and diffraction patterns were collected in the diffraction angle in the range of $2\theta = 5\text{-}70°$ at an accelerating voltage of 40 kV. PANalytical X'pert high score software was used for data analysis. Hydrodynamic diameter, zeta-potentials of nanoparticles and time dependent colloidal stability were characterized by dynamic light scattering (DLS) system (Zetasizer Nano ZEN 3600, Malvern Instruments Ltd., Worcestershire, United Kingdom)) at

25 °C. Thermogravimetric analysis of the dried samples were performed by a NETZSCH STA 409 PC/PG (Selb, Germany) at a heating rate of 10 K/min from 20 to 800 °C to monitor the mass loss of a known amount of polymer coated SPIONs. Vibrating sample magnetometer (VSM) (Lake shore 7400, United States) was employed to study the hysteresis loops and the magnetic properties of the magnetite nanoparticles at room temperature from −20000 to 20000 Oe. The iron concentration was measured by inductively coupled plasma atomic emission spectrometer (ICP) Optima 7300DV (United States). The particle size, structure and morphology of the naked and polymer coated magnetite nanoparticles were investigated by the field-emission scanning electron microscopy (FE-SEM) Mira 3-XMU (Tescan, United States).

In vitro MRI studies (Relaxometry properties of the ferrofluids)

To assess the longitudinal (R_1) and transverse (R_2) relaxation rates, clinical 1.5 T whole body magnetic resonance (MR) scanner (Siemens Healthcare Avanto Germany) was used. T_1 and T_2 weighted phantom MRI images were obtained at a series of colloidal suspension of nanoparticles with iron concentrations of 0, 25, 50, 75, 100 and 200 μM. A number of spin echo sequence with repetition times (TR) of 1600 ms and varying echo time (TE) of 10, 43, 75, 108 and 140 ms (slice thickness: 7.5 mm, field of view (FOV): 238, Turbo factor: 18, matrix: 176 × 384) was used for getting T_2 weighted images. The T_1 weighted images were obtained at various repetition times of 100, 1550, 3150, 4750 and 6400 ms with an echo time of 18 ms, slice thickness:7.5 mm, field of view (FOV): 230, and matrix: 200 × 256 [16, 17].

Signal intensity of the spin echo sequence related to TE and TR is defined as [18]:

$$I = M_0 \left[1 - \exp\left(-\frac{TR}{T_1} \right) \right] \qquad (1)$$

$$I = M_0 \exp\left(-\frac{TE}{T_2} \right) \qquad (2)$$

Where I is the signal intensity which was measured with the help of DicomWorks 1.3.5 software within a manually drawn region of interest (ROI) for each sample. Relaxation rate R_1 ($1/T_1$) and R_2 ($1/T_2$) were calculated by using the eqs. 1 and 2 via mono-exponential curve fitting of the signal intensity vs. time (TE or TR). By plotting R_1 and R_2 over Fe concentration of synthesized ferrofluids, the slope indicates the specific relaxivity, r_1 and r_2, respectively.

Results and discussion

FT-IR spectral analysis was applied to confirm the intro-duction of different coatings on SPIONs. Figure 1 shows the characteristic peaks of the naked and polymer coated SPIONs. For all the samples, a main band at 577 cm^{-1} is attributed to the vibration of Fe-O [19]. For the FT-IR spectrum of the naked SPIONs (Fig. 1a), the absorption peak at 3422 cm^{-1} corresponds to stretching vibration of OH indicating the presence of the large number of hy-droxyl groups on the surface of iron oxide particles which increase the agglomeration tendency of the synthesized SPIONs [20]. For the FT-IR spectrum of the dextran coated SPIONs, the absorption line at 1028 cm^{-1} is due to the absorption by the vibrational motion of the etheric bond (–C-O-), the signal at 3422 cm^{-1} is assignable to stretching vibration of the alcoholic hydroxyl (–OH), the peak centered at 1457 cm^{-1} is due to the bending vibra-tion of C-H bond and the peak appeared at 2923 cm^{-1} is referred to the stretching vibration of -CH$_2$- groups (Fig. 1b) [21]. FT-IR spectrum of the chitosan coated SPIONs is shown in Fig. 1c. The characteristic absorption peak at 1064 cm^{-1} can be attributed to the absorption by the vibrational motion of the C-O bond. The peak at 1387 cm^{-1} is due to the vibration of the CH$_2$ group. The characteristic absorption peak at 1623 cm^{-1} can be re-ferred to the N-H bending vibration of primary amine (NH$_2$) and corresponding high intensity and broad peak of absorption can be explained by the fact that the

hydrogen of primary amino group in chitosan form strong hydrogen bonding with the oxygen of magnetite [20]. Apparently, the above observations imply success-ful attachment of chitosan onto the surface of SPIONs. It can be seen that for mPEG-PCL coated SPIONs (Fig. 1d), the weak absorption at 1100 cm^{-1} and the small shoulder band at 1723 cm^{-1} is assignable to C-O stretching of mPEG and carbonyl stretching of ester linkages of PCL which subsequently can be con-sidered as an evidence for the copolymer attachment to the particle surface [15].

The crystalline properties of the naked and polymer coated SPIONs were analyzed by recording X-ray diffrac-tion patterns (XRD). Figure 2 shows the X-ray diffraction patterns of the naked SPIONs and the dextran, chitosan and mPEG-PCL coated SPIONs. For the naked SPIONs the multiple peaks were observed at 2θ =18.25° (1 1 1), 30.06° (2 2 0), 35.63° (3 1 1), 43.48° (4 0 0), 53.78° (4 2 2), 57.33° (5 1 1) and 63.11° (4 4 0) which are indexed as those of inverse spinal structure of magnetite (JCPDS card No. 01-088-0866) (Fig. 2a). The XRD analysis is also indi-cative of the absence of the other types of iron oxides in synthesized product [22]. Of particular note was that for the chitosan and dextran coated SPIONs, the characteris-tic peaks did not disappear and still be seen, however the peak intensities of the diffraction peaks were weakened and width was broadened (Fig. 2b, c). Whereas in the case of mPEG-PCL coated SPIONs probably due to polymer

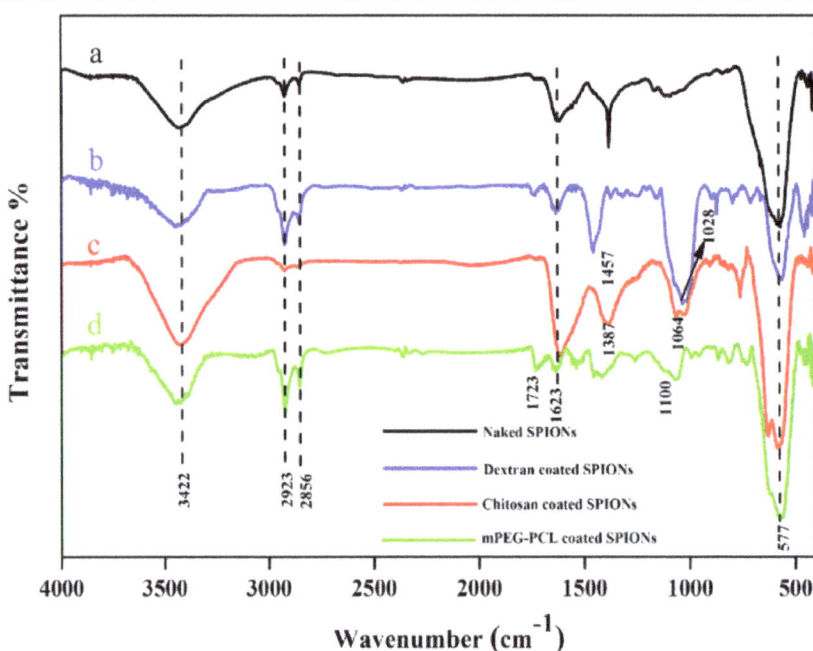

Fig. 1 FT-IR spectra of **a** naked SPIONs, **b** dextran coated SPIONs, **c** chitosan coated SPIONs, **d** mPEG-PCL coated SPIONs

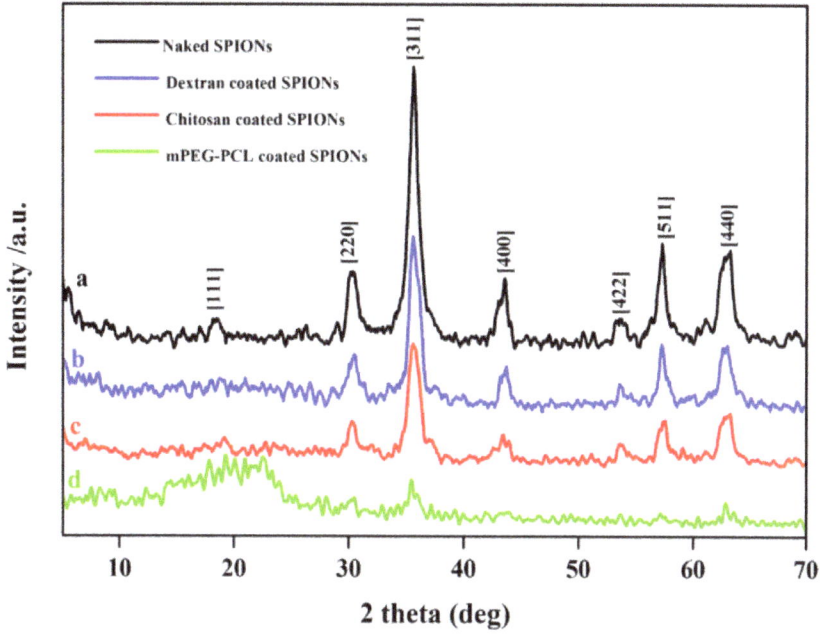

Fig. 2 X-ray diffraction (XRD) patterns of naked SPIONs **a**, dextran coated SPIONs **b**, chitosan coated SPIONs **c** and mPEG-PCL coated SPIONs **d**

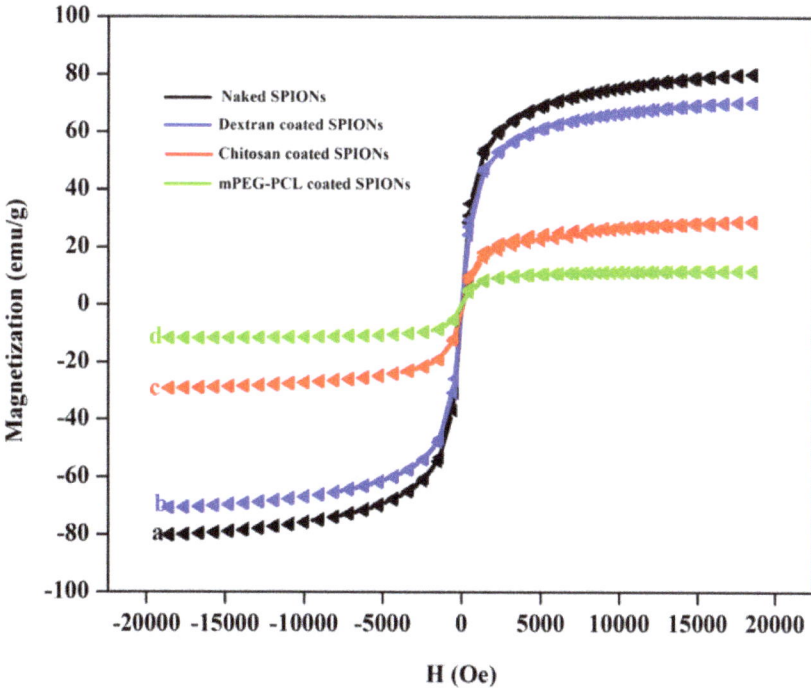

Fig. 3 Magnetization curves of naked SPIONs **a**, dextran coated SPIONs **b**, chitosan coated SPIONs **c** and mPEG-PCL coated SPIONs **d** at room temperature

amorphous properties and bilayer coverage (Fig. 2d), the characteristic peaks almost disappeared.

The average crystallite size was calculated using the Debye–Sherrer equation:

$$D = \frac{K\lambda}{\beta \cos\theta} \qquad (3)$$

Where β is the Full Width at Half Maximum (FWHM) of high intensity, K is Sherrer constant, λ is the X-ray wavelength and θ is the Bragg diffraction angle. The crystallite estimated size thus obtained from this formula were about 11, 13, 8 and 24 nm for the naked SPIONs, and the dextran, chitosan and mPEG-PCL coated SPIONs, respectively.

The magnetic properties of nanoparticles obtained via VSM technique. Figure 3 shows the hysteresis loops of the naked and various polymer coated SPIONs at room temperature. Due to fluctuation of magnetic moment by thermal energy, remanence and coercivity were about zero.

In the case of a ferrofluid the return of the magnetization to equilibrium state is determined by the sum of the Neel relaxation rate and the Brownian relaxation rate. It is believed that for a large particles, Brownian relaxation time is shorter than Neel relaxation time and subsequently, the viscous rotation determines the global relaxation. As it can be seen, for this case the magnetization curve is totally reversible because of the fast magnetic relaxation which causes the system to be remained at thermodynamic equilibrium [5]. As illustrated in the Fig. 3, all the samples exhibited a typical superparamagnetic behavior suggesting that SPIONs coated with polymeric shells can preserve their superparamagnetic properties. It could be found that the naked SPIONs presents the highest values of the magnetization (80.125 emu/g) while the saturation magnetization (M_s) was found to be 70.572, 29.085 and 11.690 emu/g at 20000 Oe, for the dextran, chitosan and mPEG-PCL coated SPIONs, respectively. The results suggest that polymer coated SPIONs demonstrated a lower level of magnetization compared to that of the naked SPIONs. The observed trend of SPIONs magnetization correlates with the size of nanoparticles. It is known that for small magnetite nanoparticles because of large surface-to-volume ratio, the spin canting effect is not negligible thus magnetization decreases [18, 21]. The low magnetic susceptibility of mPEG-PCL coated SPIONs likely arises from a double coating of magnetite core by oleic acid as hydrophobic stabilizer and polymeric layer. However, this amount of saturation magnetization is sufficient for biological applications of ferrofluids as contrast agent. The magnetic properties of the naked and the polymer coated SPIONs is displayed in Table 1.

In order to evaluate the extent of the polymer associated with the SPIONs, TGA analysis were accomplished under nitrogen atmosphere condition. As shown in Fig. 4, the TGA curves depict the changes of residual mass of the polymer coated SPIONs with temperature. As shown, for all curves a small weight loss of 2.42, 1.26, and 0.72 % for the dextran, chitosan, and mPEG-PCL coated SPIONs, respectively, within the first 150 °C which can be due to the loss of adsorbed water similar to that previously found in many systems based on polymer-coated SPIONs [23]. In the case of the dextran coated SPIONs, polymer decomposition is took place in two steps: 12.77 % between 150 and 380 °C presumably due to the breakdown of organic skeleton and 3.56 % at the range of 380–700 °C attributed to the complex degradation process. By considering these weight losses, the total amount of magnetite in sample is 81.25 %.

The TGA curve of the chitosan coated SPIONs also shows two distinct weight loss for polymer at 150–320 °C and 310–620 °C corresponding to 21.64 and 12.99 % of weight loss, respectively. The reports indicate that magnetite can be oxidized at elevated temperature up to 600 °C [24]. Thereby, the last weight loss in this thermogram can be ascribed to the magnetite oxidation which is occurred at the temperature of higher than 600 °C and subsequently indicating 42.56 % of iron oxide in the chitosan coated SPIONs. As shown in Fig. 4c, for the TGA curve of mPEG-PCL, the weight loss of 9.28 % at150–250 °C can be attributed to the evaporation of oleic acid and the weight loss of totally 33.53 % at 280–500 °C are as a result of copolymer decomposition. In this case also weight loss of 6.77 % can be related to the magnetite oxidation and consequently the residual weight of magnetite content was 50.43 %.

The average hydrodynamic diameter and size distribution of the naked and modified SPIONs were investigated by dynamic laser light scattering measurements at 25 °C in deionized water. Each measurement was repeated three times. The hydrodynamic sizes of the naked SPIONs (a), dextran coated SPIONs (b), chitosan coated SPIONs (c) and mPEG-PCL coated SPIONs (d) were 126.2 ± 9.179, 58 ± 10.594, 32.09 ± 6.766 and 42.23 ± 5.490 nm, respectively and the polydispersity indexes were 0.253 ± 0.008, 0.279 ± 0.009, 0.205 ± 0.004 and 0.264 ± 0.006, respectively. Large particle size of the naked SPIONs compared to that of polymer coated nanoparticles can be result of each nucleus surrounding by different hydrophilic polymers in the case of polymer coated SPIONs. This phenomenon ultimately forbids the addition growth of the nuclei.

The charge of the surface of nanoparticles was determined by zeta potential measurements. The naked SPIONs showed a negative zeta potential of −24.2 ± 0.494 mV. Following coating SPIONs with dextran the zeta potential

Table 1 The magnetic properties of naked SPIONs, dextran coated SPIONs, chitosan coated SPIONs and mPEG-PCL coated SPIONs

Preaperd NPs	Coercivity (Hci) G	Initial Slope emu/(gG)	Magnetization (Ms) emu/g	Negative (Hci) G	Positive (Hci) G	Retentivity (Mr) emu/g	Negative (Mr) emu/g	Positive (Mr) emu/g
Naked SPIONs	2.4059	0.023	80.152	−7.9299	−12.7420	0.16603	0.87937	0.54731
Dextran coated SPIONs	0.0850	0.021	70.572	−8.2975	−8.1267	0.00591	0.46993	0.48175
Chitosan coated SPIONs	12.5810	0.009	29.085	−31.4290	−6.2673	0.29041	0.14339	0.72421
mPEG-PCL coated SPIONs	1.2877	0.004	11.690	−0.7560	1.8194	0.01415	−0.02001	0.00830

increased to −16.9 ± 0.070 mV as a result of the interaction of the ions in aqueous dispersion with polysaccharide structure of dextran. The zeta potential of the chitosan coated SPIONs was measured to be +31.6 ± 0.919 mV. Such positive zeta potential is due to the presence of positively charged amino group of chitosan on the surface of SPIONs. mPEG-PCL coated SPIONs exhibited negative zeta potential of −21 ± 3.535 mV. Relatively high surface potential of all SPIONs could play a critical role in minimizing aggregation of particles and improvement of the colloidal stability of ferrofluid suspension.

Stability of ferrofluids plays a critical role in biofate of nanoparticles. In order to evaluate the stability of SPIONs, zeta potential of different SPIONs were followed for one month. In fact, zeta potential of nanoparticles can severely affect the stability of ferrofluids. Figure 5 illustrates the changes of zeta potential and particle size of nanoparticles for one month. As it can be seen except the naked SPIONs that showed slight variation in the size and zeta potential, the polymer stabilized nanoparticles indicated no significant changes during this time. Since magnetic dipole interaction of polymers are zero or very small, so the presence of these polymers on the surface of nanoparticles results in fine colloidal stability of polymer coated SPIONs in aqueous media [18]. Therefore, polymer coatings on SPIONs can play a critical role in minimizing aggregation of particles, and improvement of the stability and prolonging circulation times.

The surface morphology and particle size of the naked SPIONs and polymer-coated SPIONs were observed by field-emission scanning electron microscopy (FE-SEM). FE-SEM images and corresponding histograms were shown in Fig. 6. The images reveal that most of the particles are quasi-spherical and SPIONs are apt to aggregate in the solid state since the surface energy is high. The related histogram of nanoparticles shows that the mean diameter of the naked SPIONs varied from 46 to 64 nm, while average particle size of coated particles

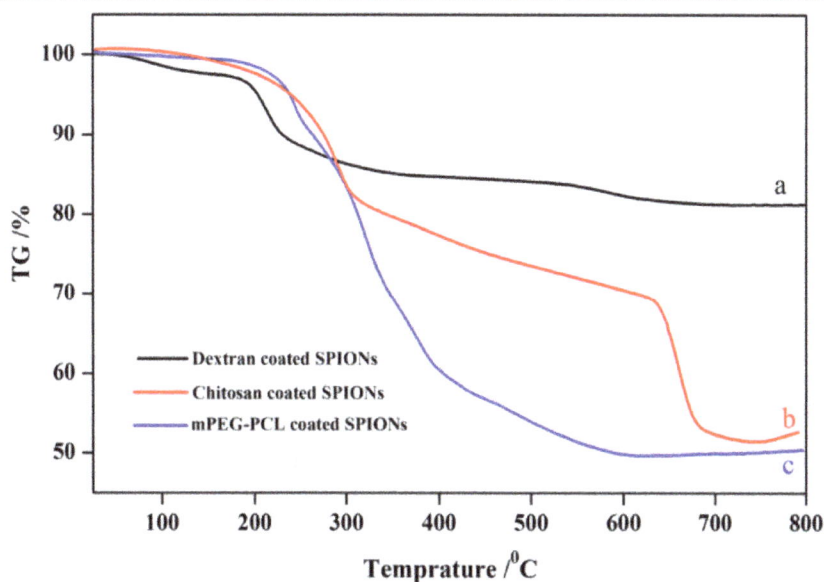

Fig. 4 TGA curve of dextran coated SPIONs **a**, chitosan-coated SPIONs **b** and mPEG-PCL SPIONs **c**

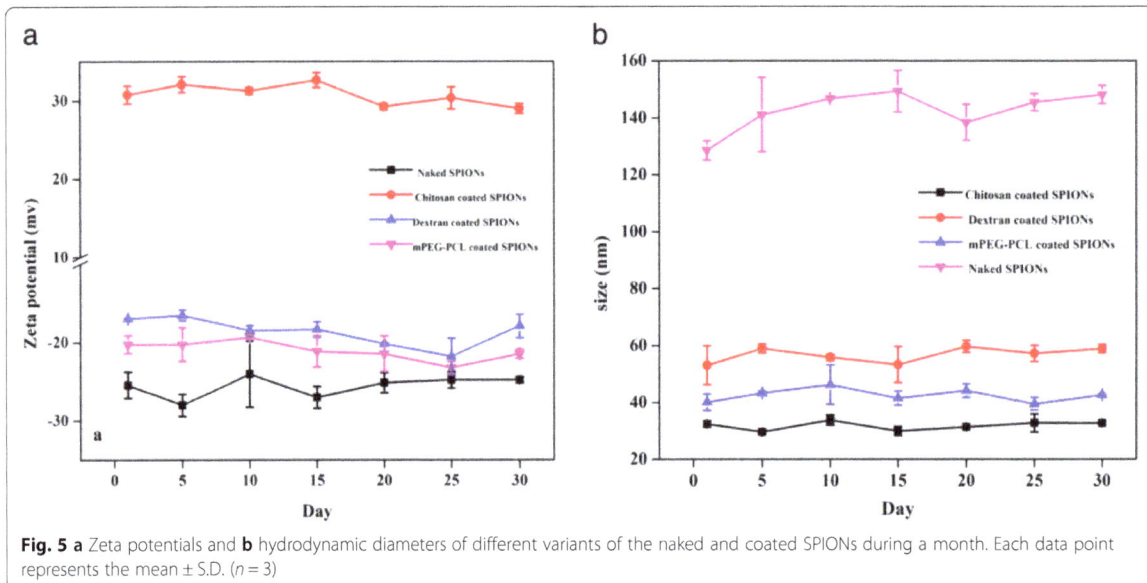

Fig. 5 a Zeta potentials and **b** hydrodynamic diameters of different variants of the naked and coated SPIONs during a month. Each data point represents the mean ± S.D. ($n = 3$)

does not approximately exceed 42 nm. By comparing the naked and polymer coated nanoparticles sizes, it can be concluded that the size of particles is significantly controlled by stabilizing agents. It is clear that the particle size obtained by DLS technique is much greater than those by FE-SEM which can be explained by the fact that in contrast to FE-SEM, DLS method measures the hydrodynamic diameter in suspension.

MRI studies and relaxometric properties

SPIONs are commonly used as T_2 MRI contrast agents and consequently they are able to decrease the MR signal intensity by dephasing of proton spins. Considering the biocompatibility of dextran, chitosan and mPEG-PCL, the effect of surface modification of SPIONs was investigated in terms of MR signal-enhancing property.

The proton relaxivity measurements of the as-prepared polymer coated magnetite nanoparticles in aqueous solution with different Fe concentrations were performed to evaluate the feasibility of polymer coated magnetite nanoparticles as T_2 MRI contrast agents. Figure 7 shows T_2-weighted MR images of dextran coated SPIONs (a), chitosan coated SPIONs (b) and mPEG-PCL coated SPIONs (c) with iron concentrations of 0, 25, 50, 75, 100 and 200 μM in deionized water.

As shown in Fig. 7, The T_2-weighted phantom images of polymer coated magnetite nanoparticles showed a significant negative dose dependent contrast enhancement which suggests them as an excellent T_2 contrast agent under the T_2-imaging sequences. From the results shown in Table 2, the images of the dextran coated SPIONs are darker than that of the chitosan and mPEG-PCL coated

SPIONs at the same Fe concentration indicating corresponding high r_2 relaxivity.

The longitudinal relaxivity (r_1, mM^{-1} s^{-1}) and transverse relaxivity (r_2, mM^{-1} s^{-1}) of polymer coated magnetite nanoparticles was calculated according to the following equation:

$$R_i = \frac{1}{T_i} = \left(\frac{1}{T_i}\right)_0 + r_i C \qquad (4)$$

Where R_i is the relaxation rate, T_{i0} is the relaxation time in the pure water, C is the concentration of the contrast agent, and r_i is relaxivity [18]. By plotting the T_1 relaxation rate ($1/T_1$) and T_2 relaxation rate ($1/T_2$) as a function of Fe concentration a linear relationships were found for both of them (Fig. 8). The calculated r_1, r_2 and r_2/r_1 values for various polymer coated SPIONs are presented in Table 2.

The T_1 relaxation rate ($1/T_1$) as a function of Fe concentration of polymer coated SPIONs is presented in Fig. 8a. The findings reveal that for all three formulations, the longitudinal relaxation decreases as the iron concentration of the magnetic fluids increases. The slope of plots give the r_1 values about 12.79, 4.708 and 4.171 mM^{-1} s^{-1} for the dextran, chitosan and mPEG-PCL coated SPIONs, respectively. Of particular note was the lower longitudinal relaxivity of mPEG-PCL coated SPIONs compared to that of dextran and chitosan coated SPIONs (Fig. 8a). It is clear that the relaxivities greatly is affect by distance of the aqueous medium from the magnetite core. On the other hand, the hydrophobicity/hydrophilicity of the coatings has an impact on the diffusion of water within

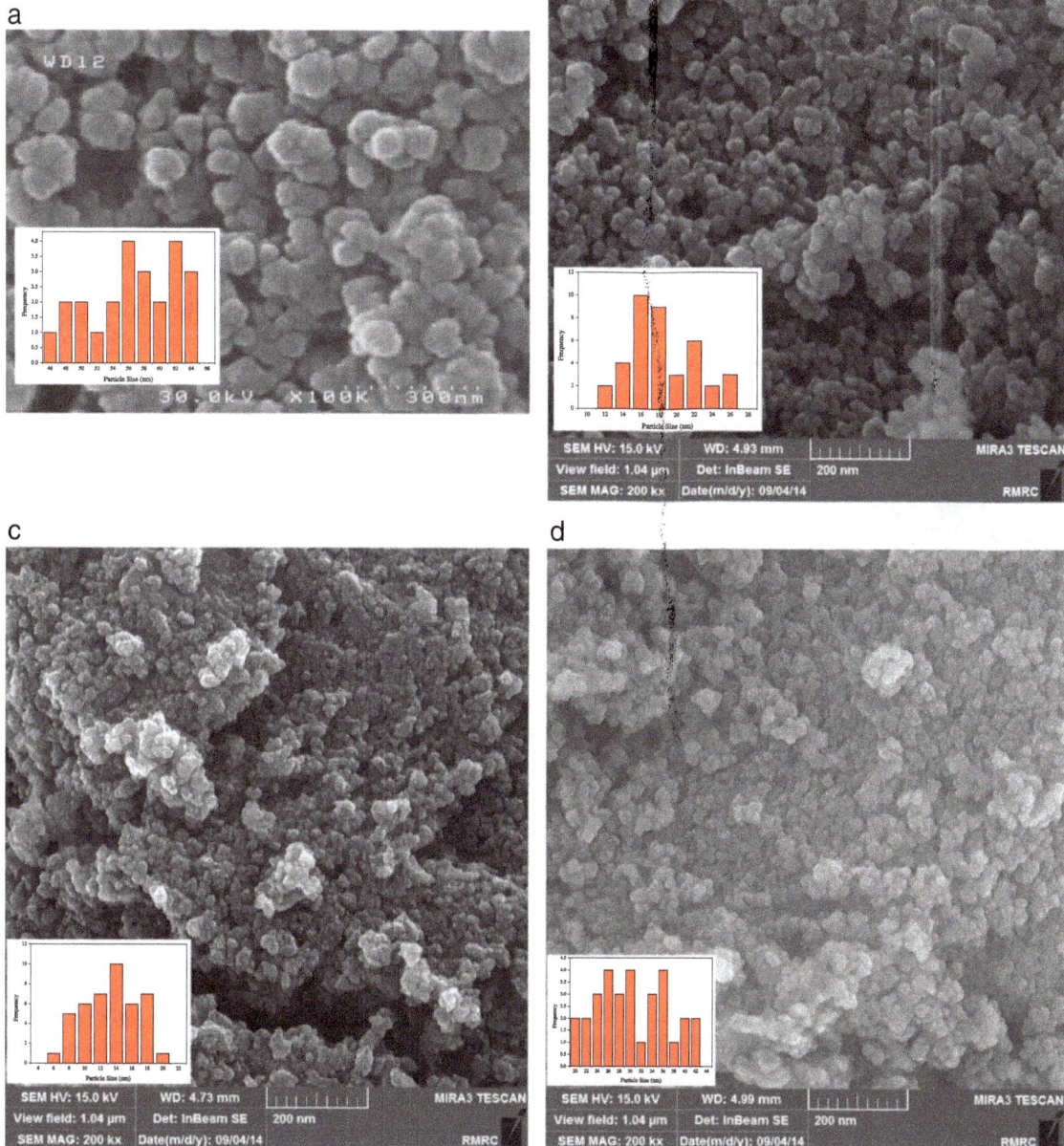

Fig. 6 Field-Emission Scanning Electron Microscopy (FE-SEM) image of **a** naked SPIONs, **b** dextran coated SPIONs, **c** chitosan coated SPIONs and **d** mPEG-PCL coated SPIONs

polymeric layer. Thereby, it can be postulated that the presence of hydrophobic inner shells of mPEG-PCL coated SPIONs including oleic acid and PCL layers will exclude water molecules and consequently extend the distance of water molecules from the magnetite core and finally result in low longitudinal relaxivity [25].

R_2 relaxivity of magnetite nanoparticles is given by the following formula:

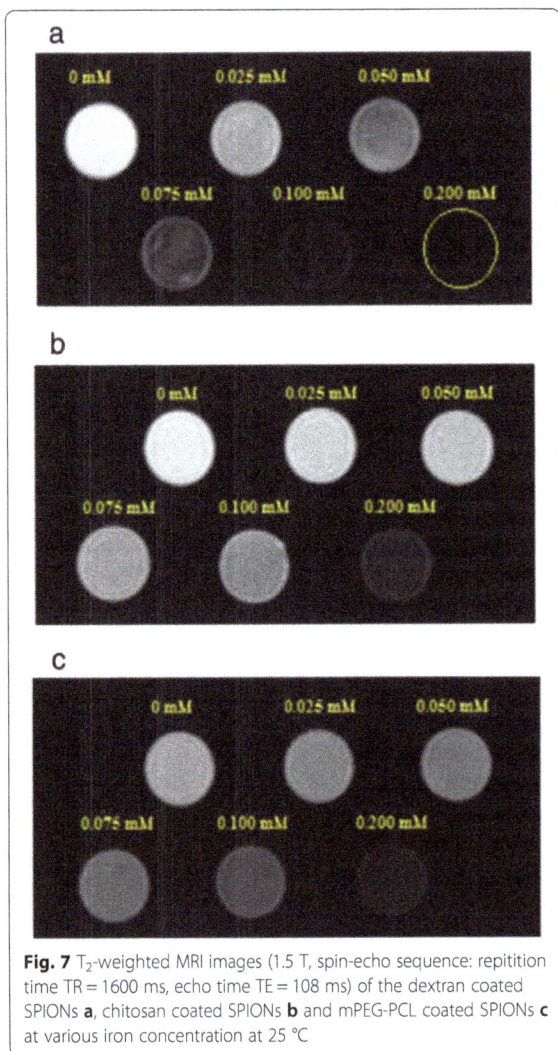

Fig. 7 T_2-weighted MRI images (1.5 T, spin-echo sequence: repitition time TR = 1600 ms, echo time TE = 108 ms) of the dextran coated SPIONs **a**, chitosan coated SPIONs **b** and mPEG-PCL coated SPIONs **c** at various iron concentration at 25 °C

$$R_2 = \frac{1}{T_2} = \frac{\left(\frac{256\pi^2\gamma^2}{405}\right)V^*M_s^2a^2}{D(1+L/a)} \qquad (5)$$

Where a is magnetite core radius, M_s is the saturation magnetization nanoparticles, V^* is the volume fraction of magnetite core and L is the thickness of an inscrutable surface coating. According to equation 5, the R_2 relaxivity decreases once coating layer thickness increases. On the other hand, surface coating affect the movement of water molecules [18]. The specific relaxivity (r_2) of the dextran coated SPIONs was calculated to be 220.20 mM^{-1} s^{-1}, which was significantly higher than that of the chitosan coated SPIONs (91.44 mM^{-1} s^{-1}) and mPEG-PCL coated SPIONs (86.46 mM^{-1} s^{-1}) (Fig. 8b). The remarkable r_2 relaxivities of dextran coated SPIONs compared to that of chitosan and mPEG-PCL coated SPIONs can be explained by its high saturation magnetizations, high crystallinity and larger hydrodynamic diameter as well as dextran hydrophilicity [5, 18]. In fact, high hydrophilicity of dextran lead to strong hydrogen bond between polymer and water molecules and prevent water molecules diffusion from the nanoparticles surface toward magnetic core which in turn can be considered as a reason for its high r_2 relaxivities. Further experimental results supporting above point can be seen elsewhere [18]. According to the DLS analysis, it can be seen that the highest r_2 relaxivities of formulations is belonged to the dextran coated SPIONs which is the largest particle according to the DLS analysis. This trend is in accordance with the literature data [5, 18]. The high r_2 relaxivities of dextran coated SPIONs can be also attributed, in part, to its high crystallinity as evidenced by the XRD data similar to that previously found [18]. The most important feature of the single monodomain is its anisotropy energy that is given by the following equation:

$$E_a = K_a V \qquad (6)$$

Where V is the crystal volume and K_a is the anisotropy constant. Clearly, the anisotropy energy increases by increasing the crystal radius, and subsequently the Neel relaxation time is influenced by the anisotropy energy [5]. It is important to note that in addition to magnetic properties of the core, hydrodynamic diameter, and crystallinity, several parameters such as composition, doping, assembly of magnetite-based nanoparticles also strongly affect the R_2 relaxivity of magnetite nanoparticles [18]. Analogously with the longitudinal relaxation results, the mPEG-PCL coated SPIONs exhibit lower r_2 values than the dextran and chitosan coated SPIONs.

Typically contrast agents with r_2/r_1 ratio of larger than 2 and up to 40 are considered as T_2 contrast agents, while for T_1 contrast agents, this ratio is relatively low [26]. The r_2/r_1 values of the prepared polymer coated magnetite nanoparticles were around 20 which is higher

Table 2 The longitudinal relaxivity (r_1, mM^{-1} s^{-1}), transverse relaxivity (r_2, mM^{-1} s^{-1}), r_2/r_1 values and R^2 of polymer coated magnetite nanoparticles was calculated by plotting the T_1 relaxation rate (1/T_1) and T_2 relaxationrate (1/T_2) as a function of Fe concentration

Preaperd NPs	r_1 (mM^{-1} s^{-1})	R^2	r_2 (mM^{-1} s^{-1})	R^2	r_2/r_1
Dextran coated SPIONs	12.790	0.967	220.20	0.981	17.21
Chitosan coated SPIONs	4.708	0.799	91.44	0.943	19.42
mPEG-PCL coated SPIONs	4.174	0.990	86.46	0.990	20.713

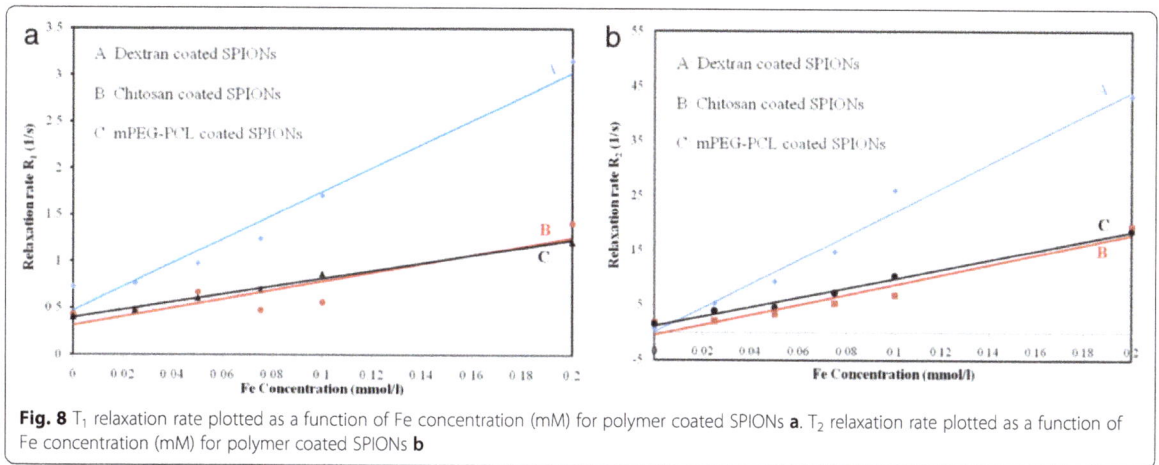

Fig. 8 T_1 relaxation rate plotted as a function of Fe concentration (mM) for polymer coated SPIONs **a**. T_2 relaxation rate plotted as a function of Fe concentration (mM) for polymer coated SPIONs **b**

than that of Resovist, commercially available MRI contrast agent [9]. From the discussion above, it can be concluded that all as prepared formulations are feasible to be used as negative MRI contrast agents. However, in view of the r_2/r_1 value of different formulations, it can be concluded that mPEG-PCL coated SPIONs compared to the chitosan and dextran coated SPIONs due to higher r_2/r_1 value, can be considered as promising candidate as T_2 contrast agent. The reason behind these results, presumably lies on presence of the hydrophobic layer on the surface of mPEG-PCL coated SPIONs. This study has hinted at the potential of mPEG-PCL coated SPIONs as T_2 contrast agent but also illustrate the need for more trials and more work.

Conclusion

Synthesis of the core – shell nanostructures composed of magnetite (Fe_3O_4) nanoparticles stabilized with various polymer coatings such as dextran, chitosan and mPEG-PCL via a simple coprecipitation method was achieved. All the as-prepared polymer coated SPIONs had excellent water dispersion and colloidal stability. FT-IR and TGA confirmed that polymer chains had been effectively coated on the surface of SPIONs. Field-emission scanning electron microscopy (FE-SEM) confirmed the formation of quasi spherical nanostructures with the average particle size about 50 nm. The VSM analysis showed that different polymer coated magnetite nanoparticles are superparamagnetic with high saturation magnetizations value (M_s) of about 70.572, 29.085 and 11.690 emu/g at 20000 Oe for the dextran, chitosan and mPEG-PCL coated SPIONs, respectively, that is sufficient for their application as MRI contrast agents. X-ray diffraction (XRD) analysis proved highly crystalline magnetite particles with an inverse spinel structure. All SPIONs exhibit high r_2 relaxivities about 220.20 mM^{-1} s^{-1}, 91.44 mM^{-1} s^{-1} and 86.46 mM^{-1} s^{-1} for the dextran, chitosan and mPEG-

PCL coated SPIONs, respectively. The value of r_2/r_1 ratios of prepared SPIONs is higher than that of some commercial contrast agents such as Resovist. The results of this study have indicated the possibility of using polymer stabilized SPIONs especially mPEG-PCL coated SPIONs as potential T_2 MRI contrast agents.

Competing interests

The authors declare that they have no competing interests.

Authors' contributions

MK carried out the experiments, helped in data analysis, and drafted the manuscript. KR conceived of the study, participated in its design and coordination and revising the manuscript. SS helped in lab work and manuscript preparation. FK cooperated in the experiments design. MN helped in MRI image acquisition. MH designed the study and revised the manuscript. All authors read and approved the final manuscript.

Acknowledgment

The project was supported by University of Zanjan, and Zanjan University of Medical Sciences. Also, authors gratefully acknowledge the cooperation of Tabesh medical imaging center (Dr. M. H. Abdkarimi) Tabriz, Iran in acquiring the MRI images.

Author details

[1]Department of Physics, Faculty of Science, University of Zanjan, Zanjan, Iran. [2]Zanjan Pharmaceutical Nanotechnology Research Center, Zanjan University of Medical Sciences, Zanjan, Iran. [3]Department of Medicinal Chemistry, School of Pharmacy, Zanjan University of Medical Sciences, Postal Code 45139-56184 Zanjan, Iran. [4]Department of Pharmaceutical Biomaterials, School of Pharmacy, Zanjan University of Medical Sciences, Zanjan, Iran. [5]Shahid Beheshti University of Medical Sciences, Tehran, Iran.

References

1. Li L, Jiang W, Luo K, Song H, Lan F, Wu Y, et al. Superparamagnetic iron oxide nanoparticles as MRI contrast agents for Non-invasive stem cell labeling and tracking. Theranostics. 2013;3(8):595–614.
2. Estelrich J, Sánchez-Martín MJ, Busquets MA. Nanoparticles in magnetic resonance imaging: from simple to dual contrast agents. Int J Nanomedicine. 2015;10:1727–41.
3. Kenouche S, Larionova J, Bezzi N, Guari Y, Bertin N, Zanca M, et al. NMR investigation of functionalized magnetic nanoparticles Fe_3O_4 as T_1–T_2 contrast agents. Powder Technol. 2014;255:60–5.

4. Sadighian S, Rostamizadeh K, Hosseini-Monfareda H, Hamidi M. Triggered Magnetic-Chitosan Nanogels (MCNs) for doxorubicin delivery: physically vs. chemically cross linking approach. Adv Pharm Bull. 2015;5(1):115–20.

5. Laurent S, Forge D, Port M, Roch A, Robic C, Vander Elst L, et al. Magnetic iron oxide nanoparticles: synthesis, stabilization, vectorization, physicochemical characterizations, and biological applications. Chem Rev. 2008;108:2064–110.

6. Neuberger T, Schöpf B, Hofmann H, Hofmann M, Von Rechenberg B. Superparamagnetic nanoparticles for biomedical applications: possibilities and limitations of a new drug delivery system. J Magn Magn Mater. 2005;293(1):483–96.

7. Branca M, Marciello M, Ciuculescu-Pradines D, Respaud M, del PuertoMorales M, Serra R, et al. Towards MRI T_2 contrast agents of increased efficiency. J Magn Magn Mater. 2015;377:348–53.

8. Xie S, Zhang B, Wang L, Wang J, Li X, Yanga G, et al. Superparamagnetic iron oxide nanoparticles coated with different polymers and their MRI contrast effects in the mouse brains. Appl Surf Sci. 2015;326:32–8.

9. Ma X, Gong A, Chen B, Zheng J, Chen T, Shen Z, et al. Exploring a new SPION-based MRI contrast agent with excellent water-dispersibility, high specificity to cancer cells and strong MR imaging efficacy. Colloids Surf B Biointerfaces. 2015;126:44–9.

10. Ahmad T, Bae H, Iqbal Y, Rhee I, Hong S, Chang Y, et al. Chitosan-coated nickel-ferrite nanoparticles as contrast agents in magnetic resonance imaging. J Magn Magn Mater. 2015;381:151–7.

11. Danafar H, Davaran S, Rostamizadeh K, Valizadeh H, Hamidi M. Biodegradable m-PEG/PCL core-shell micelles: preparation and characterization as a sustained release formulation for curcumin. Adv Pharm Bull. 2014;4:501–10.

12. Massart R, Cabuil V. Synthèse en milieu alcalin de magnétite colloïdale: contrôle du rendement et de la taille des particules. J Chim Phys. 1987;84:967–73.

13. Mohammadi-Samani S, Miri R, Salmanpour M, Khalighian N, Sotoudeh S, Erfani N. Preparation and assessment of chitosan-coated superparamagnetic Fe_3O_4 nanoparticles for controlled delivery of methotrexate. Res Pharm Sci. 2013;8(1):25–33.

14. Ahmadi R, Malek M, Hosseini HRM, Shokrgozar MA, Oghabian MA, Masoudi A, et al. Ultrasonic-assisted synthesis of magnetite based MRI contrast agent using cysteine as the biocapping coating. Mater Chem Phys. 2011;131:170–7.

15. Meerod S, Tumcharern G, Wichai U, Rutnakornpituk M. Magnetite nanoparticles stabilized with polymeric bilayer of poly(ethylene glycol) methyl ether–poly(e-caprolactone) copolymers. Polymer. 2008;49:3950–6.

16. Khalkhali M, Sadighian S, Rostamizadeh K, Khoein F, Naghibi M, Bayat N, et al. Simultaneous diagnosis and drug delivery by silymarin-loaded magnetic Nanoparticles. Nanomed J. 2015;2(3):223–30.

17. Khalkhali M, Sadighian S, Rostamizadeh K, Khoein F, Naghibi M, Bayat N, Habibizadeh M, Parsa M, Hamidi M. Synthesis and Characterization of Dextran Coated Magnetite Nanoparticles for simultaneous Diagnostics and Therapy. BI.2015;5: (doi:10.15171/bi.2015.19).

18. Lee N, Hyeon T. Designed synthesis of uniformly sized iron oxide nanoparticles for efficient magnetic resonance imaging contrast agents. Chem Soc Rev. 2012;41:2575–89.

19. Ahmad S, Riaz U, Kaushik A. Soft template synthesis of super paramagnetic Fe_3O_4 nanoparticles a novel technique. J Inorg Organomet Polymer Mater. 2009;19:355–60.

20. Sadighian S, Rostamizadeh K, Hosseini-Monfareda H, Hamidi M. Doxorubicin-conjugated core–shell magnetite nanoparticles as dual-targeting carriers for anticancer drug delivery. Colloids Surf B Biointerfaces. 2014;117:406–13.

21. Bai H, Liu Z, Delai SD. Highly water soluble and recovered dextran coated Fe_3O_4 magnetic nanoparticles for brackish water desalination. Sep Purif Technol. 2011;81:392–9.

22. Petcharoen K, Sirivat A. Synthesis and characterization of magnetite nanoparticles via the chemical co-precipitation method. Mater Sci Eng B. 2012;177:421–7.

23. Castello J, Gallardo M, Busquets MA, Estelrich J. Chitosan (or alginate)-coated iron oxide nanoparticles: a comparative study colloids surf., A. Physicochem Eng Aspects. 2015;468:151–8.

24. Rutnakornpituk M, Meerod S, Boontha B, Wichai U. Magnetic core-bilayer shell nanoparticle: a novel vehicle for entrapment of poorly water-soluble drugs. Polymer. 2009;50:3508–15.

25. Illés E, Szekeres M, Kupcsik E, Tóth IY, Farkas K, Jedlovszky-Hajdú A, et al. PEGylation of surfaced magnetite core–shell nanoparticles for biomedical application colloids surf A. : Physicochem Eng Aspects. 2014;460:429–40.

26. Casula MF, Corrias A, Arosio P, Lascialfari A, Sen T, Floris P, et al. Design of water-based ferrofluids as contrast agents for magnetic resonance imaging. J Colloid Interface Sci. 2011;357:50–5.

23

Comparison between a serum creatinine- and a cystatin C-based glomerular filtration rate equation in patients receiving amphotericin B

Iman Karimzadeh[1] and Hossein Khalili[2*]

Abstract

Serum cystatin C (Cys C) has a number of advantages over serum creatinine in the evaluation of kidney function. Apart from Cys C level itself, several formulas have also been introduced in different clinical settings for the estimation of glomerular filtration rate (GFR) based upon serum Cys C level. The aim of the present study was to compare a serum Cys C-based equation with Cockcroft-Gault serum creatinine-based formula, both used in the calculation of GFR, in patients receiving amphotericin B. Fifty four adult patients with no history of acute or chronic kidney injury having been planned to receive conventional amphotericin B for an anticipated duration of at least 1 week for any indication were recruited. At three time points during amphotericin B treatment, including days 0, 7, and 14, serum cystatin C as well as creatinine levels were measured. GFR at the above time points was estimated by both creatinine (Cockcroft-Gault) and serum Cys C based equations. There was significant correlation between creatinine-based and Cys C-based GFR values at days 0 ($R = 0.606$, $P = 0.001$) and 7 ($R = 0.714$, $P < 0.001$). In contrast to GFR estimated by the Cockcroft-Gault equation, the mean (95 % confidence interval) Cys C-based GFR values at different studied time points were comparable within as well as between patients with and without amphotericin B nephrotoxicity. Our results suggested that the Gentian Cys C-based GFR equation correlated significantly with the Cockcroft-Gault formula at least at the early time period of treatment with amphotericin B.

Keywords: Serum cystatin C, Serum creatinine, Glomerular filtration rate, Amphotericin B

Introduction

Serum cystatin C (Cys C), a 13 kDa non-glycosylated protein with cysteine protease inhibitor activity, has been proposed as an alternative marker to creatinine for assessing kidney function [1]. It lacks a number of serum creatinine drawbacks such as being influenced by non-renal factors including age, gender, muscle mass, and physical activity [2, 3]. Dose adjustment of many medications such as antibacterials depends on patients' glomerular filtration rate (GFR). Direct measurement of GFR, using urinary inulin clearance and the plasma ^{99m}Tc-DTPA or ^{125}-iothalamate is cumbersome, costly, and not readily available [4].

Besides Cys C level itself, different formulas have also been introduced in different clinical settings such as kidney transplant recipients [5], critically ill patients [6], chronic kidney disease [7], newborns [8], and the elderly [9] for the estimation of GFR, based upon Cys C serum level. In contrast to Cockcroft-Gault (CG) and Modification of Diet in Renal Disease (MDRD) formulas, which need several variables such as age and sex for calculation, Cys C-based equations are mainly dependent only on serum Cys C levels [10]. To best of our knowledge, these equations have not been investigated well enough in drug-induced acute kidney injury (AKI) conditions. The aim of the present preliminary study was to compare a serum Cys C-based equation with the classic and prominent CG serum creatinine-based formula, both used for the calculation of GFR, in patients receiving amphotericin B (AmB).

* Correspondence: khalilih@tums.ac.ir
[2]Department of Clinical Pharmacy, Faculty of Pharmacy, Tehran University of Medical Sciences, Enghelab Ave, Tehran, Iran
Full list of author information is available at the end of the article

Methods

The data of this study was extracted from a multicentre randomized, double-blinded, placebo-controlled, clinical trial (ID: IRCT201107233449N8) that assessed the effectiveness of oral N-acetylcysteine (NAC) co-treatment with AmB in preventing major features of AmB nephrotoxicity [11]. Carried out in a 15-months period, from early August 2012 to November 2013, at three university health-care settings affiliated to Tehran University of Medical Sciences, Tehran, Iran, the study included 54 adult individuals with no documented history of AKI or chronic kidney disease, having been planned to receive conventional AmB for an anticipated duration of at least 1 week for any indication. They were given either placebo or 600 mg oral NAC twice daily during the treatment course of AmB. The institutional review boards and the medical ethics committees of all hospitals approved the study and all patients or their family members signed and approved a written informed consent form.

At days 0, 7, and 14 of AmB treatment, serum Cys C as well as creatinine levels were measured. Serum creatinine level was determined by an Auto-analyzer (Biotechnica BT-3000, Italy) based on the modified Jaffe colorimetric reaction. Serum Cys C level was measured by the turbidimetric method (Gentian, Moss, Norway). GFR at days 0, 7, and 14 was calculated by the CG formula $[(140-\text{age}) \times (\text{Body weight}) \times (0.85 \text{ if female})/(\text{serum creatinine} \times 72)]$ [12]. CG values were adjusted by body surface area of relevant patients and reported as ml/min/1.73 m^2. Besides CG, GFR at the above time points was also estimated by the serum Cys C-based equation, provided in the package insert of Gentian assay kit ($79.901/\text{Serum Cys C}^{1.4389}$) [13]. AmB nephrotoxicity was defined by either a 50 % or more decline in the estimated GFR according to the CG formula or the doubling of serum creatinine from the baseline values [14].

Statistical analyses

The possible correlation between creatinine-based and Cys C-based GFR values at days 0, 7, and 14 were assessed by the Pearson correlation test. Comparison of the mean values (95 % confidence interval [CI]) of calculated creatinine-based as well as Cys C-based GFR at the above time points within and between patients with and without AmB nephrotoxicity was done by the one-way analysis of variance (ANOVA) with repeated measures. P values < 0.05 were considered statistically significant. Statistical analyses were carried out by the SPSS (Statistical Package for the Social Sciences) version 20 software.

Results

Among 54 patients randomly allocated into either placebo or NAC receiving group, 23 (42.59 %) developed AmB nephrotoxicity. The mean ± standard deviation creatinine-based GFR values at days 0, 7, and 14 were 92.94 ± 42.04, 92.21 ± 45.92, and 54.29 ± 20.63 ml/min/1.73 m^2, respectively. The Cys C-based GFR value was 73.66 ± 34.24 ml/min/1.73 m^2 at day 0, 78.19 ± 41.37 ml/min/1.73 m^2 at day 7, and 58.36 ± 25.76 ml/min/1.73 m^2 at day 14.

As depicted in Fig. 1, there was significant correlation between creatinine-based and Cys C-based GFR values at days 0 ($R = 0.606$, $P = 0.001$) and 7 ($R = 0.714$, $P < 0.001$). In contrast, the correlation of these values at day 14 was not statistically significant ($R = 0.496$, $P < 0.071$).

According to results of ANOVA with repeated measure analysis (Table 1 & Fig. 2), the mean (95 % CI) creatinine-based GFR at day 14 was significantly lower than that at day 7 in patients who developed AmB nephrotoxicity ($P = 0.024$). Furthermore, the mean (95 % CI) decrease in creatinine-based GFR values at day 14 compared to day 0 (-50.457 [-89.477 to-11.437] ml/min/1.73 m^2) as well as day 14 versus day 7 (-37.857 [-63.514 to-12.2] ml/min/1.73 m^2), were statistically significant between individuals with and without AmB nephrotoxicity ($P = 0.016$ and $P = 0.007$, respectively). In contrast to creatinine-based calculated GFR, the mean (95 % CI) Cys C-based GFR values at different studied time points were comparable within as well as between patients with and without AmB nephrotoxicity.

Discussion

Although studied extensively, Cys C-based GFR equations have not generally been introduced into routine clinical practice yet. Considerable heterogeneity between relevant GFR equations can be partially taken into account for this matter [15]. Substantial heterogeneity between Cys C-based GFR equations can be in turn attributed to four major factors including: (1) study population differences, (2) different gold standard methods of GFR measurements, (3) lack of international standardized calibration for measurement of Cys C, and (4) variation in exploited analytical techniques as well as reagents [10]. Regarding the first factor involved, elevated body mass index (BMI) can be associated with an increase in the Cys C concentration by about 10 %. Furthermore, serum Cys C concentrations have been reported to be lower in females than males (about 9 %) [15]. In the present study, no gold standard method was used for determining GFR because of both financial and technical problems.

Regarding the last two factors, three major techniques including particle-enhanced nephelometric assay (PENIA), particle enhanced turbidimetric assay (PETIA), and enzyme-linked immunosorbent assay (ELISA) are commonly used for determining Cys C. A meta-analysis on 46 articles published until December 31, 2001, revealed that immunonephelometric methods of Cys C assay produced significantly greater correlations with GFR

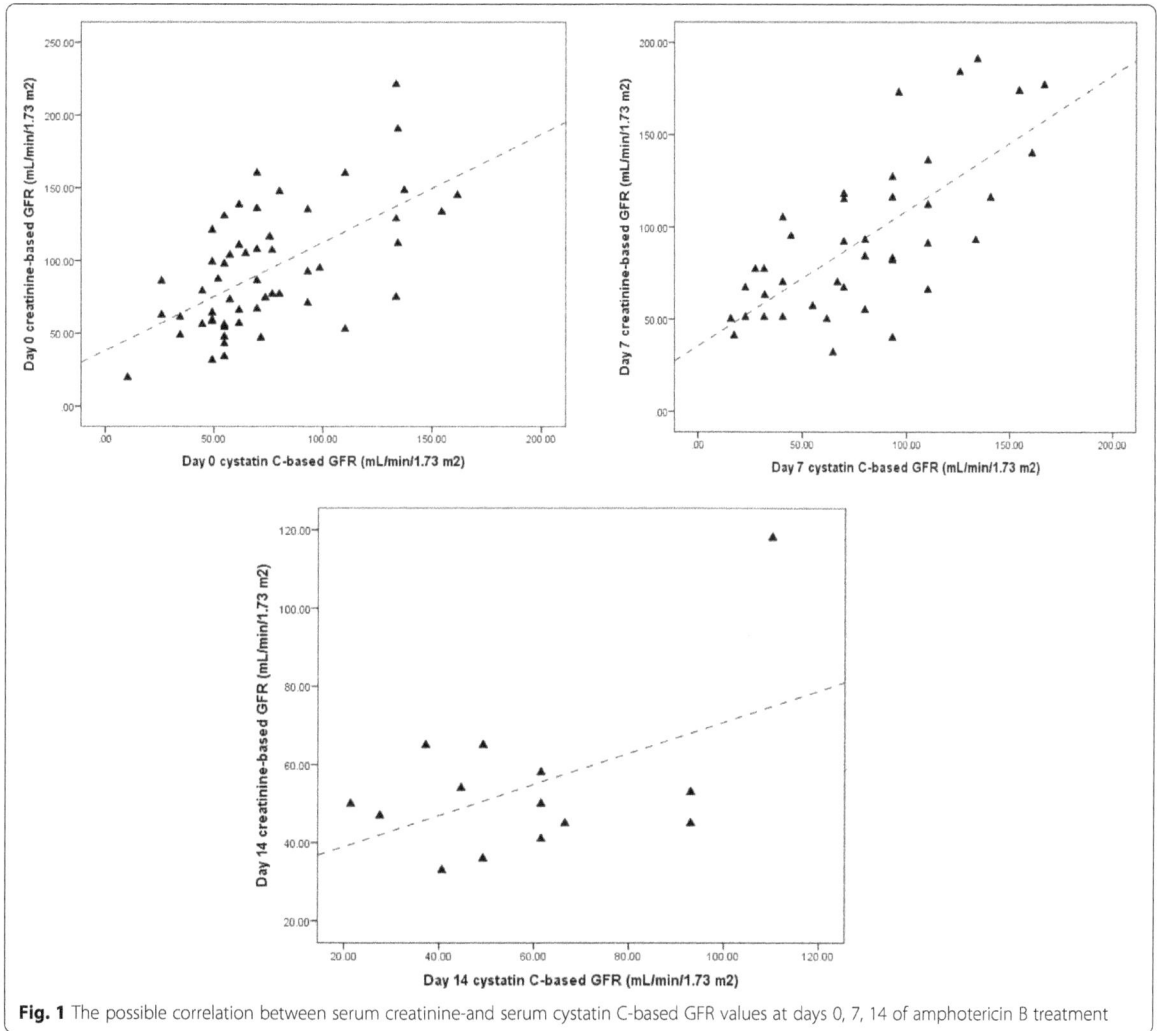

Fig. 1 The possible correlation between serum creatinine-and serum cystatin C-based GFR values at days 0, 7, 14 of amphotericin B treatment

than other assay methods ($r = 0.846$ versus $r = 0.784$, respectively; $P < 0.001$) [16]. In a study on 80 healthy volunteers and 20 patients with renal and/or heart disease, the mean difference between ELISA and PETIA or ELISA and PENIA was 0.65 ± 0.63 μg/ml and 0.58 ± 0.53 μg/ml, respectively [17]. Interestingly, Tidman et al. demonstrated that serum Cys C concentrations obtained by the Gentian method were approximately 10 % lower than the DAKO method within the normal GFR range. They also reported that among Cys C-based GFR formulas examined in 644 patients, the former Orebro-cyst Gentian equation (100/serum Cys C—14) had the highest accuracy [10].

The Cys C-based GFR equation used in our study was derived from Flodin et al. investigation on 160 patient samples aged above 15 years. Linear regression analysis showed

that there was strong correlation between Gentian Cys C assay using a chemistry instrument (Architect ci8200) and iohexol clearance ($R^2 = 0.956$) [18]. Lack of significant correlation between creatinine-based and Cys C-based GFR values only at day 14 but not days 0 and 7 of AmB treatment in our cohort, may be due to the limited number of patients (only 16) that remained in the study at this time point. It is noteworthy that considering only correlation coefficient in our survey seems inadequate and precision, accuracy, and relative difference should also be calculated to compare these two formulas properly. The pattern of Cys C-based GFR values decreased continuously during the study in patients with AmB nephrotoxicity; but these changes were not statistically significant in contrast to creatinine-based GFR values. This may be justified by the limited number of serum Cys C level measurements at

Table 1 Mean (95 % confidence interval) changes of creatinine-and serum cystatin C-based GFR values at days 0, 7 and 14 of amphotericin B treatment within and between patients with and without AmB nephrotoxicity

Time point	Day 7 vs. Day 0	Day 14 vs. Day 0	Day 14 vs. Day 7
Creatinine-based GFR (ml/min/1.73 m^2)			
Mean (95 % confidence interval) difference values in patients with nephrotoxicity [P value]	-6.258 (-82.997 to 70.480) [1]	-66.401 (-150.289 to 17.487) [0.122]	-60.143 (-110.816 to-9.470) [0.024]
Mean (95 % confidence interval) difference values in patients without nephrotoxicity [P value]	-18.942 (-70.939 to 33.055) [0.829]	-34.514 (-177.143 to 48.116) [0.656]	-15.571 (-74.111 to 42.968) [1]
Mean (95 % confidence interval) difference values between two groups [P value]	-12.6 (-43.318 to 18.118) [0.389]	-50.457 (-89.477 to-11.437) [0.016]	-37.857 (-63.514 to-12.2) [0.007]
Cystatin C-based GFR (ml/min/1.73 m^2)			
Mean (95 % confidence interval) difference values in patients with nephrotoxicity [P value]	-4.3 (-108.050 to 99.45) [1]	-42.943 (- 103.840 to 17.954) [0.179]	-38.643 (-96.965 to 19.679) [0.217]
Mean (95 % confidence interval) difference values in patients without nephrotoxicity [P value]	-19.357 (-59.401 to 20.686) [0.489]	-9.729 (-56.979 to 37.521) [1]	9.629 (-48.990 to 68.247) [1]
Mean (95 % confidence interval) difference values between two groups [P value]	-11.829 (-48.682 to 25.024) [0.498]	-26.336 (-51.878 to - 0.793) [0.44]	-14.507 (-41.909 to 12.895) [0.271]

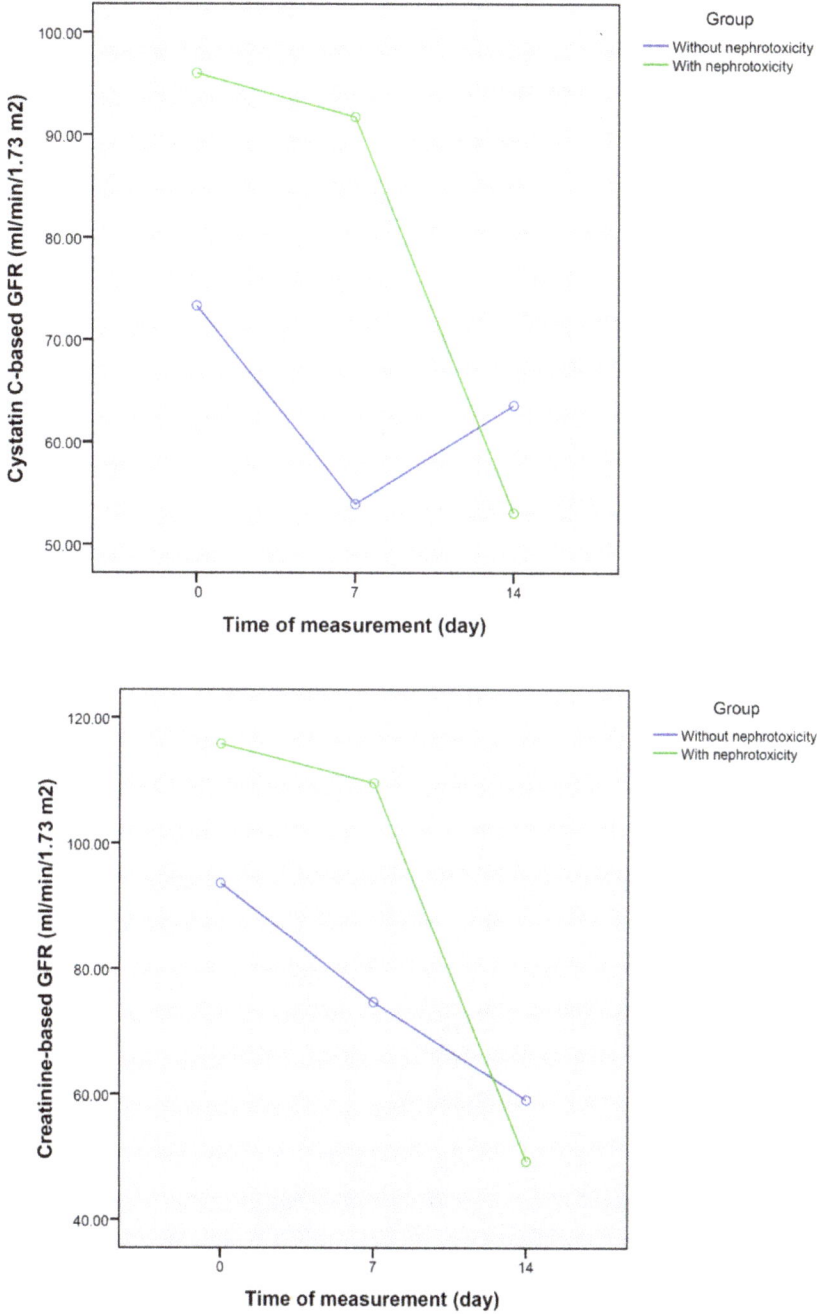

Fig. 2 Changing pattern in creatinine-and serum cystatin C-based GFR values at three time points in patients with and without amphotericin B nephrotoxicity

only three time points during AmB treatment, high intraindividual variability of serum Cys C, and absence of a gold standard method for measuring GFR.

In conclusion, our preliminary findings suggested that the Gentian Cys C-based GFR calculation equation correlated significantly with CG formula at least at the early time period of AmB treatment. However, the continuous decreasing trend in the mean (95 % CI) values of Cys C-based GFR at the studied time points was not statistically significant in patients who developed AmB nephrotoxicity. Measuring serum Cys C level at more frequent and closer time points and exploiting a gold standard method for measuring GFR can be considered for future studies in the comparison of serum Cys C-based equations with serum creatinine-based formulas used for the calculation of GFR in patients receiving nephrotoxic medications such as AmB.

Competing interests

The authors declare no conflict of interest.

Authors' contributions

IK participated in data collection, patient sampling, performing immunoassays, statistical analyses, and manuscript drafting. HK participated in study design, interperting data, and manuscript review. Both authors (IK & HK) read and approved the final manuscript.

Author details

[1]Department of Clinical Pharmacy, Faculty of Pharmacy, Shiraz University of Medical Sciences, Shiraz, Iran. [2]Department of Clinical Pharmacy, Faculty of Pharmacy, Tehran University of Medical Sciences, Enghelab Ave, Tehran, Iran.

References

1. Grubb AO. Cystatin C,–properties and use as diagnostic marker. Adv Clin Chem. 2000;35:63–99.
2. Filler G, Bokenkamp A, Hofmann W, Le Bricon T, Martinez-Bru C, Grubb A. Cystatin C as a marker of GFR–history, indications, and future research. Clin Biochem. 2005;38:1–8.
3. Royakkers AA, Van Suijlen JD, Hofstra LS, Kuiper MA, Bouman CS, Spronk PE, et al. Serum cystatin C-A useful endogenous marker of renal function in intensive care unit patients at risk for or with acute renal failure? Curr Med Chem. 2007;14:23147.
4. Hoste EA, Damen J, Vanholder RC, Lameire NH, Delanghe JR, Van den Hauwe K, Colardyn FA. Assessment of renal function in recently admitted critically ill patients with normal serum creatinine. Nephrol Dial Transplant. 2005;20:747–53.
5. Zahran A, Qureshi M, Shoker A. Comparison between creatinine and cystatin C-based GFR equations in renal transplantation. Nephrol Dial Transplant. 2007;22:2659–68.
6. Steinke T, Moritz S, Beck S, Gnewuch C, Kees MG. Estimation of creatinine clearance using plasma creatinine or cystatin C: a secondary analysis of two pharmacokinetic studies in surgical ICU patients. BMC Anesthesiol. 2015;15:62.
7. Bevc S, Hojs R, Ekart R, Završnik M, Gorenjak M, Puklavec L. Simple cystatin C formula for estimation of glomerular filtration rate in overweight patients with diabetes mellitus type 2 and chronic kidney disease. Exp Diabetes Res. 2012;2012:179849.
8. Treiber M, Pečovnik Balon B, Gorenjak M. A new serum cystatin C formula for estimating glomerular filtration rate in newborns. Pediatr Nephrol. 2015; 30:1297–305.
9. Ye X, Wei L, Pei X, Zhu B, Wu J, Zhao W. Application of creatinine-and/or cystatin C-based glomerular filtration rate estimation equations in elderly Chinese. Clin Interv Aging. 2014;9:1539–49.
10. Tidman M, Sjöström P, Jones I. A Comparison of GFR estimating formulae based upon s-cystatin C and s-creatinine and a combination of the two. Nephrol Dial Transplant. 2008;23:154–60.
11. Karimzadeh I, Khalili H, Sagheb MM, Farsaei S. A double-blinded, placebo-controlled, multicenter clinical trial of N-acetylcysteine for preventing amphotericin B-induced nephrotoxicity. Expert Opin Drug Metab Toxicol. 2015;11:1345–55.
12. Cockcroft DW, Gault MH. Prediction of creatinine clearance from serum creatinine. Nephron. 1976;16:31–41.
13. Package Insert for in vitro diagnostic use only Cystatin C Immunoassay. Available from: http://gentian.no/wp-content/uploads/2013/07/PI-Assay-CysC-AU-systems-v01-Jan13-.pdf
14. Goldman RD, Koren G. Amphotericin B nephrotoxicity in children. J Pediatr Hematol Oncol. 2004;26:421–6.
15. Harman G, Akbari A, Hiremath S, White CA, Ramsay T, Kokolo MB, Craig J, Knoll GA. Accuracy of cystatin C-based estimates of glomerular filtration rate in kidney transplant recipients: a systematic review. Nephrol Dial Transplant. 2013;28:741–57.
16. Dharnidharka VR, Kwon C, Stevens G. Serum cystatin C is superior to serum creatinine as a marker of kidney function: a meta-analysis. Am J Kidney Dis. 2002;40:221–6.
17. Hossain MA, Emara M, El Moselhi H, Shoker A. Comparing measures of cystatin C in human sera by three methods. Am J Nephrol. 2009;29:381–91.
18. Flodin M, Jonsson AS, Hansson LO, Danielsson LA, Larsson A. Evaluation of Gentian cystatin C reagent on Abbott Ci8200 and calculation of glomerular filtration rate expressed in mL/min/1.73 m (2) from the cystatin C values in mg/L. Scand J Clin Lab Invest. 2007;67:560–7.

24

Improved intraocular bioavailability of ganciclovir by mucoadhesive polymer based ocular microspheres: development and simulation process in *Wistar* rats

Usha Ganganahalli Kapanigowda[1], Sree Harsha Nagaraja[2], Balakeshwa Ramaiah[3*] and Prakash Rao Boggarapu[1]

Abstract

Background: The poor ocular bioavailability of the conventional eye drops is due to lack of corneal permeability, nasolacrimal drainage and metabolic degradation. To overcome this issue, drug encapsulated in mucoadhesive polymer based ocular microspheres have the advantages of improved drug stability, easy administration in liquid form, diffuse rapidly and better ocular tissue internalization.

Methods: The ganciclovir chitosan microspheres (GCM) were prepared by modified water-in-oil emulsification method. The formulation was optimized and characterized by investigating *in vitro* release study, release kinetics, XRD and microspheres stability. Ocular irritancy, *in vivo* ocular pharmacokinetic parameters and histopathology study was evaluated in *Wistar* rats. The use of pharmacokinetic/pharmacodynamic indices and simulation process was carried out to further ensure clinical applicability of the formulation.

Results: The *in vitro* release study showed initial burst (nearly 50 %) in first few minutes and followed Fickian ($R^2 = 0.9234$, n-value $= 0.2329$) type of diffusion release mechanism. The XRD and stability studies showed favorable results. The *Wistar* rat eyes treated with GCM showed significant increase in ganciclovir AUC ($\sim$4.99-fold) and C_{max} (2.69-fold) in aqueous humor compared to ganciclovir solution and delay in T_{max}. The C_{max}/MIC_{90}, AUC_{0-24}/MIC_{90}, AUC above MIC_{90} and T above MIC_{90} were significantly higher in GCM group. The aqueous humor concentration-time profile of ganciclovir in GCM and ganciclovir solution was simulated with every 28.1 and 12.8 h, respectively. The simulated concentration-time profile shows that in duration of 75 h, the ganciclovir solution require six ocular instillations compared to three ocular instillations of the GCM formulation. The photomicrograph of GCM and ganciclovir solution treated rat retina showed normal organization and cytoarchitecture.

Conclusions: Correlating with *in vitro* data, the formulation showed sustained drug release along with improved intraocular bioavailability of ganciclovir in *Wistar* rats.

Keywords: Franz cells, Superimposition, Release kinetics, Ocular pharmacokinetic, Simulation

* Correspondence: balupharmacy@gmail.com
[3]Department of Pharmaceutics, Karnataka College of Pharmacy, #33/2, Tirumenahalli, Hegde Nagar Main Road, Bengaluru 560064, Karnataka, India
Full list of author information is available at the end of the article

Background

Herpes simplex keratitis and cytomegalovirus retinitis have been the most common viral infections observed worldwide [1]. Recurrent and relapse of ocular viral infections can lead to corneal perforation resulting in blindness. The poor bioavailability of the conventional eye drops is due to lack of corneal permeability, nasolacrimal drainage and metabolic degradation. Hence, an optimum treatment must be considered for effective management of ocular viral diseases. Ganciclovir, a broad spectrum antiviral drug was considered to be highly active against *cytomegalovirus* and *herpes simplex virus*. Ganciclovir, an acyloguanosine derivative after *in vivo* administration gets modified into ganciclovir triphosphate. It competitively inhibits the virus deoxyribonucleic acid (DNA) polymerase by impairing the viral DNA synthesis [2].

Ganciclovir requires frequent oral administration, has it shows very poor bioavailability (6–9 %) [3]. Administration of drug via oral, intravenous or extravascular injection leads to low drug concentration at the site of infected eye [4]. This finding was supported by a study conducted by Young et al. [5], reports that the contralateral retinitis was higher in patients treated with intravenous maintenance therapy of ganciclovir (15–68 %) compared to intravitreous ganciclovir (11 %). Moreover, due to its short half-life, frequent intravitreal injections leads to risk of retinal detachments, hemorrhages, or endophthalmitis. Ganciclovir encapsulated with PLGA microspheres for ocular delivery has been investigated [6]. Reported clinical studies [2, 7, 8] found that the ganciclovir efficacy can be accomplished by formulating the drug as an ophthalmic topical preparation. Hence, a sustained intraocular drug concentration can be achieved by using a desired polymer in the form of microspheres for ocular instillation, which also seems to reduce the ocular toxicities. Ganciclovir combined with chitosan showed two fold increased oral bioavailability [9].

The inherent biological activity of chitosan [poly (β-(1 → 4)-2-amino-2-deoxy-D-glucose)] signifies its role in ocular therapeutics. With various degrees of N-acetylation of glucosamine residues, it is considered as a linear binary heteroploysaccharide composed of β-1,4-linked glucosamine. Chitosan being a promising natural biodegradable polymer with hydrophilic in nature improves stability, precorneal retention and enhances interaction with eye mucosa. Moreover, the sustained release, mucoadhesive, in situ gelling, transfection and permeation enhancing properties of chitosan are recognized as few parameters of the polymer suitable for ocular drug delivery. The unique physical properties of chitosan bring transitions in the paracellular and transcellular pathway without disturbing cellular integrity. This innate chitosan property allows the drug to be transported to the inner eye and helps the drug to get accumulated at corneal epithelia [10, 11].

Chitosan has the ability to augment intraocular drug penetration by binding with cornea and reversibly loosening the tight corneal conjunctions. Additionally, non toxic, low eye irritation and ability to release the drug at a sustainable fashion qualifies it as one of the ideal polymer for ophthalmic preparation [12, 13]. Chitosan has been used in many ophthalmic preparations such as indomethacin nanoemulsions [14]; indomethacin nanocapsules [15]; cyclosporine A nanoparticles [16]; ofloxacin microspheres [17] and acyclovir microspheres [18]. Zirgan™ and Virgan® are commercially available ganciclovir ophthalmic gels. Zirgan™ has been approved in European countries since 1995 and in 2009 it was approved in United States [1]. Additionally, the ganciclovir implant (Vitrasert) received USFDA approval for the treatment of cytomegalovirus retinitis in immunodeficiency patients.

Intraocular or periocular injections of microparticles or nanoparticles can lead to vitreous clouding and foreign body response. Due to low biodistribution coefficient, the topical administration of ganciclovir has limitations. Frequent administrations of the conventional eye drops are required due to their short retention time and decreased ocular drug bioavailability [19]. Thus, the microspheres are preferred delivery system for ocular drug delivery. The polymeric microspheres have the advantages of easy administration in liquid form, diffuse rapidly and better ocular tissue internalization. The entrapped drug in the form of monolithic-type or reservoir type in the microspheres can act as depot and sustain the release of drug. Hence, literatures [2, 3] support the use of ganciclovir as microsphere formulation for improved antiviral effectiveness.

The requirement of ganciclovir ocular preparation for topical application with better therapeutic efficacy and good safety profile was evident. Thus, this study was an attempt to investigate formulation of ganciclovir using mucoadhesive polymer intended for sustained and improved intraocular delivery. The preparation was characterized by *in vitro* drug release, release kinetics, X-ray diffraction (XRD) and stability study. Further, ocular irritancy, *in vivo* ocular pharmacokinetic, histopathology along with pharmacokinetic/pharmacodynamic indices and simulation process was utilized to identify the efficacy and tolerability of the optimized formulation.

Materials and methods

Materials

Ganciclovir was acquired as a gift sample from Dr. Reddys Laboratories, Hyderabad, India. Chitosan (93 % deactylation) was purchased from Yarrow Chem Products, Mumbai, India. Other reagents used were of analytical grade.

Analytical method

Reverse-phase high performance liquid chromatography (RP-HPLC) was used for quantitative analysis of ganciclovir

[20]. The C8 column (15 cm × 4.6 mm; 5 μ) was utilized for the analysis. The mobile phase consisted of mixture of 0.1 M sodium dihydrogen phosphate monohydrate and 0.04 M triethylamine in the ratio of 50:50 (pH maintained at 6.6). The column temperature was retained at 40 °C. The injection volume was 20 μL and the flow rate was maintained at 1 mL/min. The sample was detected using UV at 254 nm. The acyclovir was considered as an internal standard. The standard calibration curve was linear in the concentration range of 50 to 1000 ng/mL.

Experimental design
The central composite design was used to optimize ganciclovir loaded chitosan microspheres (GCM) by altering variable factors and their effect on encapsulation efficiency and 12th hour *in vitro* drug release. The model contained eight factorial points, six axial points and six centre points with total 20 experiments. The mean value was set as 0 and, +1 and –1 was considered as higher and lower levels for each factor respectively. The selected factors with their levels along with optimized levels are summarized in Tables 1 and 2.

Preparation of optimized GCM
The optimized GCMs intended for ocular sustained release were prepared by modified water-in-oil emulsification method [21]. Seven hundred and fifty milligrams of 93 % deacetylated chitosan was dissolved in 50 mL of 1 % w/v acetic acid maintained at pH 2.72. Five hundred milligrams of ganciclovir was added to the above solution with agitation and the mixture was sonicated for 10 min. The resultant mixture was centrifuged (1000 rpm, 10 min) to separate any remains of undissolved chitosan. The oil phase consisted of 20 mL of dichloromethane and 20 mL of liquid paraffin with 1 mL of 1 % v/v of Span 80. The aqueous phase was introduced slowly as drop wise in to the oil phase under continuous homogenization at 3000 rpm. Further, the water in oil emulsion was homogenized to crosslink the microspheres with 5 % v/v of glutaraldehyde. The emulsion was again added to 20 mL of pre-heated liquid paraffin at 170 °C with stirring to remove dichloromethane and aqueous solvent. The formed microspheres were filtered through 0.45 μm Millipore filters. To remove residual liquid paraffin, the

microspheres was then washed 5–6 times with 100 mL of diethyl ether and was vacuum dried for 24 h.

In vitro drug release of the optimized GCM
Using Franz diffusion cells, the *in vitro* release of ganciclovir from the microspheres was investigated. The molecular weight cut-off of the dialysis membrane was between 12,000–14,000 Da (Himedia Laborateries Pvt. Ltd, Mumbai, India). The dialysis membrane acted as a barrier to separate the donor and acceptor compartment. The simulated tear fluid (STF) was used as the dissolution medium, which was prepared by adding 0.67 % of NaCl; 0.2 % of NaHCO3; 0.008 % of $CaCl_2$. $2H_2O$ and the resultant solution pH was adjusted to 7.4. A weighed amount of microspheres dispersed in 1 mL of the STF was kept in the donor compartment. The STF (100 mL) was filled in the acceptor compartment and stirred magnetically at 100 rpm maintaining the temperature at 37 ± 0.5 °C [22]. For a period of 12 h, 1 mL of the sample was withdrawn every hour from the acceptor compartment and subjected to UV spectroscopy scanned at 254 nm. The same amount of the fresh STF was replaced into the acceptor compartment.

Release kinetics of the optimized GCM
Various models such as first order model (1); Higuchi square root model (2); Baker and Lonsdale (3); Koresmeyer-Peppas (4) and; Hixon and Crowell cube root model (5) models were used to study drug release mechanism from the microspheres. The data was fitted to these models and was analyzed using sigma plot.

$$Q_t = Q_0\, e^{-k_1 t} \tag{1}$$

$$Q_t = k_H \sqrt{t} \tag{2}$$

$$\frac{Q_t}{Q_\infty} = 1 - \frac{6}{\pi^2} exp\left(\frac{-\pi^2 \times Dt}{r^2}\right) \tag{3}$$

$$Q_t = Q_0 + a\left(\frac{t}{r^2}\right)^n + b\left(\frac{t}{r^2}\right)^{2n} \tag{4}$$

$$\sqrt[3]{Q_0} - \sqrt[3]{Q_t} = k_{HC} t \tag{5}$$

Q_t is the total amount of drug released after time (%); Q_0 the initial amount of drug (%); k_1 the first order release rate constant (h^{-1}); k_H the rate constant obtained according to the Higuchi equation ($\%h^{-1/2}$); Q_∞ is the

Table 1 Variable factors with their levels used for optimization of GCM

Variable factors	Level					Optimized level
	−1.41	−1	0	1	1.41	
Chitosan concentration (mg)	79.55	250	500	750	920.45	750
Stirring speed (rpm)	318	1000	2000	3000	3682	3000
Span 80 volume (mL)	0.20	0.40	0.70	1.0	1.20	1.00

Table 2 Response factors with expected and observed values for optimized GCM

Response factors	Expected value	Observed value	Residual value
Encapsulation efficiency (%)	81.4	80.00	−1.4
12th hour in vitro drug release (%)	77.27	78.00	0.73

percent release at infinite time; D is the diffusion coefficient in the polymer in cm^2/s; r is the radius of the sphere in cm; n and $2n$ are the release exponent for Fickian diffusion and case II transport, respectively; a and b are constants related to the drug and the structural and geometric properties of the microparticles; and k_{HC} is the rate constant obtained according to the Hixon and Crowell equation ($\%h^{-1}$) [23–25].

XRD

XRD of ganciclovir powder, chitosan and the optimized GCM was performed (Philips XPert Pro, Netherlands) at 40 kV voltage with 30 mA of the current, utilizing a nickel-filtered CuKα radiation. With 0.02° interval, the sample was scanned over a 2θ range of 10–80° at a rate of 2°/min.

Stability study of the optimized GCM

The stability study was conducted as per ICH Q1AR guideline, intended to test the stability for new substances and product. The optimized preparation was stored at 25 ± 2 °C and 60 ± 5 % RH for twelve months and at 5 ± 3 °C for a period of six months. The required volume of microsphere dispersion was stored in closed glass bottles and sealed tightly. At regular intervals, the sample was subjected for determination of encapsulation efficiency, mean particle size distribution and for any physical changes. The test was carried at three month intervals for a period of 12 months for long term storage condition at room temperature and at 0, 2, 4 and 6 months for accelerated condition at refrigeration storage.

In vivo ocular pharmacokinetic studies of the optimized GCM

Prior to the study, the ethical clearance for in vivo experimental protocol was obtained from Institutional Animal Ethics Committee (IAEC) which is registered under CPCSEA, India. The Wistar rats (male and female) free from ocular defects, 11–13 weeks older and weighing around 180–200 g was utilized for the study.

Ocular irritation

The microspheres ocular tolerability [26] was evaluated by identifying the ocular irritancy. The 1 % w/v of the sample was prepared by dispersing the microspheres in isotonic normal saline (ganciclovir solution) and was immediately used for the study. The GCM sample (25 μL)

was directly instilled into right eye of the rat and for uniform dispersion on cornea; the rats were forced to wink once. The left eye was instilled with normal saline alone and acted as a control. Post instillation, both the eyes were observed for frequency of winking in 5 min.

In vivo evaluation

A total of 32 Wistar rats were housed in standard cages and had free access to food and water. The rats were allowed for free head and eye movement. To carry out in vivo study [27], 75 μL (3 × 25 μL drops at 90 s intervals) of the GCM (1 % w/v) was freshly prepared and was immediately instilled with micropipette into lower conjunctival sac of the right eye without touching the eye. The 1 % w/v of the ganciclovir solution served as a control and as above mentioned quantity and procedure was instilled to the left eye. At 0.5 h, 1 h, 1.5 h, 2 h, 3 h, 4 h, 5 h, 6 h, 12 h, 24 h post ocular instillation, the animal was sacrificed by cervical dislocation and the entire eyes were removed. The aqueous humor from the isolated eyes was separated and was stored in micro centrifuge tubes at −20 °C until further analysis. After the process of extraction and isolation, the sample was subjected to the RP-HPLC analysis.

Extraction and isolation

The in vivo pharmacokinetic estimation of the ganciclovir in aqueous humor was performed as mentioned above by RP-HPLC method. The extracted aqueous humor (100 μL) was added to 100 μL of 50 % trichloroacetic acid, shaken well and was centrifuged at 2000 g for 10 min to deproteinize the sample. The supernatant was neutralized with 50 μL of 2 M sodium hydroxide and vortexed. Later, the sample was extracted with 5 mL of chloroform and centrifuged at 3000 g for 5 min. The extracted sample was mixed with 10 μL of the mobile phase. Finally 20 μL of the mixture and 20 μL of the acyclovir as an internal standard were injected into HPLC system [20].

Pharmacokinetic and Statistical analysis

The pharmacokinetic parameters were calculated using one compartment open model. The ganciclovir, area under the curve (AUC) in aqueous humor was determined from the beginning of the drop instillation (t_0) to the last observation (t_{last}) by linear trapezoidal rule with extrapolation to infinite time. Additionally, ganciclovir half life ($t_{1/2}$), relative bioavailability, the maximum peak concentration (C_{max})

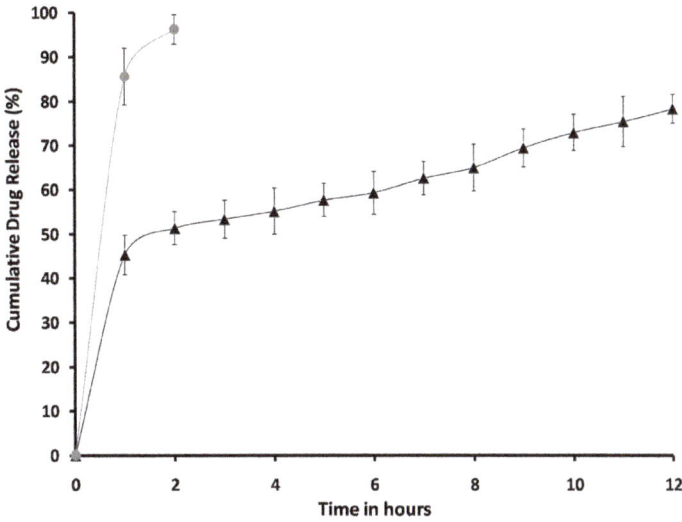

Fig. 1 Cumulative amount of drug released (▲) GCM and (●) ganciclovir solution (bars represent mean ± SD; $n = 3$)

and time to achieve maximum peak concentration (T_{max}) was also calculated. The terminal rate constant (K_e) and apparent absorption rate (K_a) of ganciclovir from aqueous humor was estimated from the terminal portions of the respective log (aqueous humor concentration) vs. time linear regression plots [28].

The Kinetica 5.0 PK/PD analysis software was also utilized for the calculation of pharmacokinetic parameters. The estimated pharmacokinetic/pharmacodynamic (PK/PD) indices such as C_{max}/MIC_{90}, AUC_{0-24}/MIC_{90}, AUC above MIC_{90} and T above MIC_{90} was calculated to determine the *in vivo* efficacy of the GCM. The principle of superimposition using Microsoft excel software was used to evaluate the simulation of aqueous humor concentration- time profile at different dosing interval [29]. Based on the time where the ganciclovir aqueous humor concentration was maintained twice the MIC_{90} (1.22 μg/mL), the subsequent dose was calculated. Student's t test ($p < 0.05$) was considered for statistical significance.

Histopathology

The isolated eyes were stored in 10 % formalin and were subjected to histopathological examination. The retina was isolated, dyed with hematoxylin-eosin and

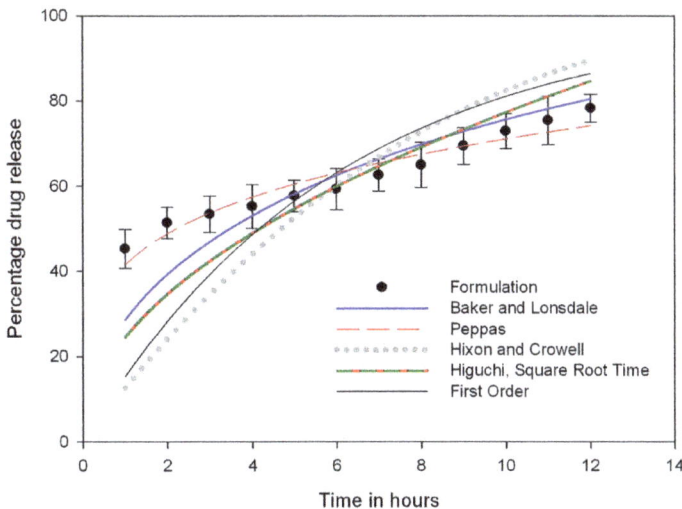

Fig. 2 *In vitro* release profile of the optimized GCM-curve fitting models (bars represent mean ± SD; $n = 3$)

Table 3 Stability test observations of the optimized GCM at room temperature

Storage	Encapsulation efficiency (%)					Mean Particle size (μm)					Physical change				
	Months					Months					Months				
25 ± 2 °C	0	3	6	9	12	0	3	6	9	12	0	3	6	9	12
	80.79	79.92	79.15	78.57	77.39	20.28	20.15	20.20	20.35	20.40	–	–	–	–	–

–: No physical change

was observed under light microscopy with 200× magnification for cytoarchitecture changes.

Results and discussion

Preparation of the optimized GCM
The modified water-in-oil emulsification method was found to be suitable and simple technique for encapsulating ganciclovir using chitosan. The degree of chitosan deacetylation and molecular weight are considered to be two fundamental parameters that influence the properties and functionality of chitosan. These parameters along with crystallinity influence chitosan degradation and ocular epithelial cell permeability. More than 60 % of deacetylation of chitosan is considered to be ideal for ocular delivery as decrease in deacetylation leads to decreased water solubility of the polymer. Interestingly, trimethylated chitosan with PEGlation a 3.4-fold increase in its mucoadhesive property was observed, but no such pronounced observation was found in respect to its permeation enhancing property [11]. However, this study used 93 % deacetylated chitosan for the purpose of encapsulation of ganciclovir. On ocular instillation, the liquid form of chitosan transforms into gel form at physiological pH of 7.4 and significantly helps in longer residence time and biodistribution of the drug on corneal surface. The negatively charged cornea and sclera interacts with positive charged amino groups of the chitosan, hence enhances the ocular bioavailability [10, 30]. A study by Mathew et al. [31], showed the increased sustained drug release by using optimum glutaraldehyde as cross linking agent. Earlier many studies [32, 33] have successfully prepared chitosan microspheres from emulsion cross-linking method.

In vitro release study of the optimized GCM
In vitro drug release of the optimized GCM and ganciclovir solution using STF was investigated separately

(Fig. 1). The in vitro data showed biphasic pattern of ganciclovir release from GCM. The initial drug loading followed by marked prolongation of drug residence time was achieved by an initial immediate burst effect (nearly 50 %) in few minutes and then slower release over few hours (up to 90 %). The appropriate physicochemical properties of the microspheres help in achieving adequate drug bioavailability and biocompatibility with ocular mucosa. The initial burst release was beneficial in attaining required therapeutic concentration of the drug in negligible time. The rapid and instantaneous initial release was due to the modified water-in-oil emulsification preparation method that resulted in deposition of drug on surface of the microspheres. The drug adhered to the surface of the microspheres are primarily released into aqueous media by desorption and diffusion causing the initial burst [29, 34]. The decrease in particle size enhances this effect as the formation of large surface area. Similar finding has been observed for different drugs encapsulated in chitosan microspheres [35]. The sustained action in the later stage was due to diffusion of ganciclovir from the polymeric matrix and biodegradation of chitosan. Genta et al., [18] has demonstrated the mucoadhesive and sustain release activity of the chitosan.

Curve fitting analysis of the optimized GCM
The Fig. 2 shows curve fitting of the optimized formulation in vitro drug release kinetics. Among the models, Koresmeyer–Peppas model was best fitted by significant regression coefficient ($R^2 = 0.9234$). Using Fick's law, Koresmeyer-Peppas model helps in investigating drug release mechanism from the polymeric system in the first 10h of the in vitro study. The n-value (0.2329, $p < 0.0001$) of the optimized formulation was less than 0.45, indicating Fickian type of diffusion mechanism of drug release. The Koresmeyer-Peppas model explains when the drug release mechanism is a combination of drug diffusion - Fickian transport-, and in Case II

Table 4 Stability test observations of the optimized GCM at refrigeration conditions

Storage	Encapsulation efficiency (%)				Mean particle size (μm)				Physical change			
	Months				Months				Months			
5 ± 3 °C	0	2	4	6	0	2	4	6	0	2	4	6
	80.79	80.62	79.89	79.00	20.28	20.19	20.24	20.30	–	–	–	–

–: No physical change

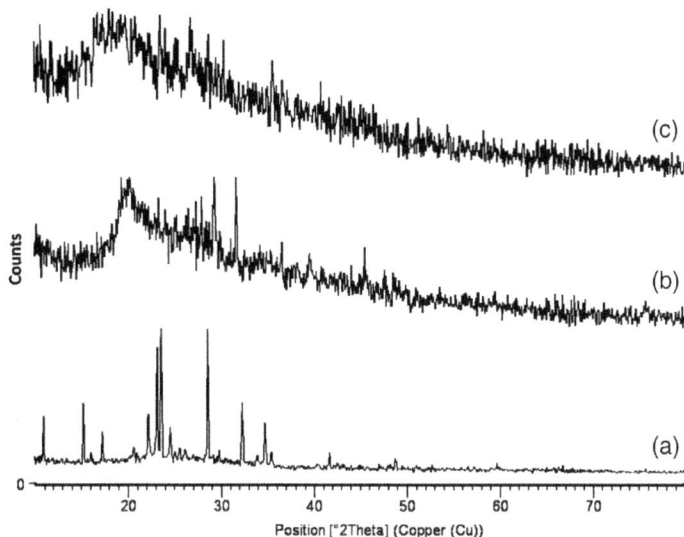

Fig. 3 XRD of (**a**) ganciclovir; (**b**) chitosan; (**c**) optimized GCM

transport - non-Fickian-, controlled by the relaxation of polymer chain. Chitosan polymeric matrix usually represents diffusion and erosion type of drug release [36]. The sustained action of the ocular delivery also depends on the surface characteristics of the microspheres. The positive zeta potential can facilitate an effective adhesion to the cornea surface and also could improve some limitations related to ocular administration, such as prevent tear washout (due to tear dynamics). Subsequently, the positive charge interact with the cell membrane leading in a structural reorganization of tight junction-associated proteins

helps in permeation of the drug through corneal surface and improves intraocular drug bioavailability [11, 37].

Stability study of the optimized GCM
The stability test observations of the optimized GCM at room temperature and refrigeration conditions are depicted in Tables 3 and 4. On storage, no major deviations were observed in the macroscopic characteristics. A slight increase in mean particle size was noted at 25 °C. The XRD spectral characteristics are shown in Fig. 3. On storage, the extent of microsphere sedimentation was not prominent, on

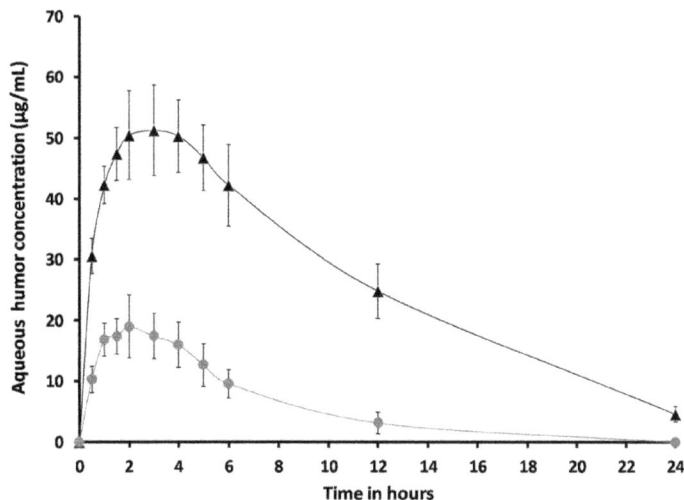

Fig. 4 Aqueous humour concentration of ganciclovir after instillation of 1 % w/v of (▲) GCM and (●) ganciclovir solution (bars represent mean ± SD; *n* = 3)

Table 5 Aqueous humor pharmacokinetics parameters after ocular instillation of GCM (1 % w/v) and ganciclovir solution (1 % w/v) in *Wistar* rat

Parameters	Units	GCM	Ganciclovir solution	P value
K_a	h^{-1}	0.7252	1.2981	0.0021
K_e	h^{-1}	0.1233	0.1662	0.6270
T_{max}	h	3.0	2.0	——
C_{max}	μgmL^{-1}	51.23	18.98	<0.0001
Relative bioavailability[a]	unitless	4.991	1.000	——
$t_{1/2}$	h	5.7654	3.5426	0.0636
AUC_{0-24}	$h\mu gmL^{-1}$	607.187	121.634	<0.0001
$AUC_{0-\infty}$	$h\mu gmL^{-1}$	645.116	137.692	<0.0001

[a]Relative bioavailability = $(AUC_{GCM} \times Dose_{ganciclovir\ solution})/(AUC_{ganciclovir\ solution} \times Dose_{GCM})$

manual agitation they were redispersed easily. XRD spectral characteristic of the ganciclovir pure drug shows many diffraction peaks, indicating the crystallinity of the drug. In contrast, the diffraction peaks were significantly reduced in GCM. XRD of chitosan shows few peaks, which indicates non crystallinity. The GCM formulation showed decreased crystallinity of ganciclovir, which was similar to that of chitosan indicating the incorporation of ganciclovir in the polymer. The increase in mean particle size could be due to increased kinetic energy of system contributing to higher rate of particle collision [26]. Thus, the optimized formula proved to be stable on long term and accelerated storage conditions as well.

In vivo ocular pharmacokinetic studies of the optimized GCM

The ocular irritation test showed that the GCM sample (12.0 ± 1.0 *vs ganciclovir solution 10.0 ± 1.0*) was well tolerated. The ocular pharmacokinetic of the optimized GCM (1 % w/v) was compared with the ganciclovir solution (1 % w/v) in *Wistar* rats. The dose volume and strength of both the samples were same. The 1 % w/v strength of both the samples would provide optimum C_{max} so as to decrease the nasolacrimal removal of ganciclovir. Subsequently, the relative hydrophilicity of the ganciclovir limits its corneal penetration. The paracellular diffusion of ganciclovir between the tight junctions of the corneal epithelial cells posses a greater challenge [1]. Peyman and Ganiban, [38] showed that the ganciclovir dose upto 400 μg/0.2 mL was found to be non toxic to the retina. Hence, to maintain higher concentration of ganciclovir, 1 % w/v of the GCM was used in this study for *in vivo* evaluation. Young et al., [5] study confirms that the injection of greater than 10 mg of ganciclovir into vitreous humor may result in retinal damage. Throughout this study, the ganciclovir concentration in aqueous humor was below the reported toxic ganciclovir concentration in eye. The 0.15 % ophthalmic gel has shown the mean ganciclovir concentration in tears

ranging from 0.92 to 6.86 μg mL^{-1} without any ocular discomfort [1].

The aqueous humor concentrations of ganciclovir after instillation of 1 % w/v of GCM and ganciclovir solution were shown in Fig. 4. The Table 5 illustrates the aqueous humor pharmacokinetic parameters. In comparison with ganciclovir solution, the GCM showed significant increase in AUC (~4.99-fold). The absorption rate constant (K_a) data showed that the GCM trans-corneal permeability was enhanced and was statistically significant than the ganciclovir solution. Subsequently, the terminal rate constant (K_e) and $t_{1/2}$ did not alter much. The C_{max} of GCM was 2.69-fold of the ganciclovir group ($p < 0.0001$) and the delay in T_{max} infers the sustained release of the GCM. The incorporation of ganciclovir into microspheres significantly increased relative bioavailability.

This finding signifies the enhanced binding force of the positively charged GCM to the eye surface. Usually, a mucus film as a thin fluid layer covers the surface of the cornea and conjunctiva. The mucin (high molecular mass glycoprotein) being a primary constituent of mucus carries negative charge at physiological pH. Hence, the positively charged chitosan interact with sialic groups and sulfonic acid substructures of mucin and act as an adhesive force to the eye surface. Upon dissolution, the protonation of amino groups (-NH$_2$) of the glucosamine to –NH$_3^+$, and the cationic polyelectrolyte readily forms electrostatic interactions with other anionic groups. Thus, the formation of hydrogen bond to the eye surface

Table 6 The estimated pharmacokinetic/pharmacodynamic (PK/PD) indices after ocular instillation of GCM (1 % w/v) and ganciclovir solution (1 % w/v) in *Wistar* rat

PK/PD indices	Units	GCM	Ganciclovir solution
C_{max}/MIC_{90}	unitless	41.991	15.560
AUC_{0-24}/MIC_{90}	h	497.694	99.700
AUC_{0-24} above MIC_{90}	$h\mu gmL^{-1}$	573.518	106.239
T above MIC_{90}	h	28.1	12.8

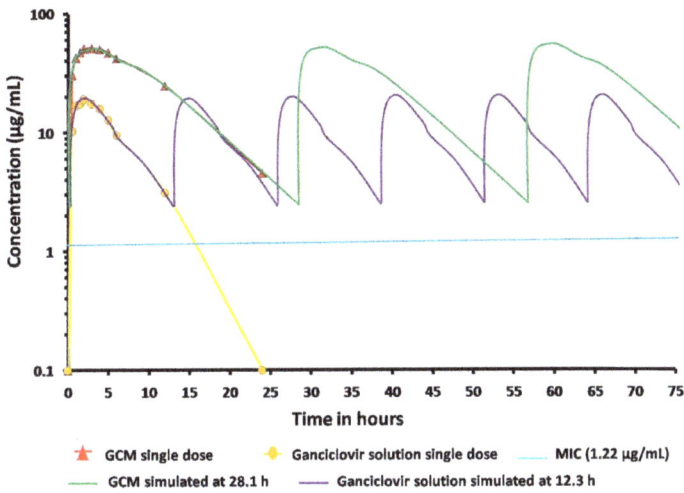

Fig. 5 Simulated ocular concentration time-profile of ganciclovir for 75 h at a dosing interval of 28.1 h for GCM and 12.3 h for ganciclovir solution

which is considerably influenced by cationic free amine and hydroxyl groups of chitosan [11, 28, 30, 39].

The estimated pharmacokinetic/pharmacodynamic (PK/PD) indices after ocular instillation of GCM and ganciclovir solution in *Wistar* rat are shown in Table 6. The PK/PD indices play an important role in treatment selection and dosage regimen of ganciclovir as its antiviral activity is concentration dependent. The minimum inhibitory concentration (MIC) solely fails to explain the *in vivo* activity of an antimicrobial agent. In this study, the C_{max}/MIC_{90} and AUC_{0-24}/MIC_{90} of GCM were maintained higher than the ganciclovir solution. The C_{max}/MIC, AUC/MIC, AUC above MIC and T above MIC were higher in the

GCM compared to ganciclovir solution and thus indicates the clinical effectiveness. Moreover, for effective antimicrobial activity, the C_{max}/MIC_{90} and AUC_{0-24}/MIC_{90} of GCM should be higher than 10 and 125, respectively which were complied with GCM formulation [29]. The simulated values also suggest the ideal dosing frequency.

Using the best fit model parameters, the aqueous humor concentration-time profile of GCM and ganciclovir solution was simulated with every 28.1 and 12.8h, respectively (Fig. 5). The simulated concentration-time profile shows that in duration of 75 h, the ganciclovir solution require six ocular instillations compared to three installations of the GCM formulation. Thus, GCM minimizes dosing

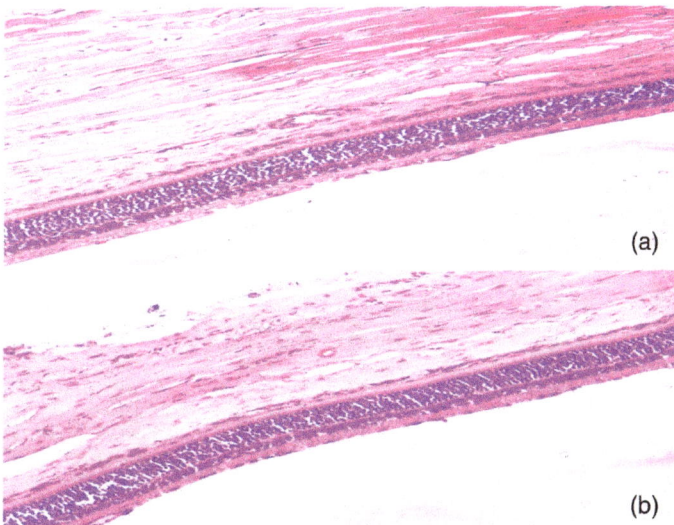

Fig. 6 Photomicrographs of histological slides of rat retina (**a**) GCM and (**b**) ganciclovir solution

frequency by sustained ganciclovir release for better efficacy. The photomicrograph of GCM and ganciclovir solution treated rat retina showed normal organization and
cytoarchitecture (Fig. 6). The photomicrograph of GCM
and ganciclovir solution showed inner layer of the retina,
which was covered by nerve fibers followed by a layer of
ganglion cells, an inner plexiform layer, inner nuclear layer,
outer plexiform layer, outer nuclear layer, inner and outer
segments of the rods, cones and sclera.

Conclusions

The development of ganciclovir loaded chitosan microspheres was found to be ideal for ocular delivery. The microspheres showed Fickian type of drug release, and the
XRD and stability studies showed favorable results. The
GCM showed significant increase in AUC and C_{max} com-
pared to ganciclovir solution. The C_{max}/MIC_{90}, AUC_{0-24}/MIC_{90}, AUC above MIC_{90} and T above MIC_{90} were higher
in the GCM. Further, the *in vivo* ocular pharmacokinetic
studies along with the histopathology report demonstrated
the efficacy and tolerability of the formulation. Hence, the
formulation significantly offered sustained drug release
and improved intraocular bioavailability of ganciclovir in
Wistar rats.

Competing interests
The authors declare that they have no competing interests.

Authors' contributions
UGK conceived the study, designed, carried out experiments and drafted the
manuscript. SN assisted in design, analysis, interpretation of the data and
manuscript plagiarism check. BR coordinated the experiments, involved in XRD,
stability studies and drafting the manuscript. PRB participated in the design of
the study, interpretation of the data, performed the statistical analysis and
revised the manuscript. All authors read and approved the final manuscript.

Acknowledgements
We are thankful to Prof. Basavaraj Ramnal, Secretary and Dr. Ramesh K,
Director, Karnataka College of Pharmacy, Bengaluru, Karnataka, India, for
valuable contribution to make this research work possible. We also thank Mr.
Lokesh Prasad, DTL, Bengaluru, Karnataka, India, for proof reading the article.

Author details
[1]Department of Pharmaceutical Technology, Karnataka College of Pharmacy,
#33/2, Tirumenahalli, Hegde Nagar Main Road, Bengaluru 560064, Karnataka,
India. [2]Department of Pharmaceutical Sciences, College of Clinical Pharmacy,
King Faisal University, Al-Ahsa 31982, Saudi Arabia. [3]Department of
Pharmaceutics, Karnataka College of Pharmacy, #33/2, Tirumenahalli, Hegde
Nagar Main Road, Bengaluru 560064, Karnataka, India.

References
1. Sahin A, Hamrah P. Acute herpetic keratitis: what is the role for ganciclovir
    ophthalmic gel? Ophthalmol Eye Dis. 2012;4:23–4.
2. Lin T, Gong L, Sun X, Zhao N, Chen W, Yuan H, et al. Effectiveness and
    safety of 0.15 % ganciclovir in situ ophthalmic gel for herpes simplex
    keratitis-a multicenter, randomized, investigator-masked, parallel group
    study in Chinese patients. Drug Des Deve Ther. 2013;7:361–8.
3. Lembo D, Cavalli R. Nanoparticulate delivery systems for antiviral drugs.
    Antivir Chem Chemother. 2010;21:53–70.
4. Moshfeghi AA, Peyman GA. Micro- and nanoparticulates. Adv Drug Deliv
    Rev. 2005;57:2047–52.

5. Young S, Morlet N, Besen G, Wiley CA, Jones P, Gold J, et al. High-dose
    (2000-µg) intravitreous ganciclovir in the treatment of cytomegalovirus
    retinitis. Ophthalmol. 1998;105:1404–10.
6. Janoria KG, Mitra AK. Effect of lactide/glycolide ratio on the *in vitro* release
    of ganciclovir and its lipophillic prodrug (GCV-monobutyrate) from PLGA
    microspheres. Int J Pharm. 2007;338:133–41.
7. Charles NC, Steiner GC. Ganciclovir intraocular implant. A clinicopathologic
    study. Ophthalmol. 1996;103(3):416–21.
8. Teoh SC, Ou X, Lim TH. Intravitreal ganciclovir maintenance injection for
    cytomegalovirus retinitis:effeicacy of a low-volume, intermediate-dose
    regimen. Ophthalmol. 2012;119:588–95.
9. Shah P, Jogani V, Mishra P, Mishra AK, Bagchi T, Misra A. Modulation of
    ganciclovir intestinal absorption in presence of absorption enhancers. L Pharm
    Sci. 2007;96:2710–22.
10. Alonso MJ, Sanchez A. The potential of chitosan in ocular drug delivery.
    J Pharm Pharmacol. 2003;55:1451–63.
11. Bernkop-Schnurch A, Dunnhaupt S. Chitosan-based drug delivery systems.
    Eur J Pharm Biopharm. 2012;81:463–9.
12. Tamboli V, Mishra GP, Mitra K. Biodegradable polymers for ocular drug
    delivery, in Mitra AK: Advances in Ocular Drug Delivery, Research signpost,
    Kerala. 2012. p. 65–86.
13. Ye T, Yuan K, Zhang W, Song S, Chen F, Yang X, et al. Prodrugs incorporated
    into nanotechnology-based drug delivery systems for possible improvement
    in bioavailability of ocular drugs delivery. Asian J Pharm Sci. 2013;8:207–17.
14. Badawi AA, El-Laithy HM, El Qidra RK. Chitosan based nanocarriers for
    indomethacin ocular delivery. Arch Pharm Res. 2008;31:1040–9.
15. Calvo P, Vila-Jato JL, Alonso MAJ. Evaluation of cationic polymer-coated
    nanocapsules as ocular drug carriers. Int J Pharm. 1997;153:41–50.
16. De Campos AM, Sanchez A, Alonso MJ. Chitosan nanoparticles: a new
    vehicle for the improvement of the delivery of drugs to the ocular surface.
    Application to cyclosporin A. Int J Pharm. 2001;224:159–68.
17. Di Colo G, Zambito Y, Brugalassi S, Serafinin A, Saettone MF. Effect of chitosan
    on *in vitro* release and ocular delivery of ofloxacin from erodible inserts on
    poly(ethylene oxide). Int J Pharm. 2002;248:115–22.
18. Genta I, Conti B, Perugini P, Pavanetto F, Spadaro A, Puglisi G. Bioadhesive
    microspheres for ophthalmic administration of acyclovir. J Pharm Pharmacol.
    1997;49:737–42.
19. Gaudana R, Ananthula HK, Parenky A, Mitra AK. Ocular drug delivery. AAPS J.
    2010;12(3):348–60.
20. Campanero MA, Sadaba B, Garcia-Quetglas E, Azanza JR. Development and
    validation of a sensitive method for the determination of ganciclovir in human
    plasma samples by reversed-phase high-performance liquid chromatography.
    J Chromatogr B. 1998;706:311–7.
21. Park J, Jin H, Kim D, Chug S, Shim W, Shim C. Chitosan microspheres as an
    alveolar macrophage delivery system of ofloxacin via pulmonary inhalation.
    Int J Pharm. 2013;441:562–9.
22. Miyazaki S, Suzuki S, Kawasaki N, Endo K, Takahashi A. In situ gelling xyloglucan
    formulations for sustained release ocular delivery of pilocarpine hydrochloride.
    Int J Pharm. 2001;229:29–36.
23. Dillen K, Vandervoort J, Mooter GV, Ludwig A. Evaluation of ciprofloxacin-
    loaded Eudragit® RS100 or RL100/PLGA nanoparticles. Int J Pharm.
    2006;314:72–82.
24. Gibaud S, Al Awwadi NJ, Ducki C, Astier A. Poly(-caprolactone) and eudragit
    microparticles containing fludracortisones acetate. Int J Pharm.
    2004;269:491–508.
25. Huang J, Wigent RJ, Bentzley CM, Schwartz JB. Nifedipine solid dispersion in
    microparticles of ammonio methacrylate copolymer and ethylcellulose
    binary blend for controlled drug delivery effect of drug loading on release
    kinetics. Int J Pharm. 2006;319:44–54.
26. Li X, Nie S, Kong J, Li N, Ju C, Pan W. A controlled-release ocular delivery
    system for ibuprofen based on nanostructured lipid carriers. Int J Pharm.
    2008;363:177–82.
27. Gavini E, Chetoni P, Cossu M, Alvarez MG, Saettone MF, Giunchedi P. PLGA
    microspheres for the ocular delivery of a peptide drug, vancomycin using
    emulsification/spray-drying as the preparation method: *in vitro/in vivo*
    studies. Eur J Pharm Biopharm. 2004;57:207–12.
28. Shen Y, Tu J. Preparation and ocular pharmacokinetics of ganciclovir liposomes.
    AAPS J. 2007;9(3):E371–7.
29. Bhatta RS, Chandasana H, Chhonker YS, Rathi C, Kumar D, Mitra K, et al.
    Mucoadhesive nanoparticles for prolonged ocular delivery of natamycin: *in
    vitro* and pharmacokinetics studies. Int J Pharm. 2012;432:105–12.

30. Elgadir MA, Uddin MS, Ferdous S, Adam A, Chowdhary AJK, Sarker MZI. Impact of chitosan composites and chitosan nanoparticle composites on various drug delivery systems: A review. J Food Drug Anal. 2014, http://dx.doi.org/10.1016/j.jfda.2014.10.008

31. Mathew ST, Devi SG, Sandhya KV. Formulation and evaluation of ketorolac tromethamine-loaded albumin microspheres for potential intramuscular administration. AAPS PharmSciTech. 2007;8(1):E1–9.

32. Kumbar SG, Kulkarni AR, Aminabhavi M. Crosslinked chitosan microspheres for encapsulation of diclofenac sodium: effect of crosslinking agent. J Microencapsul. 2002;19(2):173–80.

33. Silva CM, Ribeiro AJ, Figueiredo M, Ferreira D, Veiga F. Microencapsulation of hemoglobin in chitosan-coated alginate microspheres prepared by emulsification/internal gelation. AAPS J. 2006;7(4):E903–13.

34. Thakkar H, Sharma RK, Mishra AK, Chuttani K, Murthy RR. Albumin microspheres as carriers for the antiarthritic drug celecoxib. AAPS PharmSciTech. 2005;6(1):E65–73.

35. Bhagav P, Upadhyay H, Chandran S. Brimonidine tartrate-eudragit long-acting nanoparticles: formulation, optimization, *in vitro* and *in vivo* evaluation. AAPS PharmSciTech. 2011;12(4):1087–101.

36. Jose S, Fangueiro JF, Smitha J, Cinu TA, Chacko AJ, Premaletha K, et al. Predictive modeling of insulin release profile from cross-linked chitosan microspheres. Eur J Med Chem. 2013;60:249–53.

37. Martinac A, Filipovic-Grcic J, Voinovich D, Perissutti B, Francechinis E. Development and bioadhesive properties of chitosan-ethylcellulose microspheres for nasal delivery. Int J Pharm. 2005;291:69–77.

38. Peyman GA, Ganiban GJ. Delivery systems for intraocular routes. Adv Drug Deliv Rev. 1995;16:107–23.

39. Li N, Zhuang C, Wang M, Sun X, Nie S, Pan W. Liposome coated with low molecular weight chitosan and its potential use in ocular drug delivery. Int J Pharm. 2009;379:131–8.

25

High azithromycin concentration in lungs by way of bovine serum albumin microspheres as targeted drug delivery: lung targeting efficiency in albino mice

Balakeshwa Ramaiah[1*], Sree Harsha Nagaraja[2], Usha Ganganahalli Kapanigowda[3], Prakash Rao Boggarapu[3] and Rajarajan Subramanian[1]

Abstract

Background: Following administration, the antibiotic travels freely through the body and also accumulates in other parts apart from the infection site. High dosage and repeated ingestion of antibiotics in the treatment of pneumonia leads to undesirable effects and inappropriate disposition of the drug. By way of targeted lung delivery, this study was intended to eliminate inappropriate azithromycin disposition and to achieve higher azithromycin concentration to treat deeper airway infections.

Methods: The Azithromycin Albumin Microspheres (AAM) was prepared by emulsion polymerization technique. The optimized AAM was subjected to in vitro release study, release kinetics, XRD and stability studies. Further, in vivo pharmacokinetics and tissue distribution of azithromycin released from AAM and azithromycin solution in albino mice was investigated to prove suitability of moving forward the next steps in the clinic.

Results: The mean particle size of the optimized AAM was 10.02 μm, an optimal size to get deposited in the lungs by mechanical entrapment. The maximum encapsulation efficiency of 82.3 % was observed in this study. The release kinetic was significant and best fitted for Korsmeyer-Peppas model ($R^2 = 0.9962$, $n = 0.41$). The XRD and stability study showed favorable results. Azithromycin concentration in mice lungs (40.62 μg g^{-1}, 30 min) of AAM was appreciably higher than other tissues and plasma. In comparison with control, azithromycin concentration in lungs was 30.15 μg g^{-1} after 30 min. The azithromycin AUC (929.94 μg h mL^{-1}) and intake rate (r_e) (8.88) for lung were higher and statistically significant in AAM group. Compared with spleen and liver, the targeting efficacy (t_e) in mice lung increased by a factor of 40.15 and ~14.10 respectively. Subsequently by a factor of 8.94, the ratio of peak concentration (C_e) in lung was higher in AAM treated mice. The AAM lung tissue histopathology did not show any degenerative changes.

Conclusions: High azithromycin concentration in albino mice lung was adequately achieved by targeted drug delivery.

Keywords: Azithromycin, Albumin microspheres, Sigma plot, Targeting efficacy, Lung targeting

* Correspondence: balupharmacy@gmail.com
[1]Department of Pharmaceutics, Karnataka College of Pharmacy, #33/2,
Tirumenahalli, Hegde Nagar Main Road, Bengaluru, Karnataka 560064, India
Full list of author information is available at the end of the article

Background

Worldwide studies have revealed pneumonia to be the primary cause of death among children. Lung disorder generally affects 1 in 7 people and it is believed to be the major cause of death in the United States [1, 2]. The antimicrobial therapy has considerably reduced the outbreak of pneumonia, but there are instances reported on the failure of antimicrobial therapy. This was primarily owing to the increased antimicrobial-resistant pathogenic microorganisms, which resulted in the administration of ineffective treatments [3]. Following administration, drug travels freely through the body and also accumulates in other parts apart from the infection site. High dosage and repeated ingestion of antibiotics in the treatment of pneumonia leads to undesirable effects and inappropriate disposition of the drug.

The sub-therapeutic antibiotic concentration at the infection site and prolong usage of antibiotic has led to antibiotic resistance [4]. These issues facilitate the requirement of a targeted drug delivery model to maximize the therapeutic efficacy against pneumonia. Drug targeting at the site of infection minimizes dosage of the drug required to achieve the optimum serum concentration leading to obtain the desired pharmacological action. The role of drug targeting was found to be evident considering various parameters such as pharmaceutical, biopharmaceutical, pharmacokinetic, pharmacodynamic and clinical [5]. Additionally, development of targeted drug for treatment of pneumonia improves health care and promises survival of the patient [1].

Azithromycin, (9-deoxo-9a-aza-9a-methyl-9a-homoerythromycin A) dihydrate, a macrolide antiobiotic used as a broad spectrum antibiotic was proved to be efficacious in the treatment of pneumonia. It is primarily active against *Haemophilus influenza, Moraxella catarrhalis, Streptococcus pneumonia, Chlamydophila (Chlamydia) pneumonia* and *Mycoplasma pneumonia* [6]. Azithromycin has high affinity towards the 50S ribosomal subunit of the organism and blocks its protein synthesis. Several unique pharmacokinetic properties such as excellent tissue penetration, high volume of distribution and prolong half life has lead the use of azithromycin for the treatment of pneumonia. Azithromycin has very large volume of distribution (2100 L) results in good tissue penetration and a long half-life (40–60 h) [4]. The antimicrobial activity of azithromycin against pneumonia pathogens depends on its relative concentration at the infection site. Therefore increasing localized azithromycin tissue concentration will clear the pathogen more rapidly and reduce the possibility of drug resistance.

The tissue minimum inhibitory concentration (MIC_{90}) breakpoint of azithromycin susceptibility against major organisms in US citizens was found to be ≤ 4 μg mL^{-1} [6]. As though to support this theory, clinical studies [7, 8] showed the azithromycin coverage in lungs was high with extended release of single or double dose microspheres. The better dosage regimen has improved azithromycin concentration especially in lower respiratory tract. The only novel marketed azithromycin microsphere (Zmax in USA) had proven to increase the plasma concentration by two to threefold to that of the conventional preparations [4]. The antimicrobial and post antibiotic effect (PAE) of azithromycin are characterized as concentration dependent [9]. By drug targeting, azithromycin concentration at the site of infection will be higher when compared to serum [6]. On intravenous administration, microspheres with 7–15 μm particle range are capable of being entrapped by lung capillaries [10].

In the recent past, a great deal of awareness has been observed in the preparation of microspheres using albumin for targeted drug delivery. The rationale was to specifically deliver the drug to the target tissues or cells by evading other tissue from undesirable effect [11]. A drastic increase, in the use of albumin in drug delivery was observed since 1970s proving albumin as a drug carrier and depicting greater attention in drug delivery system [12]. Albumin microspheres are nontoxic, physically and chemically stable, moreover they have specific receptor affinity in lungs. Albumin has numerous binding sites for exogenous ligands such as antibiotics and the properties of acidic, solubility, stability in pH range of 4–9 and preferential uptake by inflamed cells allows it to be chosen as ideal polymer. Bovine Serum Albumin (BSA) microspheres by phagocytosis are rapidly removed from the vascular system. On digestion of the albumin by lysosomal enzymes leads to release of free drug. Various drugs such as streptomycin, ofloxacin, clarithromycin and sodium cromoglicate when used with albumin microspheres, has significantly proven to be efficacious in lung targeting [13].

The microspheres intended as targeted delivery, injected via intravenous route enables to treat the deep lung disorders from the vascular side eliminating the need to traverse the mucus/surfactant and mucosal layers. At situations of compromised lung capacity and inhalation is not a viable option, use of injecting drug via intravenous route would be particularly helpful. It is evident that higher drug disposition in lungs and prolonged retention may translate into reduced doses, less frequent administration and lower bioavailability variability. Hence, the main purpose of this study was to prepare, develop and in vivo characterization of lung targeting efficiency to achieve high azithromycin concentration in lungs by way of Azithromycin Albumin Microsphere (AAM) as targeted drug delivery. The excellent tissue penetration enables azithromycin to get inappropriately deposit in various tissues such as liver and spleen apart from the infected lungs. Thus, the minimization of inappropriate azithromycin disposition and maintenance of higher azithromycin concentration in lungs can effectively combat the deeper lung tissue infections.

Methods

Materials

Azithromycin was acquired as a gift sample from Karnataka Antibiotic Pharmaceutical Limited, Bengaluru, India. BSA fraction V was purchased from SD Fine-CHEM limited, Mumbai, India. The Tween 80, heavy liquid paraffin, n-hexane, glutaraldehyde, petroleum ether, sodium bisulphite and Span 80 were obtained from Merck Specialties Pvt. Ltd, India. All the ingredients were of analytical grade.

Experimental design

The central composite design was used to optimize azithromycin loaded albumin microspheres (AAM) by altering albumin, glutaraldehyde and Span 80 concentrations. The independent variable factors effect on mean particle size of the microspheres along with encapsulation efficiency and 6th hour in vitro drug release was investigated. The model contained eight factorial points, six axial points and six centre points with total 20 experiments. The mean value was set as 0 and, +1 and −1 was considered as higher and lower levels for each factor respectively. The selected factor constraints with their levels along with optimized levels are summarized in Tables 1 and 2.

Preparation of AAM intended for lung targeting

Azithromycin microspheres were prepared using albumin, a biodegradable polymer by emulsion polymerization technique [14]. Initially, BSA was dissolved in distilled water (22.24 %) and 0.5 mL of Tween 80 was added to the aqueous phase. Secondly, finely triturated 250 mg of azithromycin was added into the aqueous phase with bath sonication (3 min) for consistent dispersion. While stirring at 2500 rpm, 1 mL of the above solution was slowly incorporated in to 30 mL of heavy liquid paraffin containing a lipophillic surfactant, Span 80. The mixture was homogenized for 10 min to form water/oil emulsion. To crosslink the albumin, the emulsion was homogenized by adding glutaraldehyde. Further, the emulsion was homogenized for 5 min with addition of 5 mL n-hexane for hardening the formed microspheres. The microspheres were then centrifuged at 1000 rpm at room temperature for 1 min and washed with petroleum ether to remove the heavy liquid paraffin. To remove the residual glutaraldehyde, the microspheres were dispersed in 10 mL of 5 % w/v sodium bisulphite solution and stirred on a magnetic stirrer for 5 min. The microspheres were filtered through Whatmann filter paper with pore size of 0.45 μm and again washed with 100 mL of water to completely remove residual glutaraldehyde. At room temperature, the microspheres were dried and were stored in a dessicator.

Particle size measurement of the optimized AAM

The particle size analysis [15] was carried out by photon correlation spectroscopy in Malvern Meta sizer, UK (He-Ne laser beam at wavelength of 633 nm and 90^0 scattering angle). Ten milligram of the preparation was dispersed in 0.1 % of tween 80 containing 10 mL of water and was subjected to mean particle size determination. The mean particle size was averaged after three reading of the samples. The PCS software (Malvern Instruments Inc.) was used for processing of the data.

Estimation of azithromycin

Reverse phase high performance liquid chromatography (RP-HPLC) was used as analytical tool for quantitative estimation of azithromycin [16]. Stainless steel column (25 cm × 4.6 mm) with end-capped octadecylsilyl amorphous organosilica polymer, 5 μm (Waters Xterra) was used for analysis. Mobile phase in the ratio of 40:60 consisted of 0.18 % w/v anhydrous disodium hydrogen phosphate solution (pH adjusted to 8.9) and a mixture of methanol (25 volumes) with acetonitrile (75 volumes), respectively. The injection volume was 50 μL with flow rate of 1 mL/min. At 60 ^{0}C column temperature, UV detector was set at 210 nm. The retention time of the drug peak was observed at 5.916 min.

Estimation of drug encapsulation efficiency of the optimized AAM

The encapsulation efficiency was estimated by solvent extraction method [11]. Ten milligram of the microspheres was dispersed in 0.5 mL of methylene dichloride. Later, 4.5 mL of ethanol was added to precipitate the polymer. After stirring at 14,500 rpm for 10 min, the supernatant was separated and diluted with 10 times by PBS (pH 6.8, 50 mM). By previously mentioned RP-

Table 2 Response factor constraints with expected and observed values for optimized AAM

Response factors	Constraints	Expected value	Observed value	Residual value
Mean particle size (μm)	Target of 8 μm	9.04	10.02	0.98
Encapsulation efficiency (%)	In range	81.4	80.00	−1.4
6th hour in vitro drug release (%)	In range	77.27	78.00	0.73

Table 1 Variable factors with their levels used for optimization of AAM

Variable factors	Level					Optimized level
	−1.41	−1	0	1	1.41	
Albumin concentration (%)	16.59	20	25	30	33.41	22.24
Glutaraldehyde volume (%)	0.16	0.3	0.50	0.7	0.84	0.58
Span 80 volume (mL)	0.20	0.4	0.70	1.0	1.20	1.0

HPLC, the quantification of the drug was performed. Equations (1) and (2) were utilized to determine the drug encapsulation efficiency.

$$Drug\ loading\ (\%) = \frac{D_t}{M_t} \times 100 \qquad (1)$$

$$Encapsulation\ efficiency\ (\%) = \frac{L_a}{L_t} \times 100 \qquad (2)$$

D_t: amount of encapsulated drug in microspheres; M_t: microsphere quantity; L_a: actual drug content and L_t: theoretical drug content.

X-ray diffraction (XRD) analysis

The XRD analysis of azithromycin powder, BSA and AAM formulation (Pre and post stability studies at refrigeration and accelerated conditions) was performed using Philips X'Pert Pro, Netherlands at 40 KV voltages and applied 30 mA of current (nickel-filtered CuKα radiation). The sample was scanned over a 2θ range of 10–800 with an interval of 0.020 at the rate of 20/min.

In vitro study and curve fitting analysis of the optimized AAM

Azithromycin release from AAM was estimated using Franz diffusion cells. The cell consisted of a dialysis membrane with MW cut-off of 12,000–14,000 Da (Himedia Laboratories Pvt. Ltd, Mumbai, India). This membrane acted as a barrier between donor and acceptor compartment. Hundred milligram of the microspheres dispersed in 1 mL of phosphate saline buffer (PBS) was placed in the donor compartment. The PBS was prepared by dissolving 0.2 g of potassium chloride, 1.44 g of disodium hydrogen phosphate, and 0.24 g of dihydrogen potassium phosphate in 800 mL of distilled water. The pH was maintained at 7.4 and the volume was made upto 1000 mL [17]. At $37 \pm 0.5\ ^0C$, 200 mL of PBS was placed in the acceptor compartment and stirred on a magnetic stirrer at 200 rpm. At specified time, 1 mL of the solution was pipetted out from the acceptor compartment and was replaced with the same volume of PBS. The drug content was determined utilizing the formerly mentioned RP-HPLC method. After three runs, the data was utilized to determine release kinetics.

Using Sigma plot, the release kinetics of the optimized AAM was fitted to various models such as first order model (3), Higuchi square root model (4), Baker and Lonsdale (5), Koresmeyer-Peppas (6) and Hixson and Crowell cube root model (7) to study the release of drug from the microspheres.

$$Log\ (100-Q_t) = log Q_0 - \frac{K_t}{2.303} \qquad (3)$$

$$Q_t = k_H \sqrt{t} \qquad (4)$$

$$\frac{Q_t}{Q_\infty} = 1 - \frac{6}{\pi^2} \exp\left(\frac{-\pi^2 \times Dt}{r^2}\right) \qquad (5)$$

$$Q_t = Q_0 + a\left(\frac{t}{r^2}\right)^n + b\left(\frac{t}{r^2}\right)^{2n} \qquad (6)$$

$$\sqrt[3]{Q_0} - \sqrt[3]{Q_t} = k_{HC}t \qquad (7)$$

Q_t is the total amount of drug release after t time (%); Q_0 is the initial amount of drug (%); K is the first order release rate constant (h^{-1}); k_H is the rate constant obtained according to the Higuchi equation ($\%h^{-1/2}$); Q_∞ is the percent release at infinite time; D is the diffusion coefficient in the polymer in cm^2/s; r is the radius of the sphere in cm; n and $2n$ are the release exponent for Fickian diffusion and case II transport, respectively; a and b are constants related to the drug and the structural and geometric properties of the microparticles; and k_{HC} is the rate constant obtained according to the Hixon and Crowell equation ($\%h^{-1}$) [18–20].

Stability study of the optimized AAM

The stability study was conducted as per ICH Q1AR guideline, intended to test the stability for new substances and product. The optimized preparation was stored at $5 \pm 3\ ^0C$ for twelve months and at $25 \pm 2\ ^0C$ and 60 ± 5 % RH for a period of six months. The required volume of microsphere dispersion was stored in closed glass bottles and sealed tightly. At regular intervals, the sample was subjected for determination of encapsulation efficiency, mean particle size distribution and for any physical changes. The test was carried at 3 month intervals for a period of 12 months for long term storage condition under refrigeration and at 0, 2, 4 and 6 months for accelerated condition at room temperature. To confirm the stability of the drug in the formulation, the samples were also subjected to XRD analysis.

In vivo pharmacokinetic studies in albino mice

The animal experiments were carried out in accordance to the protocol approved by the Institutional Animal Ethics Committee formed under CPCSEA guidelines. Prior to the study, thirty six adult male and female, Swiss Albino mice, weighing 20 ± 3 g was kept starving for 12 h with free access to water. AAM microspheres were dispersed in saline with 1 % of Tween 80 and vortexed for 5 s. The control group received azithromycin (in saline) solution containing a dose of 50 μg g^{-1} injected intravenously via tail vein, while the AAM group was injected with equivalent content of azithromycin in AAM.

Blood or organ isolation and extraction

At specified intervals (0.5 h, 1 h, 3 h, 6 h, 8 h and 12 h), the blood samples were collected from the ocular artery directly from each mouse after eye ball removal and placed into heparinized test tubes. By centrifugation (4000 g) for 15 min, the plasma was immediately separated. The animals were then sacrificed by cervical dislocation. The plasma and tissue samples of targeted organs such as lung, liver and spleen were isolated and stored at $-20\ ^{0}$C for 24 h. To determine the targeted release, the azithromycin concentration in each organ was determined by subjecting 1 g (after removal of surface water) of the tissue sample through extraction process. The normal saline (0.1 mg mL^{-1}) was added to the isolated organs and homogenized. To precipitate protein, 2 mol L^{-1} perchloric acid (100 μL) was added to the plasma sample and homogenized tissues. Subsequently, 300 μL of plasma or homogenized tissues suspension was added to 450 μL methanol. The mixture was vortexed for 60 s and then centrifuged at 10,000 g for 5 min [17]. The supernatant was collected and filtered through a 0.22 μm pore size Phenomenex filter. The azithromycin concentration in the processed samples was quantitatively analyzed by above mentioned RP-HPLC method.

Pharmacokinetic parameters

Change in azithromycin concentration with time was monitored in blood, lung, liver and spleen. Based on the analysis of parameters and model, the two compartment model could best describe the in vivo pharmacokinetics of microspheres in blood. The azithromycin, area under the curve (AUC$_{0-\infty}$) was determined from the beginning of the intravenous injection (t$_0$) to the last observation (t$_{last}$) by linear trapezoidal rule with extrapolation to infinite time. Additionally, azithromycin half life (t$_{1/2}$ α and β), distribution rate constants (K$_{21}$, K$_{10}$ and K$_{12}$), clearance (CL) and apparent volume of distribution at steady state (V$_{SS}$) were also calculated. The Kinetica 5.0 PK/PD analysis software was also utilized for the calculation of pharmacokinetic parameters.

Lung targeting characteristics and histopathological studies

The lung targeting efficiency of AAM was evaluated by using intake rate (r$_e$), targeting efficacy (t$_e$) and peak concentration ratio (C$_e$) [21]. At the end of the study (12 h post sample administration), the animals were subjected to experimenting process by excess anesthesia. To examine the tissue tolerability of the formulation specified organs (lungs, liver and spleen) were washed with cold saline. Later, the organs were pressed between filter pads and weighed. Using 10 % formalin, the tissues were fixed and stained with hematoxylin and eosin. Under light microscopy with 200 × magnification, the tissue samples were examined for any cytoarchitecture changes.

Statistical analysis

Statistical analysis was carried out by using Student's t test with a P value less than 0.05 was considered as statistically significant.

Results and discussion

Preparation of AAM

Compared to other macrolides, azithromycin enhances extended spectrum and potency especially against pneumonia [5]. The biocompatibility, low toxicity, non antigenicity and physicochemical property of the BSA influenced to select it as an ideal polymer in this study. The preparation of

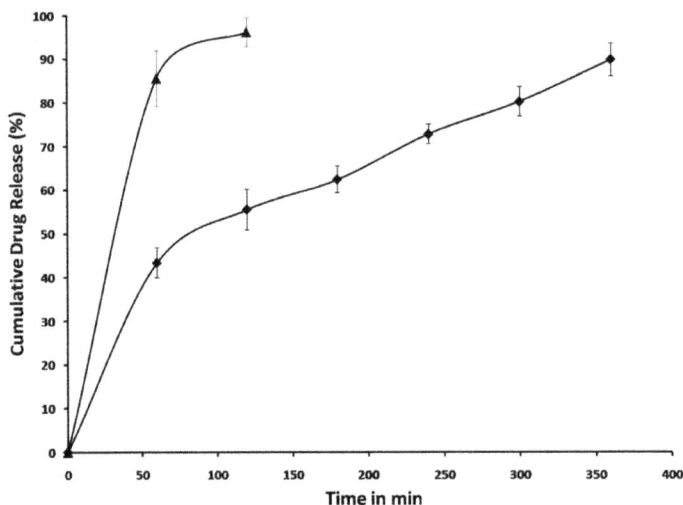

Fig. 1 Cumulative amount of drug released (▲) optimized AAM and (●) azithromycin solution (bars represent mean ± SD; $n = 3$)

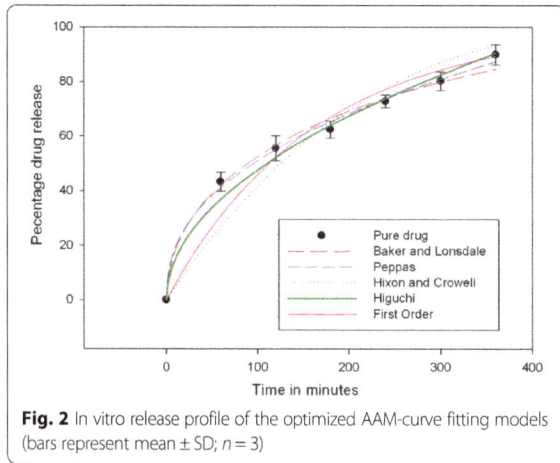

Fig. 2 In vitro release profile of the optimized AAM-curve fitting models (bars represent mean ± SD; n = 3)

albumin microsphere involved suspending an aqueous solution of albumin in an external non-polar phase. The nuclei formation due to the micronized azithromycin induces small droplet formation during emulsification resulting in smaller microsphere until steady state droplet size distribution. Glutaraldehyde a five-carbon dialdehyde, chemically cross links with albumin lysines. The glutaraldehyde as a fixative enhances covalent stabilization of the albumin producing stable and biocompatible microspheres. However, the residual glutaraldehyde could be toxic and was

removed by bisulphate wash. The carbonyl group pi bond of glutaraldehyde was subjected to nucleophilic addition of bisulphate resulting in organic sulphite (water soluble sodium salt), which was further removed by water washing. Many earlier studies [22, 23] have successfully used emulsion polymerization for albumin microsphere preparations. This method was found to be advantageous, as the microspheres from the high molecular weight polymers are usually shaped at a faster rate and at low temperature.

Mean particle size and drug encapsulation efficiency

Albumin microspheres in the range of 1–100 µm influence its biodistribution characteristics. Particle size was found to be a significant factor to distinguish between soluble carrier and particulate systems. The particle size being an important parameter for drug targeting with microspheres, as the size helps in discharge of drug in controlled manner and uptake of drugs into the tissues. In this study, the particle size ranged from 3.9–19.8 µm and the mean particle size of the optimized AAM was 10.02 µm. Various other studies [17, 22, 24] have reported similar particle size for albumin microspheres. Following intravenous administration, 7–15 µm particle size range of microspheres gets deposited in the lungs by mechanical entrapment [10]. To support this hypothesis, Kutscher et al. [25] proved that 10 µm sized microspheres were uniformly distributed throughout the lung

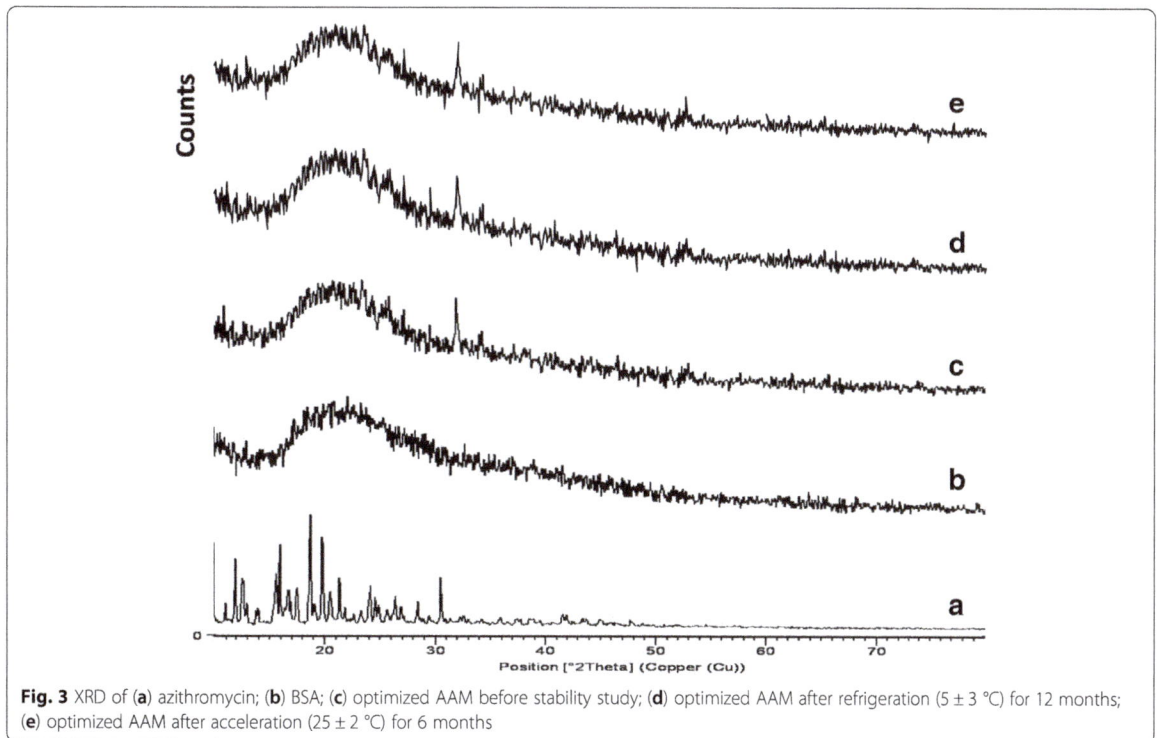

Fig. 3 XRD of (**a**) azithromycin; (**b**) BSA; (**c**) optimized AAM before stability study; (**d**) optimized AAM after refrigeration (5 ± 3 °C) for 12 months; (**e**) optimized AAM after acceleration (25 ± 2 °C) for 6 months

Table 3 Stability test observations of the optimized AAM at refrigeration for long term storage condition

Storage	Encapsulation efficiency (%)					Mean particle size (μm)					Physical change				
5 ± 3^0C	Months					Months					Months				
	0	3	6	9	12	0	3	6	9	12	0	3	6	9	12
	68.1	67.5	66.8	66.0	65.0	10.02	09.98	10.01	10.02	10.02	–	–	–	–	–

–: No physical change

capillaries to that of 3 μm sized microspheres, which usually pass through the lungs.

The injected microspheres primarily get lodged in alveolar capillaries that have diameters considerably less than those of the microspheres and thus, the concept of mechanical entrapment offers a unique opportunity for passive targeting of microspheres to lungs. Since there is a possibility of larger microspheres occluding larger capillaries leading to blockage of small downstream vessels may result in augmentation of potential toxic effect. To resolve this issue and avoid embolism due to injected microspheres, the USP has stated that ">90 % of microspheres must have a size between 10–90 μm and no microspheres may be larger than 150 μm". A study by Glenny et al. [26] reported that the blood flow in rat lungs was not significantly affected by 15 μm particle size of the microspheres and neither emboli nor tissue infarction was observed. The same study states that these microspheres will occlude only a small fraction of capillaries (0.5–0.7 %) and significantly do not alter local vascular resistance. Within the capillaries, red blood cells can continue to flow past lodged microspheres.

In fact, the lung at rest only uses approximately 30 % of its capacity and is therefore able to recruit other capillaries to avoid massive increases in the arterial pressure when blockages do occur. Additionally, the lung utilizes variety of ways such as recruiting unused vessels and use of arteriovenous shunts to improve the blood circulation in the pulmonary capillaries. Microspheres with 1–3 μm particle size passes through the lung and will be removed by reticuloendothelial system and, usually accumulate in liver and spleen, excrete through the feces or sequestration by macrophages in other organ systems [25].

The maximum encapsulation efficiency of 82.3 % was observed in this study. The high encapsulation efficiency may also have contributed to low partition coefficient of azithromycin. Studies done by Bozdag et al. [24] and Jones et al. [27] stated that the albumin microspheres can be sustained and the encapsulation efficiency can be increased by escalating glutaraldehyde volume. The swelling, encapsulation efficiency and drug release profile can be controlled by cross linking density.

In vitro study and curve fitting analysis
AAM in vitro release study (Fig. 1) showed a minimum of 40.34 % and a maximum of 94.63 % of azithromycin release at the end of 1st hour and 6th hour, respectively. AAM showed biphasic in vitro drug release viz, an initial burst followed by sustained release at the end. The initial burst was due to the dispersed drug close to the microsphere surface and additionally, high encapsulation also contributes to this effect. The diffusion of dispersed drug in the polymeric matrix and BSA erosion would lead to the sustained release of the microspheres. Initial burst effect was required to provide the loading dose of the drug to combat the high bacterial load which usually seen during the initial phase of pneumonia.

The release pattern of the optimized formulation on sigma plot has been represented in Fig. 2. The regression coefficient of Korsmeyer-Peppas model ($R^2 = 0.9962$) was significant. The Korsmeyer-Peppas model illustrates the drug release mechanism from polymeric devices. To describe the drug release process, the n-value can be obtained by fitting data into Korsemeyer Peppas model. The n-value was found to be 0.41, indicating Fickian diffusion type of release. Due to dispersion of the azithromycin in polymeric matrix, the dissolution may not be rate limiting step, but the diffusion of the drug through polymeric matrix considered to be the slowest step for drug release. A study [14] showed similar behavior for albumin microspheres.

XRD analysis
XRD of the pure azithromycin, albumin and AAM (Pre and post stability studies at refrigeration and accelerated conditions) are shown in Fig. 3. XRD spectral characteristic of the azithromycin pure drug shows many diffraction peaks, indicating the crystallinity of the drug. In contrast,

Table 4 Stability test observations of the optimized AAM at room temperature for accelerated condition

Storage	Encapsulation efficiency (%)				Mean particle size (μm)				Physical change			
25 ± 2^0C	Months				Months				Months			
	0	2	4	6	0	2	4	6	0	2	4	6
	68.1	67.8	67.3	66.9	10.02	10.02	10.01	10.01	–	–	–	–

–: No physical change

Table 5 Pharmacokinetic parameters after intravenous injection of AAM and azithromycin solution (control) in albino mice

Pharmacokinetic Parameters	AAM	Azithromycin solution
$AUC_{0-\infty}$ (μg h mL^{-1})	32.73	88.70
$t_{1/2}$ (α) (h)	0.950	0.522
$t_{1/2}$ (β) (h)	11.38	10.32
K_{21} (h^{-1})	0.400	0.940
K_{10} (h^{-1})	0.111	0.940
K_{12} (h^{-1})	1.88	0.360
CL (h^{-1})	0.102	0.061
V_{ss} (L)	9.49	1.26
C_0 (μg mL^{-1})	6	11

Data are represented as means $\pm$ SD ($n = 3$)

the diffraction peaks was significantly reduced in AAM. XRD of BSA shows one peak, which indicates non crystallinity. The AAM formulation showed decreased crystallinity of azithromycin, which was similar to that of BSA indicating the incorporation of azithromycin in the polymer.

Stability study

The stability test observations of the optimized AAM at room temperature and refrigeration conditions are depicted in Tables 3 and 4. On storage, no major deviations were observed in the macroscopic characteristics. There were no changes in mean particle size of the optimized formulations stored at 25 ^{0}C. On storage, the extent of microsphere sedimentation was not prominent, on manual agitation they were redispersed easily. Even though, there was slight decrease in the encapsulation efficiency (3.1 %), but was within the acceptable range. Thus, the optimized formula proved to be stable on long term and accelerated storage conditions as well.

In vivo pharmacokinetic studies

Based on the analysis of parameters and model, the two compartment model could best describe the in vivo pharmacokinetics of microspheres in blood. The pharmacokinetic parameters are illustrated in Table 5. The decisive parameters for the penetration into biological fluids and tissues are the drug molecular weight, lipophilicity and protein binding [13]. Compared to control, AAM altered in vivo azithromycin distribution and the half-life of azithromycin released from AAM intravenous injection ($t_{1/2}$ (α) = 0.950 h, $t_{1/2}(\beta)$ = 11.38 h) were prominently higher than the intravenous injection of azithromycin solution ($t_{1/2}$ (α) = 0.522 h, $t_{1/2}(\beta)$ = 10.32 h). This data proves the sustained release efficacy of AAM. Azithromycin concentration in mice lungs (40.62 μg g^{-1}, 30 min) of AAM was appreciably higher than other tissues and plasma. In comparison with control, azithromycin concentration in lungs was 30.15 μg g^{-1} after 30 min. A clinical study [28] has shown that the initial high upfront release of azithromycin from the microspheres helps in achieving higher azithromycin concentration required to act against the early bacterial burden at the infection site in lungs.

After intravenous injection of AAM and azithromycin solution preparations, the distribution of azithromycin with time was estimated in lung, liver, spleen (μg mL^{-1}) and blood (μg g^{-1}). Azithromycin concentration in blood and other organs was considered as 100 %. The targeting parameters are shown in Table 6. The semilogarithmic plot showing azithromycin distribution in mice after intravenous injection of AAM and azithromycin solution (control) are shown in Fig. 4a and b, respectively. Azithromycin tissue distribution was found to be higher than plasma concentration in all time points. Azithromycin concentration in lungs considered to be a vital factor in achieving an effective clinical treatment. The capillary blockade (as a function of particle size) resulting in mechanical filtration leads to accumulation of microspheres in lung.

AAM showed the highest value of AUC (929.94 μg h mL^{-1}) and re (8.88) for lung, and the difference was statistically significant ($p = 0.0011$). The AAM targeting efficacy (t_e) of lung increased by a factor of 40.15 (compared with spleen) and ~14.10 (compared with liver). The targeting ratio of AAM increased by a factor of 46.39 (compared to spleen) and ~16.21 (compared to liver). Additionally, compared with control the ratio of peak concentration in lung (C_e) increased by a factor of 8.94. Literatures state that PAEs are

Table 6 Lung-targeting parameters after intravenous administration of AAM and azithromycin solution (control) in albino mice

Parameters	AUC^a		r_e	t_e		$(t_e)_{AAM}/(t_e)_{Control}$	C_p^a		C_e
	AAM	Control		AAM	Control		AAM	Control	
Blood	32.73	88.69	0.369	28.42	1.18	24.06	5.60	10.80	0.519
Liver	65.97	120.45	0.547	14.10	0.870	16.21	7.75	12.00	0.646
Spleen	23.16	121.01	0.191	40.15	0.866	46.39	2.94	18.27	0.160
Lung	929.94	104.75	8.88	1.00	1.00	1.00	93.65	10.47	8.94

r_e = $(AUC)_{AAM}/(AUC)_{Control}$
t_e = $(AUC)_{lung\ targeted}/(AUC)_{untargeted}$
C_p: peak concentration (μg mL^{-1} or μg g^{-1}) C_e = $(C_p)_{AAM}/(C_p)_{Control}$
^{a}unit of AUC: μg h mL^{-1} or μg h g^{-1}

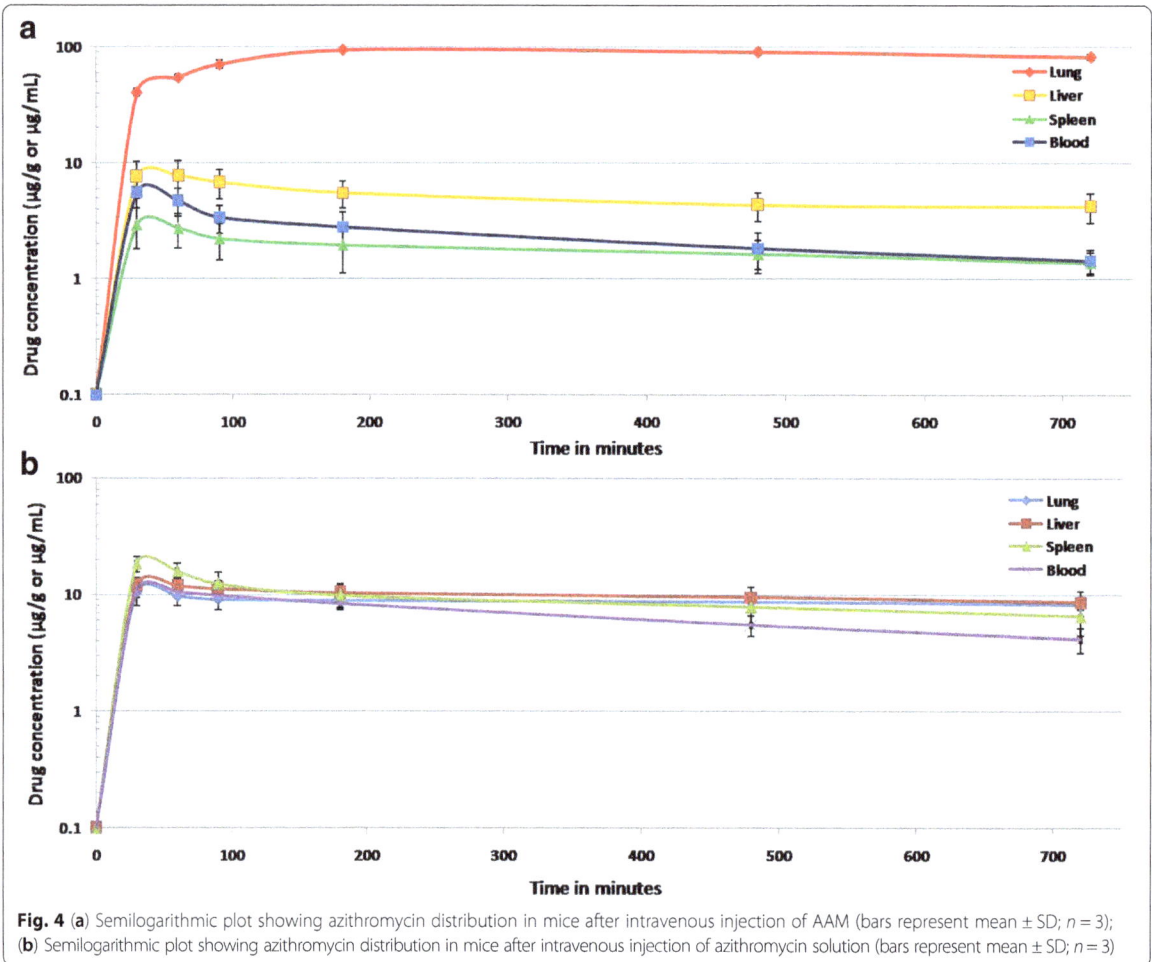

Fig. 4 (**a**) Semilogarithmic plot showing azithromycin distribution in mice after intravenous injection of AAM (bars represent mean ± SD; $n = 3$); (**b**) Semilogarithmic plot showing azithromycin distribution in mice after intravenous injection of azithromycin solution (bars represent mean ± SD; $n = 3$)

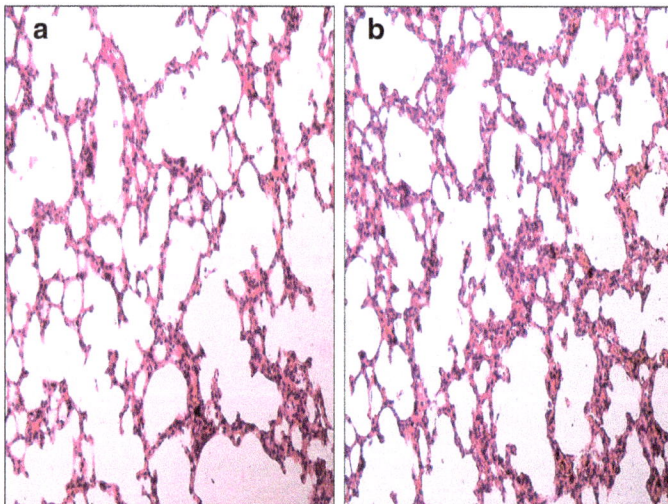

Fig. 5 (**a**) Cytoarchitecture of albino mice lung (*azithromycin solution*); (**b**) Cytoarchitecture of albino mice lung (AAM)

usually investigated at ten times the MIC and in this study the azithromycin concentration was all time maintained above MIC. Among macrolides, the longer retain time (t > MIC) at the target site and strongest PAE up to 2.3–4.7 h of azithromycin results in relatively short treatment period [9].

Albumin microsphere improves circulatory half-lives of the drug by inhibiting drug uptake by reticuloendothelial system [14]. In this study, the albumin microsphere certainly has further influenced the accumulation of azithromycin particularly in lungs. The presence of specific albumin binding protein in alveolar epithelial cells further increases affinity to albumin leading to higher azithromycin concentration especially in lungs [29]. The protection of microspheres from opsonization and decreased urinary clearance of BSA (67 kDa) considered to be also a beneficial effect [30]. High azithromycin loading in lung tissues by AAM compared to control confirms the alteration in biodistribution of the azithromycin thus, the lung targeting characteristic of AAM was evident.

The tissue tolerability considered to be a major concern as in microsphere based targeted system due to accumulation of the drug and excipients in the targeted organs. The histopathology of the mice lungs (Fig. 5a and b) did not show any degenerative changes in the AAM formulation compared to control group. This proves the safety and biocompatibility of the AAM as a parenteral formulation for lung targeting.

Conclusions

Currently a single dose extended release azithromycin formulation has been found to be the only FDA approved antibiotic for the treatment of pneumonia. This study successfully formulated azithromycin incorporation into albumin microspheres. The particle size, encapsulation efficiency, in vitro study, release kinetics, XRD and stability study showed the suitability of the microspheres for lung targeting. In comparison with control, AAM showed better azithromycin concentration in lungs, higher AUC, the ratio of peak concentration (C_e) and intake rate (r_e). The favorable in vivo pharmacokinetics, lung targeting efficacy and histopathology proved applicability of the microspheres as targeted drug delivery to lungs.

Competing interests
The authors declare that they have no competing interests.

Authors' contributions
BR conceived the study, designed, carried out experiments and drafted the manuscript. SN assisted in design, analysis, interpretation of the data and manuscript plagiarism check. UGK coordinated the experiments, involved in XRD, stability studies and drafting the manuscript. PRB and RS participated in the design of the study, interpretation of the data, performed the statistical analysis and revised the manuscript. All authors read and approved the final manuscript.

Acknowledgements
We are thankful to Prof. Basavaraj Ramnal, Secretary and Dr. Ramesh K, Director, Karnataka College of Pharmacy, Bengaluru, Karnataka, India, for valuable contribution to make this research work possible. We also thank Mr. Lokesh Prasad, DTL, Bengaluru, Karnataka, India, for proof reading the article.

Author details
[1]Department of Pharmaceutics, Karnataka College of Pharmacy, #33/2, Tirumenahalli, Hegde Nagar Main Road, Bengaluru, Karnataka 560064, India. [2]Department of Pharmaceutical Sciences, College of Clinical Pharmacy, King Faisal University, Al-Ahsa 31982, Saudi Arabia. [3]Department of Pharmaceutical Technology, Karnataka College of Pharmacy, #33/2, Tirumenahalli, Hegde Nagar Main Road, Bengaluru 560064, Karnataka, India.

References
1. Giordano RJ, Edwards JK, Tuder RM, Arap W, Pasqualini R. Combinatorial ligand-directed lung targeting. Proc Am Thorac Soc. 2009;6:411–5.
2. Hittinger M et al. Preclinical safety and efficacy models for pulmonary drug delivery of antimicrobials with focus on in vitro models. Adv Drug Deliv Rev. 2014. http://dx.doi.org/10.1016/j.addr.2014.10.011
3. Zhang Z, Zhu Y, Yang X, Li C. Preparation of azithromycin microcapsules by a layer-by-layer self-assembly approach and release behaviors of azithromycin. Colloids Surf A Physicochem Eng Asp. 2010;362:135–9.
4. Blasi F, Aliberti S, Tarsia P. Clinical applications of azithromycin microspheres in respiratory tract infections. Int J Nanomed. 2007;2:551–9.
5. Zhang Y, Wang X, Lin X, Liu X, Tian B, Tang X. High azithromycin loading powders for inhalation and their in vivo evaluation in rats. Int J Pharm. 2010;395:205–14.
6. Harrison TS, Keam SJ. Azithromycin extended release-a review of its use in the treatment of acute bacterial sinusitis and community-acquired pneumonia in the US. Drugs. 2007;67:773–92.
7. Amrol D. Single-dose azithromycin microsphere formulation: a novel delivery system for antibiotics. Int J Nanomed. 2007;2:9–12.
8. Lucchi M, Damle B, Fang A, De Caprariis PJ, Mussi A. Pharmacokinetics of azithromycin in serum, bronchial washings, alveolar macrophages and lung tissue following a single oral dose of extended or immediate release formulations of azithromycin. J Antimicrob Chemother. 2008;61:884–91.
9. Levison ME. Pharmacodynamics of antimicrobial drugs. Infect Dis Clin N Am. 2004;18:451–65.
10. Ozkan Y, Dikmen N, Isimer A, Gunhan O, Aboul-Enein HY. Clarithromycin targeting to lung: characterization, size distribution and in vivo evaluation of the human serum albumin microspheres. Il Farmaco. 2000;55:303–7.
11. Li X, Chang S, Du G, Li Y, Gong J. Encapsulation of azithromycin into polymeric microspheres by reduced pressure-solvent evaporation method. Int J Pharm. 2012;433:79–88.
12. Elsadek B, Kratz F. Impact of albumin on drug delivery—New applications on the horizon. J Contr Rel. 2012;157:4–28.
13. Saroglou M, Ismailos G, Tryfon S, Liapakis I, Papalois A, Bouros D. Penetration of azithromycin in experimental pleural empyema fluid. Eur J Pharmacol. 2010;626:271–5.
14. Thakkar H, Sharma RK, Mishra AK, Chuttani K, Murthy RR. Albumin microspheres as carriers for the antiarthritic drug celecoxib. AAPS PharmSciTech. 2005;6:E65–73.
15. Zeng XM, Martin GP, Marriott C. Preparation and in vitro evaluation of tetrandrine-entrapped albumin microspheres as an inhaled drug delivery system. Eur J Pharm Sci. 1995;3:87–93.
16. Ghari T, Kobarfard F, Mortazavi SA. Development of a simple RP-HPLC-UV method for determination of azithromycin in bulk and pharmaceutical dosage forms as an alternative to the USP method. Iranian J Pharm Res. 2013;12:57–63.
17. Harsha S, Chandramouli R, Rani S. Ofloxacin targeting to lungs by way of microspheres. Int J Pharm. 2009;380:127–32.
18. Dillen K, Vandervoort J, Mooter GV, Ludwig A. Evaluation of ciprofloxacin-loaded eudragit® RS100 or RL100/PLGA nanoparticles. Int J Pharm. 2006;314:72–82.
19. Gibaud S, Al Awwadi NJ, Ducki C, Astier A. Poly(-caprolactone) and eudragit microparticles containing fludracortisones acetate. Int J Pharm. 2004;269:491–508.
20. Huang J, Wigent RJ, Bentzley CM, Schwartz JB. Nifedipine solid dispersion in microparticles of ammonio methacrylate copolymer and ethylcellulose

binary blend for controlled drug delivery effect of drug loading on release kinetics. Int J Pharm. 2006;319:44–54.

21. Lu B, Zhang JQ, Yang H. Lung-targeting microspheres of carboplatin. Int J Pharm. 2003;265:1–11.

22. Gulsu A, Ayhan H, Ayhan F. Preparation and characterization of ketoprofen loaded albumin microspheres. Turk J Biochem. 2012;37:120–8.

23. Mathew ST, Devi SG, Sandhya KV. Formulation and evaluation of ketorolac tromethamine-loaded albumin microspheres for potential intramuscular administration. AAPS PharmSciTech. 2007;8:E1–9.

24. Bozdag S, Çalis S, Kas HS, Ercan MT, Peksoy I. In vitro evaluation and intra-articular administration of biodegradable microspheres containing naproxen sodium. J Microencapsul. 2001;18:443–56.

25. Kutscher HL, Chao P, Deshmukh M, Singh Y, Hu P, Joseph LB, et al. Threshold size for optimal passive pulmonary targeting and retention of rigid microparticles in rats. J Contr Rel. 2010;144:31–7.

26. Glenny RW, Bernard S, Lamm WJ. Hemodynamic effects of 15-mm-diameter microspheres on the rat pulmonary circulation. J Appl Physiol. 2000;89:499–504.

27. Jones C, Burton MA, Gray BN. Albumin microspheres as vehicles for the sustained and controlled release of doxorubicin. J Pharm Pharmacol. 1989; 41:813–6.

28. Blumer JL. Evolution of a new drug formulation: the rationale for high-dose, short-course therapy with azithromycin. Int J Antimicrob Agents. 2005;26:S143–7.

29. Todoroff J, Vanbever R. Fate of nanomedicines in the lungs. Curr Opin Colloid Interface Sci. 2011;16:246–54.

30. Yamashita F, Hashida M. Pharmacokinetic considerations for targeted drug delivery. Adv Drug Deliv Rev. 2013;65:139–47.

26

Protection by beta-Hydroxybutyric acid against insulin glycation, lipid peroxidation and microglial cell apoptosis

Manijheh Sabokdast[1,5], Mehran Habibi-Rezaei[1,2*], Ali Akbar Moosavi-Movahedi[3,4], Maryam Ferdousi[1], Effat Azimzadeh-Irani[1] and Najmeh Poursasan[3]

Abstract

Background: Diabetes mellitus is characterized jointly by hyperglycemia and hyperinsulinemia that make insulin more prone to be glycated and evolve insulin advanced glycation end products (Insulin- AGE). Here, we report the effect of beta-hydroxy butyrate (BHB) (the predominant ketone body) on the formation of insulin-AGE, insulin glycation derived liposomal lipid peroxidation and insulin-AGE toxicity in microglial cells.

Methods: The inhibitory effect of BHB was monitored as a result of insulin incubation in the presence of glucose or fructose using AGE-dependent fluorescence, Tyr fluorescence as well as anilinonaphthalenesulfonate (ANS) andthioflavin T (ThT) binding, and circular dichroism (CD) investigations. To study lipid peroxidation induced by insulin glycation, thiobarbituric acid (TBA) assay and thiobarbituric acid reactive substance (TBARS) monitoring were used. The effect of insulin–AGE on microglial viability was investigated by 3-(4, 5 dimethylthiazol-2-yl)—2, 5-diphenyltetrazoliumbromide (MTT) cell assay and Annexin V/propidium iodide (PI) staining.

Results: Here we are reporting the inhibitory effect of BHB on insulin glycation and generation of insulin-AGE as a possible explanation for insulin resistance. Moreover, the protective effect of BHB on consequential glycation derived liposomal lipid peroxidation as a causative event in microglial apoptosis is reported.

Conclusion: The reduced insulin fibril formation, structural inertia to glycation involved conformational changes, anti-lipid peroxidation effect, and increasing microglia viability indicated the protective effect of BHB that disclose insight on the possible preventive effect of BHB on Alzheimer's disease.

Introduction

Type 1 Diabetes is generally characterized by raised level of blood sugar (hyperglycemia) due to imperfection in insulin secretion, type 2 diabetes is characterized by insulin resistance that results in both of hyperglycemia and hyperinsulinemia and finally type 3 diabetes is characterized with neurodegeneration linked with insulin resistance. Although, increasing evidences in the literature pointing toward strong correlation between insulin resistance and Alzheimer's disease (AD) [1, 2] but, that correlation has not been yet formally recognized.

Under hyperglycemic condition almost all proteins are prone to be glycated in a nonenzymatic fashion. It is established that protein glycation, oxidative stress, and lipid peroxidation are key processes in diabetes and related complications [3, 4]. Due to the glucose auto-oxidation and protein glycation, hyperglycemia result in increased production of reactive oxygen species (ROS) that originates oxidative stress as an imbalance between radical- generating and radical-scavenging systems [5].

Protein glycation is whereby labile Schiff base is formed by nonenzymatic reaction between annomeric carbonyl group of an open ring carbohydrate and amino group(s) of the protein molecule followed by molecular rearrangement to form stable Amadori products that provoke the formation of advanced glycation end products (AGE) after additional dehydration reaction and further molecular rearrangements [6]. Following the protein glycation, a series

* Correspondence: mhabibi@ut.ac.ir
[1]School of Biology, College of Science, University of Tehran, Tehran, Iran
[2]Nano-Biomedicine Center of Excellence, Nanoscience and Nanotechnology Research Center, University of Tehran, Tehran, Iran
Full list of author information is available at the end of the article

of events occur covering α-helix to β-sheet transformation, cross β structure formation, and generation of soluble amyloid prefibrils [7]. Membrane lipids are mainly prone to oxidation by ROS owing to their polyunsaturated fatty acid content [8]. That is why prefibriles and ROS initiate membrane involved events or damages, that consequently induce apoptotic response and cell death [9]. Hence, antioxidants suppose to effectively protect against glycation derived free radicals and considered as a therapeutic potential for the inhibition of ROS involved processes [10].

Ketone bodies (KB) comprise 3-beta-hydroxybutyrate (BHB), acetoacetate (AcAc), and acetone while the later is the least abundant one. They are always present in the blood and their levels increase during fasting and prolonged exercise [11]. They are also found in the blood of neonates and pregnant women. However, type 1 diabetes is the most common pathological cause of raised blood ketones due to increased lipid catabolism under hypoinsulinemia. In such a condition, the BHB: AcAc ratio arises from normal, 1:1 to as high as 10:1. It has been a decade that BHB is reported to be useful against cell apoptosis [12], adipocyte lipolysis inhibition [13], and considered as a treatment for various diseases including epilepsy, Huntington's, Parkinson's, and Alzheimer's [14, 15]. Concurrency of hyperglycemia and hyperinsulinemia in type 2 diabetes, make insulin prone to be glycated. Here we are reporting the inhibitory effect of BHB on insulin glycation and generation of insulin advance glycation end product (insulin-AGE) as a possible explanation for insulin resistance. Moreover, the protective effect of BHB on consequential glycation derived liposomal lipid peroxidation as causative events in microglial apoptosis are reported.

Materials and methods
Material
Newborn rats (Wistar strain) were obtained from the University of Tehran animal facilities. The Annexin-V-FITC apoptosis assay kit was from Molecular Probes Inc., UK. Human recombinant insulin was gifted by Exir pharmaceutical company (Iran). Thioflavin T was from Merck Company and other chemicals used in this study were obtained from Sigma Aldrich (USA). All solutions were prepared using double—distilled water.

Sample preparation
Insulin at a final concentration of 0.5 mg.ml^{-1} was dissolved in phosphate buffer (50 mM, pH 7. 4) and incubated with 16.5 mM D-glucose or D-fructose in either the presence or absence of 14.4 mM β-hydroxy butyrate (BHB) which is close concentration in individuals with post prolonged fasting (mM) or ketoacidosis, based on literature [16–19]. All solution was filtered using 0.2 μm membrane filter (Milipore, USA) under sterile condition.

All samples were incubated under physiological conditions (at dark and 37 °C) for 0 to 96 h, and then stored at −20 °C until using for further analysis.

Fluorescence measurement
The Cary Eclipse fluorescence spectrophotometer (Varian, Australia) was used for monitoring the AGE dependent fluorescence, the changes in the environment of the Tyr residue in insulin and for probing the available hydrophobic portion of protein (ANS) and ELISA reader fluorescence H4 (Synergy H4, Bio Tek, USA) was used for ThT binding analysis. Protein intrinsic (Tyr) fluorescence was analyzed at 307 nm after excitation at 276 nm. AGE dependent fluorescence intensity measurement of glycated insulin in the presence or absence of BHB was carried out at 384 nm excitation wavelength and emission spectra were recorded in the wavelength range of 384–500 nm. The protein concentration was 0.5 mg.ml^{-1}.

For ANS fluorescence measurement, 200 μL from the incubated mixtures (0.2 mg.ml^{-1} insulin) in the presence or absence of BHB (14.4 mM) at 37 °C were added to fresh solution of ANS (3 μM in 50 mM phosphate buffer pH 7.4) and incubated for 30 min in the dark, then the emission intensity was measured after excitation at 463 nm at room temperature to study the kinetics of change in solvent-exposed hydrophobic pockets due to the generation of partially folded intermediates during insulin glycation, aggregation, and AGE formation. For ThT assay 20 μL aliquots of 0.5 mg.ml^{-1} samples were added to 180 μL solution containing 25 μM ThT (in 50 mM phosphate buffer pH 7.4), then fluorescence emission was determined at 490 nm using a H4 spectrometer. Fluorescence emission intensities were plotted against time after excitation at 440 nm. The emission values of the buffer and fresh insulin were used as background correction and control, respectively. The averages of triplicate measurements were used for each sample.

Circular dichroism (CD) spectroscopy
Far-UV CD was used for analyzing secondary structure during fibrillation. The CD measurements were obtained using a CD spectropolarimeter (J-810, Jasco, Japan) with 1-mm path length of a quartz cuvette at 25 °C and data were scanned from 190 nm to 260 nm at 1 nm intervals. The final protein concentration was 0.2 mg.ml^{-1} in 50 mM phosphate buffer pH 7.4. The bandwidth was set at 1 nm. The spectrum of phosphate buffer was subtracted from sample spectra for data analysis. All CD spectra converted to mean residue ellipticity using the following relationship:

$$[\theta] = (\theta/10)\,(MRM/LC)$$

Where $[\theta]$ is ellipticity (deg.cm^2.dmol^{-1}) at wavelength λ, θ is the observed ellipticity in millidegree, MRW is the mean residue weight, L is the path length (in cm), and C is the protein concentration (mg.ml^{-1}). The percentage of secondary structure was obtained using CDNN software.

Preparation of liposome and lipid peroxidation assay

Liposomes were made using a modification of the method of Bangham [20]. Briefly, a solution of soybean phosphatidylcholine/cholesterol in the weight ratio of 4:1 in chloroform was dried under reduced pressure using a rotary evaporator at <50 °C to provide a thin homogenous film, which was placed in a desiccator for next 24 h. The film was then dispersed in phosphate buffer and stirred for 15 min. The mixture was sonicated to achieve a homogeneous suspension of liposomes. Lipid peroxidation was used as an indicator of tissue injury induced by reactive oxygen species. It was measured using the thiobarbituric acid assay (TBA) based on thiobarbituric acid reactive substance (TBARS) monitoring. The amount of tissue TBARS was measured by the method described by Buege and Aust [21]. In brief, 250 µl of sample at incubation time periods (10, 30, 50, 70, and 90 h) was added to an aliquot of liposomes and then incubated at 37 °C for 24 h. Then 50 µL of TCA (50 %) and 100 µL of TBA (0.35 g) were added to the reaction mixture. It absolutely was then incubated for a quarter-hour at boiling water bath and TBARS was identified at 532 nm.

Cell culture and cell viability assay

The microglia from neocortex of newborn rats (Wistar strain) were cultured from mixed glia cultures according to the procedure by Giulian and Baker with some modifications [22]. Briefly, the cerebellum was detached, meninges were dissected, and brain cortex tissue was minced in a nutrient medium. Then cells were dissociated by triturating with sterile pipettes to obtain a cell suspension. The cell suspension from each brain was separated into two 75 ml tissue culture flasks (Falcon) in DMEM and 20 % FCS at 37 °C with 5 % CO_2 for 24 h. After 24 h, the medium was half changed to reach 10 % FCS for the rest of the day. The cells were fed every 4 days with a fifty percent spent medium. After 2 weeks, cultures contained glial cells, including rounded microglial cells mostly localized on the top of the monolayer. The loosely adherent microglial cells were recovered by gentle shaking by hand for 2 min. The cell suspension was then cultured on 96 multiwell plates at a density of 3×10^4 cell/cm2, in 10 % FCS supplemented DMEM medium (total volume 200 µl) for 24 h, to enter the ramified phase. To treat the cells, the culture medium was replaced with the insulin (6.25, 12.5, 25, 50, 75,125, 200, and 375 µg/ml, the final concentration of the glycated insulin was determined according to the final

volume of 200 µl) which was glycated in the presence or absence of BHB for a series of incubation time (0, 10, 30, 50, 70, and 90 h). Treated cells were kept in this medium for 24 h, after which the effect of AGE on the viability of the cells was evaluated via the MTT assay [23]. This assay measures the mitochondrial function and is most frequently used to detect loss of cell viability [24]. Nevertheless, this assay can underestimate the cell death because it works best to detect the later stages of apoptosis when the metabolic activity of the cells is strictly reduced [25]. The treated cultured cells were incubated with 10 % of MTT per well for four hours (from the stock solution of 5 mg.ml^{-1} of MTT in PBS, which was filtered through 0.2 µm syringe filter and kept all the time in dark condition), after which the whole media were replaced with 100 µl DMS solution to dissolve the MTT formazan crystals. The optical density (OD) at 580 nm was determined using an EIA Multiscan MS micro-plate reader.

Cell survival was calculated as a percentage by dividing the absorbance values of the experimental group (treated cells) by the absorbance values of the control group (untreated cells). Each assay was repeated six times, to ensure the reproducibility of the results. Moreover, apoptosis analysis was performed using Annexin V-FITC and propidium iodide (PI) dual staining according to the manufacturer's instructions. Briefly after a period of treatment, cells were harvested and washed in cold phosphate-buffered saline (PBS) followed by centrifugation at $900 \times g$ for 10 min. The pellet re-suspend in 200 µL annexin binding buffer to prepare a cell density of 1×10^6 cell.ml^{-1}. Then 5 µl of Alexa Fluor 488 annexin V and 5 µl of the 50 µg.ml^{-1} propidium iodide (PI) solutions was added. After 15 min incubation at room temperature, 300 µl of 1× annexin binding buffer was added and samples were kept on ice. Then the cells were analyzed by flowcytometry, measuring the fluorescence emission at 530 nm (e.g. FL1) and 575 nm (e.g. FL2). After staining apoptotic, necrotic and live cells show green, red and no fluorescence, respectively [26]. All procedures were performed in accordance with institutional guidelines for animal care and use, which adhered to the international principles of Laboratory Animal Care (NIH publication #85-23, revised in 1985).

Statistical analysis

Data were expressed as mean ± SD. static analysis between treatments was made using one-way ANOVA (analysis of variance) followed by Duncan's new multiple range tests for multiple comparisons. P-value <0.01 was considered statistically significant.

Results

Intrinsic and extrinsic fluorescence analysis Conformational change, the formation of glycation products, and increasing surface hydrophobicity of insulin alone as a control, insulin in the presence of Glc or Fru and in the presence or absence of BHB were examined using intrinsic tyrosine (excitation at 280 nm), AGE-dependent (excitation at 384 nm), and ANS-binding fluorescence (excitation at 460 nm), respectively (Fig. 1). Fig. 1a illustrates increase in the intensity of AGE-dependent fluorescence (λ_{ex} 370 nm; λem425 nm) to detect the formation of AGE [27] upon glycation by Glc or Fru also the inhibitory effect of BHB has been presented. The kinetics of Tyr fluorescence of insulin under glycation in the presence of Glc or Fru and presence or absence of

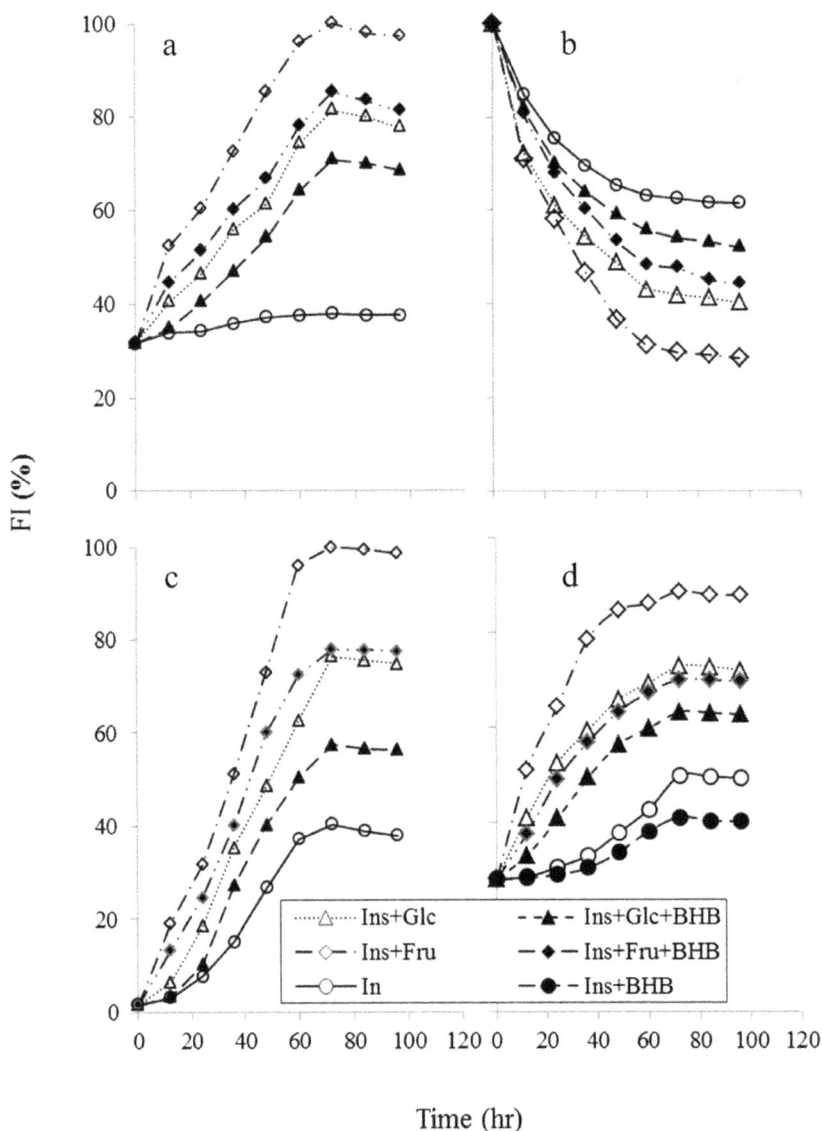

Fig. 1 The kinetics of changes in the fluorescence of glycated insulin in the presence or absence of BHB. **a** AGE-related auto-fluorescence of insulin and modified insulin (Ins + Glc, Ins + Glc + BHB, Ins + Fru, Ins + Fru + BHB) was monitored in emission wavelength range of 384–500 nm. After excitation at 370 nm. Insulin, glucose, fructose and BHB were alone used as a control. **b** Changes in the intrinsic fluorescence (λex 276 nm; λem 307 nm) of insulin incubated with Glc or Fru in the presence or absence of BHB was used to assess the change in surface hydrophobicity of insulin. Aliquots of the incubated insulin were added to 3 μM ANS and the spectra recorded after 30 min. The excitation was performed at 350 nm and fluorescence spectra were obtained from 405 nm to 550 nm. **d** The β-sheet content of insulin was determined with Thiflavin T fluorescence. Excitation and emission wavelength was 450 nm and 490 nm respectively

BHB has been depicted in Fig. 1b. Fluorescence at 280 nm region is commonly used to study conformational alterations of a protein in solution [28]. The intrinsic fluorescence of insulin decreased markedly during incubation with glucose or fructose that was diminished by BHB which indicates an inhibitory effect of BHB on glycation-induced insulin conformation change (Fig. 1b). ANS fluorescence was employed to study the kinetics of change in solvent exposed hydrophobic pockets of insulin in the presence of insulin and Glc or Fru and presence or absence of BHB to characterize partially folded intermediates during insulin glycation, aggregation, and AGE formation (Fig. 1c). The fluorescence intensity enhancement of ANS in glycated insulin with glucose or fructose indicates the increase in solvent-exposed hydrophobic regions, originating from partially folded intermediates. BHB was approved to decrease glycation-involved ANS fluorescence.

Thioflavin T fluorescence test resulted less β-sheet content in the samples glycated by Glc or Fru in the presence of BHB than the samples in the absence of BHB (Fig. 1d).

Circular dichroism (CD) analysis

Figure 2 represents glycation-induced insulin secondary structure transformation by Glc (2a) or Fru (2b), using circular dichroism (CD) for the products of 72 h incubation; inhibitory effect of BHB was also included. Glycation by Glc or Fru brings about 9.7 and 15.1 percent decrease in α-conformation, respectively. BHB not only inhibited all, 7.9 % decreasing in α-conformation due to glycation by Glc, but also caused even 0.9 % increasing of this conformation for insulin incubated alone for 72 h (BHB treatment similarly diminished increase in β-conformation from 3.82 % to 0.2 %). Under glycation by Fru, BHB diminished α-decrease or β-increase from 13.3 % to 6.7 % and 8.12 % to 2.8 %, respectively (Table 1). These results support a protective effect of BHB against glycation-induced sheet formation, proceeding less fibril formation, and indicates on a structural inertia to glycation induced conformational changes due to the BHB.

Lipid peroxidation analysis

In order to investigate the preventive effect of BHB on lipid peroxidation potential, TBARs assay was performed. Figure 3 shows the level of lipid peroxidation marker, malondialdehyde (MDA) at 532 nm as a function of time. The level of MDA as an end product of lipid peroxidation was markedly increased in the presence of insulin glycation by glucose or fructose that was

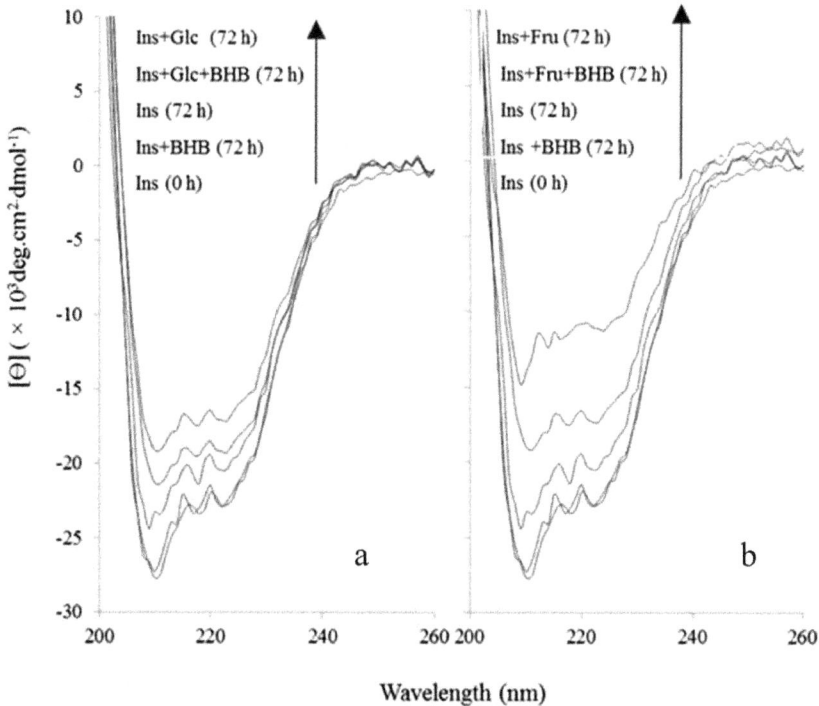

Fig. 2 3-β hydroxybutyrate (BHB) inhibits the secondary structure change in glycated protein. **a** The secondary structure percentage of insulin and modified insulin (Ins + Glc, Ins + Glc + BHB) in 50 mM sodium phosphate buffer pH 7.4 containing 0.1 mM sodium azide incubated at 37 °C for 72 h. **b** CD spectra of insulin glycated with fructose in the presence or absence of BHB

Table 1 The relative percentages of the secondary structures were estimated using the CDNN CD spectra deconvolution software. The results are expressed as mean ± S.D. from three independent experiments

Sample	α-Helix	β-Sheet	β-Sheet	β-Turn	Random-coil
Ins 0 h	39.2 ± 0.2	5.8 ± 0.05	7.7 ± 0.03	15.5 ± 0.0	31.4 ± 0.06
Ins 72 h	37.4 ± 0.1	6 ± 0.1	8 ± 0.03	15.5 ± 0.09	32.7 ± 0.3
Ins + Glc 72 h	29.5 ± 0.2	8.42 ± 0.1	9.4 ± 0.05	16 ± 0.03	36.4 ± 0.1
Ins + Fru 72 h	24.1 ± 0.05	10.5 ± 0.3	11.7 ± 0.5	16.7 ± 0.3	38.1 ± 0.9
Ins + BHB 72 h	36.3 ± 0.1	732 ± 0.2	8.1 ± 0.2	16.1 ± 0.1	32.0 ± 0.08
Ins + Glc + BHB 72 h	38.3 ± 0.1	5.9 ± 0.1	7.8 ± 0.03	15.5 ± 0.05	32.0 ± 0.08
Ins + Fru + BHB 72 h	30.7 ± 0.08	7.6 ± 0.8	9.2 ± 0.03	15.7 ± 0.03	36.5 ± 0.08

effectively inhibited by BHB (Fig. 3), most probably or as a reason of preventive effect of BHB on insulin glycation or pertained antioxidative property.

Microglial cell survival assay

Random images were obtained and semi-confluent ramified microglial culture was observed to confirm the right phenotype of the isolated cells. The effect of insulin-AGEs as the products of insulin glycation by glucose or

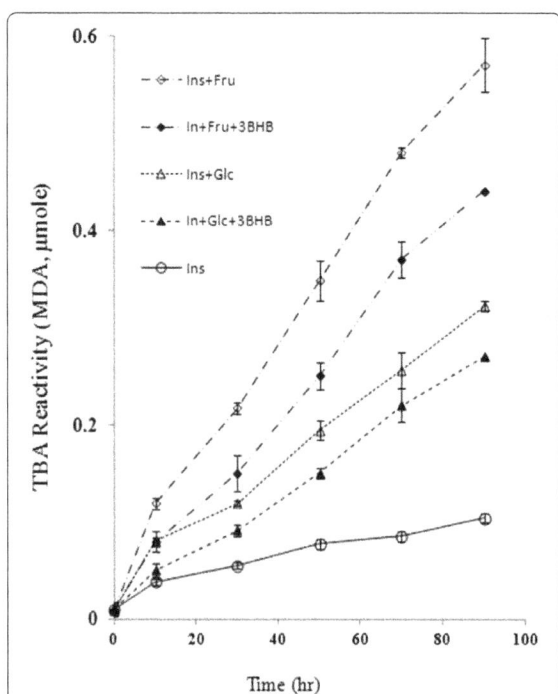

Fig. 3 The liposomal lipid peroxidation derived by insulin glycation and reduced by BHB. It was measured using TBA assay based on MDA and TBARS monitoring. MDA formation was determined at 532 nm against the time of incubation of glycated insulin by Glc or Fru in the presence or absence of BHB. Results are expressed as mean ± S.D. from three independent experiments

fructose on rat microglial viability was studied using MTT assay according to the conventional protocols with at least 5 repeats [23]. As shown in Fig. 4a, when culture medium was replaced with medium supplemented with products of insulin glycation in the absence of BHB for different period of time (0, 10, 30, 50, 70 and 90 h), the cell viability was dramatically affected by the presence of insulin–AGEs and as depicted, fructation derived insulin-AGEs were 1.4–1.8 folds more effective than the glycation products of Glc on decreasing cell viability in the absence of BHB (Fig. 4a). However, in the presence of BHB the cell viability was improved at more than 1.5 folds. Besides, the indices of rat microglial apoptosis were determined using Annexin V/PI staining [29]. The flow cytometry (FACS) analysis was carried out on microglial cells that were treated with glycated insulin for 72 h in the presence or absence of BHB against corresponding control (Fig. 4b). The percentage of cell apoptosis were significantly increased when microglial culture was treated with insulin glycation products, especially by fructose BHB decreased apoptotic cells about 5.3 and 8.2 folds corresponding to the cells treated with glycation products of glucose or fructose, respectively.

Discussion

Nowadays, protein aggregation diseases such as Alzheimer's, Parkinson's, cataract, mad cow diseases and physiological aging have attained particular attention. Moreover, protein aggregation turns out to play a significant role in cancer i.e. p53 aggregation (as an important tumor suppressor protein) leads to uncontrolled cell growth [30]. One of the causative conditions in protein aggregation known to be protein glycation [31] which not only makes friend proteins disabilities, but also makes them toxic and foe. In protein glycation after a nonenzymatic reaction between reducing sugars and protein, a series of glycation products are consecutively generated, including soluble prefibriles and non-soluble fibrils that are collectively called advance glycated end products or AGEs. Considerable evidences indicate that under

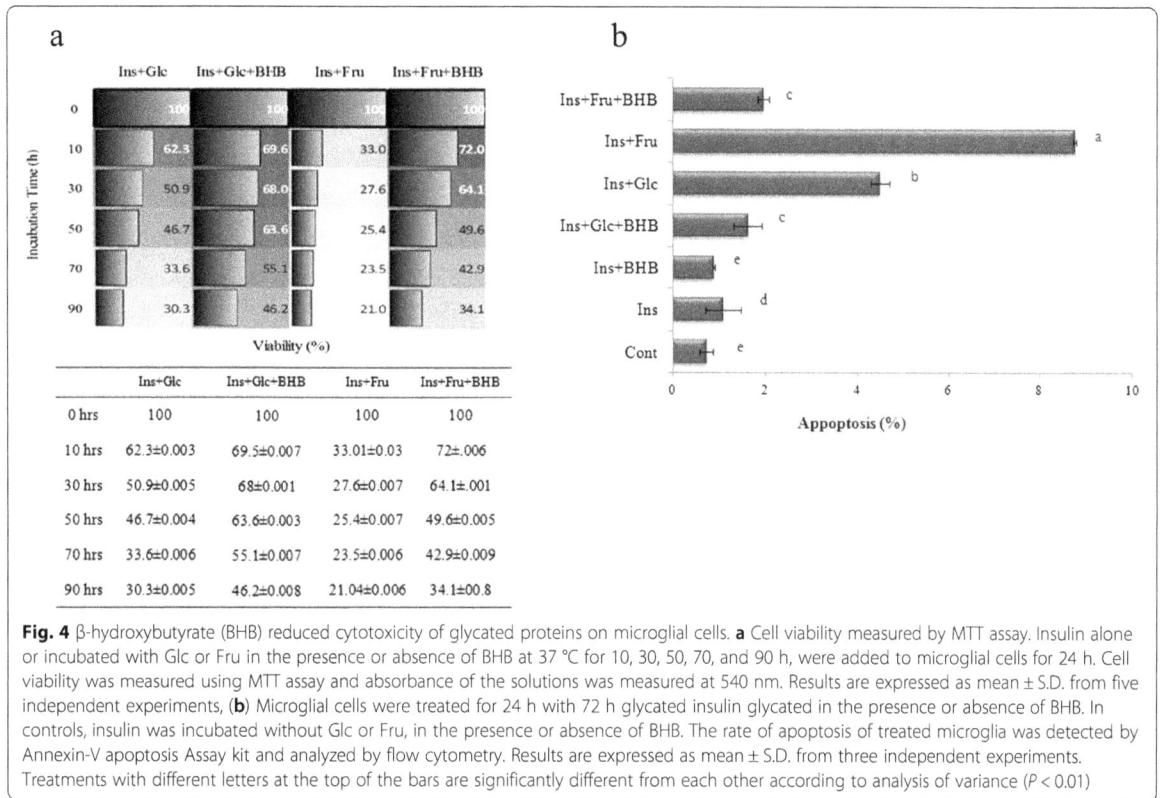

Fig. 4 β-hydroxybutyrate (BHB) reduced cytotoxicity of glycated proteins on microglial cells. **a** Cell viability measured by MTT assay. Insulin alone or incubated with Glc or Fru in the presence or absence of BHB at 37 °C for 10, 30, 50, 70, and 90 h, were added to microglial cells for 24 h. Cell viability was measured using MTT assay and absorbance of the solutions was measured at 540 nm. Results are expressed as mean ± S.D. from five independent experiments, (**b**) Microglial cells were treated for 24 h with 72 h glycated insulin glycated in the presence or absence of BHB. In controls, insulin was incubated without Glc or Fru, in the presence or absence of BHB. The rate of apoptosis of treated microglia was detected by Annexin-V apoptosis Assay kit and analyzed by flow cytometry. Results are expressed as mean ± S.D. from three independent experiments. Treatments with different letters at the top of the bars are significantly different from each other according to analysis of variance ($P < 0.01$)

hyperglycemia, protein glycation and AGE generation are important determinants of complications often observed in type 1 and type 2 diabetes, including nephropathy, retinopathy, neuropathy and cardiovascular disease (CVD) [32]. Although, almost all proteins could be targets for glycation, but more specifically, concurrency of hyperglycemia and hyperinsulinemia in type 2 diabetes makes insulin prone to be glycated to generate ROS and produce insulin-AGEs. Insulin is glycated even in the pancreas which has been considered in the pancreas of various animal models of type 2 diabetes [33, 34]. Prevention of protein glycation and its consecutive symptoms are of great importance. We are reporting the inhibitory effect of BHB on insulin-AGE formation and insulin-AGE toxicity in microglial cells. When insulin was incubated in the presence of glucose or fructose, insulin was glycated and AGE-dependent fluorescence was increased by the time, followed by a protein conformational change monitored by decreasing Tyr or increasing ANS fluorescence intensities; while BHB inhibited all three mentioned cases. Since most AGEs (such as N-carboxymethyl lysine; CML and N-carboxyethyl lysine; CEL, and cross links such as pentosidine, methylglyoxal lysine dimmer; MOLD, and threosidine) have a characteristic fluorescence, with an excitation maximum at 360, and

emission around 460 nm, detection through fluorescence spectroscopy is a widely available method. Insulin-AGEs formation and inhibitory effect of BHB were collectively monitored using AGEs fluorescence (ex360 nm, em460 nm) as a result of insulin incubation in the presence of Glc or Fru in Fig. 1a. Insulin has three glycation prone positions, the N-terminals of both chains (Gly1 and Phe1) and residue Lys29 of B-chain. As a result, three forms of insulin glycation products have been reported (mono, di, and tri-glycated forms) [35]. Most probably, the effect of BHB on preventing insulin glycation is due to BHB binding to glycation prone residues in protein to diminish the glycation susceptibility. In addition, proteins present their intrinsic fluorescence because of their main flourophore residues; tryptophan (Trp, W), tyrosine (Tyr, Y) and phenylalanine (Phe, F), but only Trp and Tyr are used experimentally because their quantum yields are high enough to give a good fluorescence signal [36]. In insulin as a special case, Tyr dominates the fluorescence excitation at 280 nm in the absence of Trp. It has been found that insulin denaturation results in (or brought about) a decrease in Tyr fluorescence, suggesting that in insulin, Tyr residues were translocated from hydrophobic pockets to the aqueous environment and were effectively quenched [37]. As a result of glycation process over the period of 96 h, further fluorescence quenching was observed when insulin was incubated in the presence of Glc and far more in the presence of Fru. Such conformational changes were also monitored using ANS fluorescence (Fig. 1c). The presence of BHB interestingly and successfully protected insulin against glycation-involved conformational changes. Insulin glycation ended in protein fibrillation that exhibited increased β-sheets (Fig. 1d) and decreased α-conformation (and increased β-conformation) (Fig. 2) relative to the non-glycated and non-fibrillar form reporting by CD analysis and ThT binding fluorescence, respectively. The CD is a powerful tool for investigating glycation dependent α- to β-conformational changes in proteins [38]. However, ThT can bind to β-sheets due to its geometric fitness [39], stochiometrically emits after excitation at 440 nm. As expected, Fru changed secondary structure and developed β-sheet more effectively than the Glc; however, the preventive effect of BHB was observed in both cases. Glycation has reported to cause a decrease in α-helix content in various proteins, e.g. human serum albumin (HSA) [40], bovine serum albumin (BSA) [41], and hemoglobin (Hb) [42]. More recently, we observed that BHB can preserve the secondary structure of HSA against Glc using CD [43]. Interestingly, BHB not only prevents glycation—derived sheet development, but also presents a stabilizing effect on insulin in the absence of Glc or Fru (Fig. 1d). Our results show that insulin-AGEs induce liposomal lipid peroxidation in a time dependent manner, nonetheless, BHB can effectively reduce these effects (Fig. 3). The relationship between the level of glycated hemoglobin and lipid peroxidation in erythrocytes of both diabetic and healthy subjects have been reported [44] and higher lipid peroxidation in seminal plasma of diabetic than non-diabetic subjects has been reported [45]. We assume that insulin glycation not only can explain insulin resistance, but also can play a role in cell death through lipid peroxidation more importantly glial cells. Also, we are reporting the anti-lipid peroxidation effect of BHB that can explain its protection on microglial apoptosis. To continue, the effects of products of insulin glycation by glucose or fructose on rat microglial survival as well as the protective effect of BHB on microglial cells were estimated using MTT assay and flow cytometry using Annexin V/PI staining.

These observations confirmed the cytotoxic effects of insulin glycation products, especially by fructose, on microglial cells (Fig. 4). Since microglia are implicated in cascades causing neuronal loss and cognitive decline in Alzheimer's disease (AD), insulin–AGEs formation, especially in type 2 diabetes, are most probably involved in AD that is proposed as type 3 diabetes. However, BHB diminished the extent of toxicity evolved by insulin glycation on microglial cells or probably inhibited microglial cell apoptosis. Shan Chenga et al. has reported preventive effect of BHB on apoptotic and necrotic cell death by serving as a metabolic fuel for cells [46]. Because of the fact that BHB can cross the blood brain barrier (BBB), arriving at neurons and glial cells [47], the inhibitory effect of BHB on insulin-glycation, insulin-AGEs formation, and insulin-AGEs derived liposomal lipid peroxidation are collectively offer a possible explanation on protective effect of BHB on microglial apoptosis under diabetic condition.

Conclusion

Insulin glycation by Glc and more effectively by Fru results in insulin-AGEs formation and lipid peroxidation that may involve in insulin resistance. Moreover, the toxic effect of insulin-AGEs on cultured microlia are reported in which, the glycation product of insulin by Fru presented more toxic effect than glycation product of insulin by Glc. Microglial apoptosis may involved in neurodegenerative diseases such as AD. The observed protective effects of BHB in insulin glycation and insulin-AGEs induced microglial apoptosis, disclose the new insights of BHB action against type 3 diabetes or AD.

Competing interests
The authors declare that they have no competing interests.

Authors' contributions
MHR conceived the studies. MS and MHR wrote the manuscript, MS, MF, NP and MHR designed experiments. MS, MHR, EAI and AAMM analysed data and contributed to the acquisition and interpretation of data. All authors approved the final manuscript. MHR is the guarantor of this work.

Acknowledgements
We are grateful to Dr. Sarrafnejhad, Tehran University of Medical Sciences for providing access to his FACS. Also, we thank Dr. Ali Akbar Saboor and Farhad Jadidi-Niaragh for their helps in FACS analysis. The support of the University of Tehran and Iran National Science foundation (INSF), UNESCO Chair of Interdisciplinary Research in Diabetes (University of Tehran, Tehran, Iran) are gratefully acknowledged

Author details
[1]School of Biology, College of Science, University of Tehran, Tehran, Iran. [2]Nano-Biomedicine Center of Excellence, Nanoscience and Nanotechnology Research Center, University of Tehran, Tehran, Iran. [3]Institute of Biochemistry and Biophysics, University of Tehran, Tehran, Iran. [4]Center of Excellence in Biothermodynamics, University of Tehran, Tehran, Iran. [5]Present address: Department of agronomy, and plant breeding, College of Agriculture & Natural Resources, University of Tehran, Karaj, Iran.

References
1. Association AD. Diagnosis and classification of diabetes mellitus. Diabetes Care. 2008;31:S55–60.
2. Suzanne M, Wands JR. Alzheimer's disease is type 3 diabetes—evidence reviewed. J Diabetes Sci Technol. 2008;2:1101–13.
3. Moussa S. Oxidative stress in diabetes mellitus. Rom J Biophys. 2008;18:225–36.

4. Bonnefont-Rousselot D, Bastard J, Jaudon M, Delattre J. Consequences of the diabetic status on the oxidant/antioxidant balance. Diabetes Metab. 2000;26:163–77.

5. Halliwell B, Gutteridge JM. Free radicals in biology and medicine. Oxford: Oxford university press; 1999.

6. Turk Z. Glycotoxines, carbonyl stress and relevance to diabetes and its complications. Physiol Res. 2010;59:147–56.

7. Chiti F, Webster P, Taddei N, Clark A, Stefani M, Ramponi G, et al. Designing conditions for in vitro formation of amyloid protofilaments and fibrils. Proc Natl Acad Sci. 1999;96:3590–4.

8. Aruoma OI. Free radicals, oxidative stress, and antioxidants in human health and disease. J Am Oil Chem Soc. 1998;75:199–212.

9. Chiti F, Dobson CM. Protein misfolding, functional amyloid, and human disease. Annu Rev Biochem. 2006;75:333–66.

10. Ceriello A, Giugliano D, Quatraro A, Donzella C, Dipalo G, Lefebvre PJ. Vitamin E reduction of protein glycosylation in diabetes: new prospect for prevention of diabetic complications? Diabetes Care. 1991;14:68–72.

11. Le Maho Y, Van Kha HV, Koubi H, Dewasmes G, Girard J, Ferre P, et al. Body composition, energy expenditure, and plasma metabolites in long-term fasting geese. Am J Physiol Endocrinol Metab. 1981;241:E342–54.

12. Cheng B, Yang X, Hou Z, Lin X, Meng H, Li Z, et al. D-β-hydroxybutyrate inhibits the apoptosis of PC12 cells induced by 6-OHDA in relation to up-regulating the ratio of Bcl-2/Bax mRNA. Auton Neurosci. 2007;134:38–44.

13. Taggart AK, Kero J, Gan X, Cai T-Q, Cheng K, Ippolito M, et al. (D)-β-hydroxybutyrate inhibits adipocyte lipolysis via the nicotinic acid receptor PUMA-G. J Biol Chem. 2005;280:26649–52.

14. Kashiwaya Y, Takeshima T, Mori N, Nakashima K, Clarke K, Veech RL. d-β-Hydroxybutyrate protects neurons in models of Alzheimer's and Parkinson's disease. Proc Natl Acad Sci. 2000;97:5440–4.

15. Lim S, Chesser AS, Grima JC, Rappold PM, Blum D, Przedborski S, et al. D-β-Hydroxybutyrate Is Protective in Mouse Models of Huntington's Disease. Plos one. 2011;6:e24620.

16. Bohlooli M, Moosavi-Movahedi A, Taghavi F, Habibi-Rezaei M, Seyedarabi A, Saboury, et al. Thermodynamics of a molten globule state of human serum albumin by 3-β-hydroxybutyrate as a ketone body. Int J Biol Macromol. 2013;54:258–63.

17. Laffel L. Ketone bodies: a review of physiology, pathophysiology and application of monitoring to diabetes. Diabetes Metab Res Rev. 1999;15:412–26.

18. Xie J, García-Pérez E, Méndez JD. In vitro Glycation of Hemoglobin by Acetone and-hydroxibutirate. World Appl Sci J. 2007;2:099–106.

19. Aguilar-Hernández M, Méndez JD. In vitro glycation of brain aminophospholipids by acetoacetate and its inhibition by urea. Biomed Pharmacother. 2007;61:693–7.

20. Bangham A, Standish M, Watkins J. Diffusion of univalent ions across the lamellae of swollen phospholipids. J Mol Biol. 1965;13:238–IN27.

21. Buege JA. Microsomal lipid peroxidation. Methods Enzymol. 1978;52:302–10.

22. Giulian D, Baker TJ. Characterization of ameboid microglia isolated from developing mammalian brain. J Neurosci. 1986;6:2163–78.

23. Mosmann T. Rapid colorimetric assay for cellular growth and survival: application to proliferation and cytotoxicity assays. J Immunol Methods. 1983;65:55–63.

24. Green LC, Wagner DA, Glogowski J, Skipper PL, Wishnok JS, Tannenbaum SR. Analysis of nitrate, nitrite, and nitrate in biological fluids. Anal Biochem. 1982;126:131–8.

25. Petty RD, Sutherland LA, Hunter EM, Cree IA. Comparison of MTT and ATP-based assays for the measurement of viable cell number. J Biolumin Chemilumin. 1995;10:29–34.

26. Van Engeland M, Nieland LJ, Ramaekers FC, Schutte B, Reutelingsperger CP. Annexin V-affinity assay: a review on an apoptosis detection system based on phosphatidylserine exposure. Cytometry. 1998;31:1–9.

27. Schmitt A, Schmitt J, Münch G, Gasic-Milencovic J. Characterization of advanced glycation end products for biochemical studies: side chain modifications and fluorescence characteristics. Anal Biochem. 2005;338:201–15.

28. Gorinstein S, Goshev I, Moncheva S, Zemser M, Weisz M, Caspi A, et al. Intrinsic tryptophan fluorescence of human serum proteins and related conformational changes. J Protein Chem. 2000;19:637–42.

29. Yan SD, Schmidt AM, Anderson GM, Zhang J, Brett J, Zou YS, et al. Enhanced cellular oxidant stress by the interaction of advanced glycation end products with their receptors/binding proteins. J Biol Chem. 1994;269:9889–97.

30. Xu J, Reumers J, Couceiro JR, De Smet F, Gallardo R, Rudyak S, et al. Gain of function of mutant p53 by coaggregation with multiple tumor suppressors. Nat Chem Biol. 2011;7:285–95.

31. Adrover M, Mariño L, Sanchis P, Pauwels K, Kraan Y, Lebrun P, et al. Mechanistic insights in glycation-induced protein aggregation. Biomacromolecules. 2014;15:3449–62.

32. Yan SF, Ramasamy R, Schmidt AM. Mechanisms of disease: advanced glycation end-products and their receptor in inflammation and diabetes complications. Nat Rev Endocrinol. 2008;4:285–93.

33. Abdel-Wahab YH, O'Harte FP, Ratcliff H, McClenaghan NH, Barnett CR, Flatt PR. Glycation of insulin in the islets of Langerhans of normal and diabetic animals. Diabetes. 1996;45:1489–96.

34. Abdel-Wahab Y, O'Harte F, Boyd A, Barnett C, Flatt P. Glycation of insulin results in reduced biological activity in mice. Acta Diabetol. 1997;34:265–70.

35. Guedes S, Vitorino R, Domingues MRM, Amado F, Domingues P. Mass spectrometry characterization of the glycation sites of bovine insulin by tandem mass spectrometry. J Am Soc Mass Spectrom. 2009;20:1319–26.

36. Arutyunyan A, L'vov K, Mnatsakanyan A, Oganesyan V, Shakhnazaryan N. Light quenching of fluorescence of aromatic amino acids. J Appl Spectrosc. 1985;43:992–4.

37. Swamy MJ, Surolia A. Studies on the tryptophan residues of soybean agglutinin. Involvement in saccharide binding. Biosci Rep. 1989;9:189–98.

38. Khazaei MR, Bakhti M, Habibi-Rezaei M. Nicotine reduces the cytotoxic effect of glycated proteins on microglial cells. Neurochem Res. 2010;35:548–58.

39. Nilsson MR. Techniques to study amyloid fibril formation in vitro. Methods. 2004;34:151–60.

40. Khan MWA, Rasheed Z, Khan WA, Ali R. Biochemical, biophysical, and thermodynamic analysis of in vitro glycated human serum albumin. Biochem (Moscow). 2007;72:146–52.

41. Khazaei MR, Habibi-Rezaei M, Karimzadeh F, Moosavi-Movahedi AA, Sarrafnejhad AA, Sabouni F, et al. Microglial cell death induced by glycated bovine serum albumin: nitric oxide involvement. J Biochem. 2008;144:197–206.

42. Sen S, Kar M, Roy A, Chakraborti AS. Effect of nonenzymatic glycation on functional and structural properties of hemoglobin. Biophys Chem. 2005;113:289–98.

43. Bohlooli M, Moosavi-Movahedi A, Taghavi F, Saboury A, Maghami P, Seyedarabi A, et al. Inhibition of fluorescent advanced glycation end products (AGEs) of human serum albumin upon incubation with 3-β-hydroxybutyrate. Mol Biol Rep. 2014;41:3705–13.

44. Varashree B, Bhat GP. Correlation of Lipid Peroxidation with Glycated Haemoglobin Levels in Diabetes Mellitus. Online J Health Allied Sci. 2011;10.

45. Karimi J, Goodarzi M, Tavilani H, Khodadadi I, Amiri I. Relationship between advanced glycation end products and increased lipid peroxidation in semen of diabetic men. Diabetes Res Clin Pract. 2011;91:61–6.

46. Cheng S, Chen G-Q, Leski M, Zou B, Wang Y, Wu Q. The effect of d, β-hydroxybutyric acid on cell death and proliferation in L929 cells. Biomater. 2006;27:3758–65.

47. Thaler S, Choragiewicz TJ, Rejdak R, Fiedorowicz M, Turski WA, Tulidowicz-Bielak M, et al. Neuroprotection by acetoacetate and β-hydroxybutyrate against NMDA-induced RGC damage in rat—possible involvement of kynurenic acid. Graefes Arch Clin Exp Ophthalmol. 2010;248:1729–35.

Permissions

The contributors of this book come from diverse backgrounds, making this book a truly international effort. This book will bring forth new frontiers with its revolutionizing research information and detailed analysis of the nascent developments around the world.

We would like to thank all the contributing authors for lending their expertise to make the book truly unique. They have played a crucial role in the development of this book. Without their invaluable contributions this book wouldn't have been possible. They have made vital efforts to compile up to date information on the varied aspects of this subject to make this book a valuable addition to the collection of many professionals and students.

This book was conceptualized with the vision of imparting up-to-date information and advanced data in this field. To ensure the same, a matchless editorial board was set up. Every individual on the board went through rigorous rounds of assessment to prove their worth. After which they invested a large part of their time researching and compiling the most relevant data for our readers.

The editorial board has been involved in producing this book since its inception. They have spent rigorous hours researching and exploring the diverse topics which have resulted in the successful publishing of this book. They have passed on their knowledge of decades through this book. To expedite this challenging task, the publisher supported the team at every step. A small team of assistant editors was also appointed to further simplify the editing procedure and attain best results for the readers.

Apart from the editorial board, the designing team has also invested a significant amount of their time in understanding the subject and creating the most relevant covers. They scrutinized every image to scout for the most suitable representation of the subject and create an appropriate cover for the book.

The publishing team has been an ardent support to the editorial, designing and production team. Their endless efforts to recruit the best for this project, has resulted in the accomplishment of this book. They are a veteran in the field of academics and their pool of knowledge is as vast as their experience in printing. Their expertise and guidance has proved useful at every step. Their uncompromising quality standards have made this book an exceptional effort. Their encouragement from time to time has been an inspiration for everyone.

The publisher and the editorial board hope that this book will prove to be a valuable piece of knowledge for researchers, students, practitioners and scholars across the globe.

List of Contributors

Hamid Reza Monsef-Esfahani and Zahra Tofighi
Department of Pharmacognosy, Faculty of Pharmacy, Tehran University of Medical Sciences, Tehran, Iran

Mohsen Amini
Department of Medicinal Chemistry, Faculty of Pharmacy, Tehran University of Medical Sciences, Tehran, Iran

Fatemeh Saiedmohammadi
Department of Pharmacognosy, Faculty of Pharmacy, Tehran University of Medical Sciences, Tehran, Iran
Department of Pharmacology and Toxicology, Faculty of Pharmacy, Tehran University of Medical Sciences, Tehran, Iran

Navid Goodarzi
Department of Pharmaceutics, Faculty of Pharmacy, Tehran University of Medical Sciences, Tehran, Iran
Nanotechnology Research Centre, Faculty of Pharmacy, Tehran University of Medical Sciences, Tehran, Iran

Mohammad Hossein Ghahremani
Nanotechnology Research Centre, Faculty of Pharmacy, Tehran University of Medical Sciences, Tehran, Iran
Department of Pharmacology and Toxicology, Faculty of Pharmacy, Tehran University of Medical Sciences, Tehran, Iran

Reza Hajiaghaee
Pharmacognosy & Pharmaceutics Department of Medicinal Plants Research Center, Institute of Medicinal Plants, ACECR, Karaj, Iran

Mohammad Ali Faramarzi
Department of Pharmaceutical Biotechnology, Faculty of Pharmacy & Biotechnology Research Center, Tehran University of Medical Sciences, Tehran, Iran

Songhee Jeon
Dongguk University Research Institute of Biotechnology, Seoul 100-715, Republic of Korea

Chia-Hung Lee and Quan Feng Liu
Department of Neuropsychiatry, Graduate School of Oriental Medicine, Dongguk University, Gyeongju, Republic of Korea

Geun Woo Kim
Department of Korean Neuropsychiatry, Dongguk University Bundang Oriental Hospital, Sungnam, Republic of Korea

Byung-Soo Koo
Department of Korean Neuropsychiatry, Dongguk University Ilsan Oriental Hospital, Goyang, Republic of Korea

Sok Cheon Pak
School of Biomedical Sciences, Charles Sturt University, Bathurst, NSW 2795, Australia

Hasan Vakili-Arki
Student Research Committee, Department of Medical Informatics, Faculty of Medicine, Mashhad University of Medical Sciences, Mashhad, Iran

Ehsan Nabovati
Student Research Committee, Department of Medical Informatics, Faculty of Medicine, Mashhad University of Medical Sciences, Mashhad, Iran
Department of Health Information Management/Technology, School of Allied Health Professions, Kashan University of Medical Sciences, Kashan, Iran

Zhila Taherzadeh
Neurogenic Inflammation Research Center, Faculty of Medicine, Mashhad University of Medical Sciences, Mashhad, Iran
Targeted Drug Delivery Research Center, School of Pharmacy, Mashhad University of Medical Sciences, Mashhad, Iran

Saeid Eslami
Pharmaceutical Research Center, School of Pharmacy, Mashhad University of Medical Sciences, Mashhad, Iran
Department of Medical Informatics, Faculty of Medicine, Mashhad University of Medical Sciences, Mashhad, Iran
Department of Medical Informatics, Academic Medical Center, University of Amsterdam, Amsterdam, The Netherlands

Mohammad Reza Hasibian
Department of Medical Informatics, Faculty of Medicine, Mashhad University of Medical Sciences, Mashhad, Iran

Ameen Abu-Hanna
Department of Medical Informatics, Academic Medical Center, University of Amsterdam, Amsterdam, The Netherlands

Jamileh Moghimi
Department of Internal Medicine, School of Medicine, Semnan University of Medical Sciences, Semnan, Iran

Daryiush Pahlevan and Maryam Azizzadeh
Research Center for Social Determinants of Health, Semnan University of Medical Sciences, Semnan, Iran

Hamid Hamidi
Department of Dermatology, School of Medicine, Arak University of Medical Sciences, Arak, Iran

Mohsen Pourazizi
Students' Research Committee, Semnan University of Medical Sciences, Semnan, Iran

Sahabjada Siddiqui and Mohammad Arshad
Molecular Endocrinology Laboratory, Department of Zoology, University of Lucknow, Lucknow 226007, India

Rouzbeh Jahanbakhsh and Zahra Sobhani
Department of Pharmaceutics, Faculty of Pharmacy, Tehran University of Medical Sciences, Tehran 14174, Iran

Rassoul Dinarvand and Fatemeh Atyabi
Department of Pharmaceutics, Faculty of Pharmacy, Tehran University of Medical Sciences, Tehran 14174, Iran
Nanotechnology Research Centre, Faculty of Pharmacy, Tehran University of Medical Sciences, Tehran 14174, Iran

Saeed Shanehsazzadeh
Department of Biomedical Physics and Engineering, School of Medicine, Tehran University of Medical Sciences, Tehran, Iran

Mohsen Adeli
Department of Chemistry, Sharif University of Technology, Tehran, Iran
Department of Chemistry, Faculty of Science, Lorestan University, Khoramabad, Iran

Azadeh Manayi, Mahdieh Kurepaz-mahmoodabadi, Ahmad R Gohari and Soodabeh Saeidnia
Medicinal Plants Research Center, Faculty of Pharmacy, Tehran University of Medical Sciences, P.O. Box 14155–6451, Tehran, Iran

Yousef Ajani
Institute of Medicinal Plants (IMP), Iranian Academic Centre for Education, Culture and Research (ACECR), Karaj, Iran

Tahereh Hosseinabadi, Hossein Vahidi and Bahman Nickavar
Department of Pharmacognosy and Biotechnology, School of Pharmacy, Shahid Beheshti University of Medical Sciences, Vali-e Asr Ave., Niayesh Junction, Tehran 1996835113, Iran

Farzad Kobarfard
Department of Medicinal Chemistry, School of Pharmacy, Shahid Beheshti University of Medical Sciences, Vali-e Asr Ave., Niayesh Junction, Tehran 1996835113, Iran

Maryam Payan and Mohammad Reza Rouini
Biopharmaceutics and Pharmacokinetics Division, Department of Pharmaceutics, School of Pharmacy, Tehran University of Medical sciences, Tehran, Iran

Nader Tajik
Cellular and Molecular Research Center (CMRC), Iran University of Medical Sciences, Tehran, Iran

Mohammad Hossein Ghahremani
Department of Pharmacology and Toxicology, School of Pharmacy, Tehran University of Medical sciences, Tehran, Iran

Reza Tahvilian
Department of pharmaceutics, School of Pharmacy, Kermanshah University of Medical Sciences, Kermanshah, Iran

Ghazal Labbeiki, Hossein Attar and Amir Heydarinasab
Department of Chemical Engineering, Science and Research Branch, Islamic
Azad University(IAU), Tehran, Iran

Sayed Sorkhabadi
Department of Pharmacology, School of Advanced Sciences and Technologies in Medicine, Tehran University of Medical Sciences, Tehran, Iran
Department of Toxicology and Pharmacology, Islamic Azad University of Pharmaceutical Sciences Branch, Tehran, Iran

Alimorad Rashidi
Catalyst and Nanotechnology Division, Research Institute of Petroleum Industry, Tehran, Iran

Nasser Nassiri Koopaei, Akbar Abdollahiasl and Shekoufeh Nikfar
Department of Pharmacoeconomics and Pharmaceutical Administration, Faculty of Pharmacy, Tehran University of Medical Sciences, P.O. Box 14155–6451, Tehran 14174, Iran

Abbas Kebriaeezadeh
Department of Pharmacoeconomics and Pharmaceutical Administration, Faculty of Pharmacy, Tehran University of Medical Sciences, P.O. Box 14155–6451, Tehran 14174, Iran

Department of Toxicology and Pharmacology, Faculty of Pharmacy, Tehran University of Medical Sciences, P.O. Box 14155–6451, Tehran 14174, Iran

Nafiseh Mohamadi
Management Information System Division, Osvah Pharmaceutical Company, Tehran, Iran

Mohsen Vosooghi and Armin Dadgar
Department of Medicinal Chemistry, Faculty of Pharmacy, Tehran University of Medical Sciences, Tehran, Iran

Loghman Firoozpour and Abolfazl Rodaki
Drug Design and Development Research Center, Tehran University of Medical Sciences, Tehran, Iran

Mahboobeh Pordeli and Sussan K Ardestani
Institute of Biochemistry and Biophysics, University of Tehran, PO Box 13145–1384, Tehran, Iran

Maliheh Safavi
Department of Biotechnology, Iranian Research Organization for Science and Technology, Tehran, Iran

Ali Asadipour and Mohammad Hassan Moshafi
Neuroscience Research Center, Institute of Neuropharmacology, Kerman University of Medicinal Sciences, Kerman, Iran

Alireza Foroumadi
Neuroscience Research Center, Institute of Neuropharmacology, Kerman University of Medicinal Sciences, Kerman, Iran
Pharmaceutical Sciences Research Center, Tehran University of Medical Sciences, Tehran, Iran

Fatemeh Sadat Hoseini
Department of Anatomy and Reproductive Biology, School of Medicine, Tehran University of Medical Sciences, Tehran, Iran

Seyed Mohammad Hossein Noori Mugahi
Departments of Histology, School of Medicine, Tehran University of Medical Sciences, Tehran, Iran

Firoozeh Akbari-Asbagh
Department of Obstetrics and Gynecology, Tehran Women General Hospital, School of Medicine, Tehran University of Medical Sciences, Tehran, Iran

Poopak Eftekhari-Yazdi
Department of Embryology at Reproductive Biomedicine Research Center, Royan Institute for Reproductive Biomedicine, ACECR, Tehran, Iran

Behrouz Aflatoonian
Lab director Assisted Conception Units, Laleh Hospital, Tehran, Iran and Madar Hospital, Yazd, Iran

Seyed Hamid Aghaee-Bakhtiari
Department of Molecular Biology and Genetic Engineering, Stem Cell Technology Research Center, Tehran, Iran and Molecular Medicine Department, Biotechnology Research Center, Pasteur Institute of Iran, Tehran, Iran

Reza Aflatoonian
Department of Endocrinology and Female Infertility at Reproductive Biomedicine Research Center, Royan Institute for Reproductive Biomedicine, ACECR, Tehran, Iran

Nasser Salsabili
Department of Physiotherapy, School of Rehabilitation of Tehran University of Medical Sciences, Tehran, Iran; Lab director Assisted Conception Unit, Tehran Women General Hospital, Tehran University of Medical Sciences, Tehran, Iran

Elham Ghasemian, Alireza Vatanara, Abdolhossein Rouholamini Najafabadi, Mohammad Reza Rouini, Kambiz Gilani and Majid Darabi
Pharmaceutics Department, Faculty of Pharmacy, Tehran University of Medical Sciences, Tehran, Iran

Masoomeh Yosefifard and Majid Hassanpour-Ezatti
Department of Biology, Sciences School, Shahed University, Tehran, IRAN

Nasser Nassiri-Koopaei
Department of Pharmacoeconomics and Pharmaceutical Administration, Faculty of Pharmacy, Tehran University of Medical Sciences, Tehran, Iran

Abbas Kebriaeezadeh and Shekoufeh Nikfar
Department of Pharmacoeconomics and Pharmaceutical Administration, Faculty of Pharmacy, Tehran University of Medical Sciences, Tehran, Iran
Pharmaceutical Policy Research Center, Faculty of Pharmacy, Tehran University of Medical Sciences, Enqelab Square, Tehran, Iran

Reza Majdzadeh Saharnaz Nedjat
Knowledge Utilization Research Centre and School of Public Health, Tehran University of Medical Sciences, Tehran, Iran
Pharmaceutical Policy Research Center, Faculty of Pharmacy, Tehran University of Medical Sciences, Enqelab Square, Tehran, Iran

Arash Rashidian
Knowledge Utilization Research Centre and Department of Health Management and Economics, School of Public Health, Tehran University of Medical Sciences, Tehran, Iran

Mojtaba Tabatabai Yazdi
Department of Pharmaceutical Biotechnology, Faculty of Pharmacy, Tehran University of Medical Sciences, Tehran, Iran

Paria Motahari, Majid Sadeghizadeh, Mehrdad Behmanesh and Fatemeh Zolghadr
Faculty of Biological Sciences, Department of Molecular Genetics, School of Biological Sciences, Tarbiat Modares University, Jalal Ale Ahmad Highway, PO Box 14115-111, Tehran, Iran

Shaghayegh Sabri
Department of Medical Genetics, School of Medical Sciences, Tarbiat Modares University, Tehran, Iran

Leila Jalaly and Gholamreza Sharifi
Department of Exercise Physiology, Isfahan (Khorasgan) Branch, Islamic Azad University, Isfahan, Iran

Mohammad Faramarzi
Associate Professor in Exercise Physiology,Shahrekord University, Shahrekord, Iran

Alireza Nematollahi
Subspecialist of Cardiology and Assistant Professor, Shahrekord Univercity of Medical Sciences, Shahrekord, Iran

Mahmoud Rafieian-kopaei
Medical Plants Research Center, Shahrekord Univercity of Medical Sciences, Shahrekord, Iran

Masoud Amiri
Health Research Center, Shahrekord Univercity of Medical Sciences, Shahrekord, Iran

Fariborz Moattar
School of Pharmacy and Pharmaceutical Sciences, Isfahan University of Medical Sciences and Health Services, Isfahan, Iran

Clarence S. Yah
Department of Biochemistry and Microbiology, Nelson Mandela Metropolitan University, Port Elizabeth, South Africa
Department of Epidemiology, Johns Hopkins Bloomberg School of Public Health, E7146, 615 N. Wolfe Street, Baltimore 21205, MD, USA

Geoffrey S. Simate
School of Chemical and Metallurgical Engineering, University of the Witwatersrand, P/Bag 3, Wits2050, Johannesburg, South Africa

Javad Motaharinia, Azadeh Moghaddas and Mojtaba Mojtahedzadeh
Department of Pharmacotherapy, Faculty of Pharmacy, Tehran University of Medical Sciences, 16 Azar Ave, Enghelab Sq, Tehran, Iran

Farhad Etezadi
Department of Anesthesiology & Critical Care, Sina Hospital, Tehran University of Medical Sciences, Tehran, Iran

Waheed Asghar, Elliot Pittman and Fakhreddin Jamali
Faculty of Pharmacy and Pharmaceutical Sciences, University of Alberta, 11361 – 87 Avenue, Edmonton, AB T6G 2E1, Canada

Maryam Khalkhali and Farhad Khoeini
Department of Physics, Faculty of Science, University of Zanjan, Zanjan, Iran

Mehrdad Hamidi
Zanjan Pharmaceutical Nanotechnology Research Center, Zanjan University of Medical Sciences, Zanjan, Iran

Kobra Rostamizadeh
Zanjan Pharmaceutical Nanotechnology Research Center, Zanjan University of Medical Sciences, Zanjan, Iran
Department of Medicinal Chemistry, School of Pharmacy, Zanjan University of Medical Sciences, Postal Code 45139-56184 Zanjan, Iran

Somayeh Sadighian
Zanjan Pharmaceutical Nanotechnology Research Center, Zanjan University of Medical Sciences, Zanjan, Iran
Department of Pharmaceutical Biomaterials, School of Pharmacy, Zanjan University of Medical Sciences, Zanjan, Iran

Mehran Naghibi
Shahid Beheshti University of Medical Sciences, Tehran, Iran

Iman Karimzadeh
Department of Clinical Pharmacy, Faculty of Pharmacy, Shiraz University of Medical Sciences, Shiraz, Iran

Hossein Khalili
Department of Clinical Pharmacy, Faculty of Pharmacy, Tehran University of Medical Sciences, Enghelab Ave, Tehran, Iran

Usha Ganganahalli Kapanigowda and Prakash Rao Boggarapu
Department of Pharmaceutical Technology, Karnataka College of Pharmacy, #33/2, Tirumenahalli, Hegde Nagar Main Road, Bengaluru 560064, Karnataka, India

Sree Harsha Nagaraja
Department of Pharmaceutical Sciences, College of Clinical Pharmacy, King Faisal University, Al-Ahsa 31982, Saudi Arabia

Balakeshwa Ramaiah
Department of Pharmaceutics, Karnataka College of Pharmacy, #33/2, Tirumenahalli, Hegde Nagar Main Road, Bengaluru 560064, Karnataka, India

Balakeshwa Ramaiah and Rajarajan Subramanian
Department of Pharmaceutics, Karnataka College of Pharmacy, #33/2, Tirumenahalli, Hegde Nagar Main Road, Bengaluru, Karnataka 560064, India

Sree Harsha Nagaraja
Department of Pharmaceutical Sciences, College of Clinical Pharmacy, King Faisal University, Al-Ahsa 31982, Saudi Arabia

Usha Ganganahalli Kapanigowda and Prakash Rao Boggarapu
Department of Pharmaceutical Technology, Karnataka College of Pharmacy, #33/2, Tirumenahalli, Hegde Nagar Main Road, Bengaluru 560064, Karnataka, India

Maryam Ferdousi and Effat Azimzadeh-Irani
School of Biology, College of Science, University of Tehran, Tehran, Iran

Manijheh Sabokdast
School of Biology, College of Science, University of Tehran, Tehran, Iran
Present address: Department of agronomy, and plant breeding, College of Agriculture & Natural Resources, University of Tehran, Karaj, Iran

Mehran Habibi-Rezaei
School of Biology, College of Science, University of Tehran, Tehran, Iran
Nano-Biomedicine Center of Excellence, Nanoscience and Nanotechnology Research Center, University of Tehran, Tehran, Iran

Najmeh Poursasan
Institute of Biochemistry and Biophysics, University of Tehran, Tehran, Iran

Ali Akbar Moosavi-Movahedi
Institute of Biochemistry and Biophysics, University of Tehran, Tehran, Iran
Center of Excellence in Biothermodynamics, University of Tehran, Tehran, Iran

Index

www.ingramcontent.com/pod-product-compliance
Lightning Source LLC
Chambersburg PA
CBHW061938190326
41458CB00009B/2772